Adults With Disabilities

International Perspectives
in the Community

Adults With Disabilities

International Perspectives in the Community

Edited by
PAUL RETISH
The University of Iowa
SHUNIT REITER
The University of Haifa

Routledge
Taylor & Francis Group
LONDON AND NEW YORK

First published 1999 by Lawrence Erlbaum Associates, Inc.

2 Park Square, Milton Park, Abingdon, Oxon OX14 4RN
711 Third Avenue, New York, NY 10017, USA

Routledge is an imprint of the Taylor & Francis Group, an informa business

First issued in paperback 2016

Transferred to digital printing 2010 by Routledge

Cover design by Kathryn Houghtaling Lacey

Library of Congress Cataloging-in-Pu0blication Data

Adults with disabilities : international perspectives in the
community / edited by Paul Retish and Shunit Reiter.
    p.   cm.
Includes bibliographical references and index.
ISBN 978-0-8058-2424-7
1. Handicapped—Social conditions. 2. Handicapped—
Services for. 3. Handicapped—Cross-cultural studies. I.
Retish, Paul. II. Reiter, Shunit.
HV1568.A36   1999
362.4—dc21   98-35593
                                             CIP

ISBN 978-0-8058-2424-7 (hbk)
ISBN 978-1-138-96601-7 (pbk)

Contents

v

Introduction

Paul Retish
The University of Iowa

This book concerns the process of transition that we all make throughout our lifetimes: the first time a child leaves the house, the first day at school, the first time going to a social event, junior or senior high school, and so on. For this text, we are concerned with the necessary skills individuals with disabilities need to function outside of school; not just when they graduate, but on a daily basis, from the time they enter the school to when they finish. Each of these times are steps in transition. With what is known about schools today, we may infer that, more often than not, the school teaches pupils how to go to school and not how to make the transitions necessary for functioning on a daily basis. This seems to be true for all students—not just those with a disability (Skrtic, 1991).

To complicate the matter further, we also have evidence that the programs are in existence are not adequate in the preparations for individuals to take their place in society. Sitlington and Easterday (1992) have both shown that the key factor in job success outside of school for persons with disabilities is to have connections with individuals who can employ someone with disabilities. This group is usually composed of relatives and friends who are willing to hire the individual without regard to their disability.

The concept of *transition* in the United States is also complicated by the strong academic movement in schools that attempts to raise the standards for graduation for all students (Goals 2000). This process along with cost factors, have led to a deterioration of specific programs that assist students to become more work ready and community oriented. Secondary schools in America are very often judged by the numbers who go to prestigious colleges or postsecondary institutions. Where does this leave the student who wishes to find employment after high school? There is a great gap in this area that at present is not being filled.

As the editors of this text travel to different countries, these countries are often intent on imitating program designs and delivery systems that they perceive as being of the highest quality. In many cases, they want to Americanize their system without concern as to whether this would be appropriate for the local or national culture.

Each of the authors of this text try to discuss their own work and place it an international perspective. The reader can then determine the validity of the transfer, if it exists, and what more needs to be accomplished in order for transition to occur successfully. What is to be learned from the world we live in? Can we discuss the processes of what is done to assist those with disabilities and learn from each other? Are we so heavily tied into cultural differences and superiority that this puts blinders on how we view each other? Individuals, communities, organizations, parents, professionals and governments all over the world have tried a variety of processes to assist persons with disabilities. We may have data that could help in not making the same mistakes over and over again. This streamlining of the process can speed the time when persons with disabilities can enter into all societies as equal members. No matter where one travels, being different is an uncomfortable position to be in and leads to misunderstandings, frustration and anger.

For instance Dave, who was going blind, had some residual vision in each eye. He could only see out of the corners of each of his eye so when he played cards he held the cards in an awkward manner and the others in the game did not know what to say as the cards were always in front of them. Simply "putting the problem on the table" for all to discuss solved this dilemma and the game preceded. David also would stand on a corner looking at the sights (he was 18, and the sights were female students) when someone would come along, and grab him to take him across the street. Dave's humor which helps him cope, handled the situation by saying that he has crossed so many streets, he was getting tired and didn't want to cross them anymore.

Therefore, the problems of transition are not just for persons with disabilities but for everyone in society. Acceptance of differences, understanding that our perceptions of others' needs may not be accurate, and just the ability to be honest with one another may be a reasonable amount of accommodation necessary to assist transition. We as individuals, societies, and organizations need to continually ask ourselves how we can assist all people to use the system. We can never be satisfied as to where we are but we must continually look at improving. In looking at improvement, we need to be sure that we have access to information that gives us the broadest possible information to digest and cultivate for our own use. The rationale for this process is one of equal rights, but it is also based upon the economic reactions to not doing this transition process. Dependency or the lack of productivity is expensive for the taxpayer, the government, and business. The more we assist in the process of transition, the better all of us will be in a humanistic and monetary sense.

We have wasted a great deal of time and money not moving ahead. How to begin, how to adapt, and how to continue to adapt are the yard sticks we need to use to proceed.

REFERENCES

Skrtic, T., (1991). Behind special education: A critical analysis of professional culture and school organization. Denver: Love.

Sitlington, P., & Easterday, J. (1992). An analysis of employer incentive rankings relative to the employment of persons with mental retardation. *Education and Training in Mental Retardation, 27*, 75–80.

Preface

When we first discussed writing a text together, we tried to determine what we, as two professionals in Special Education, had in common. We found distinct areas of commonalty: We both have done a great deal of traveling in the area of special education. We had met very fine scholars with similar interests and that interest was concerned with the process of transition. We decided to combine all of the areas and ask various scholars to give an international perspective on dimensions of transition as they saw it. They would then write in the perspective of who they are rather than trying to translate to an American perspective.

We felt and continue to feel that we who are members of the world community interested in persons with special needs have a great deal to learn from one another. We can learn from successes and failures, laws and cultural norms and discussions that have been held and that are being held. Willingness to learn also means enhancing the skills of listening, and accepting the experiences and conclusions of others who are accomplished in vastly different ways than we are. Initially, we had to assure ourselves, and then the perspective authors, that there would be no hierarchy of power regarding which group has accomplished the most and who needed to learn from whom.

In our international travels and consultation, we are often in the position of being asked how to aid the process of transition; or people tell us how to do it the way they feel is best. We sometimes reject these positions as being unfriendly because we are unaware of local norms, customs, and realities. Therefore, we are asking all of our readers to have an open mind, to read thoroughly before reacting, and to try to understand the context of how transition processes come about in the culture described and to look for a common thread. We believe that similarity can be found through the fact that these accomplishments are written by people who are trying to do the best possible with, and for people, with disabilities.

This text is geared to any and all people who are interested in persons with special needs in the community. Therefore, we are emphasizing work, sexuality, leisure, access to systems, medical concerns, technology, and rights of citizenship. These various views should give the reader information that initiates new ideas on how to be accessible to those with disabilities and to reinforce what has already begun in many systems. We have purposefully not written or geared this text to any one profession. We are interested in professionals and nonprofessionals using this text as a resource as they work their way through, making systems more open and accepting. Therefore, we would hope that parents, employers, medical personnel, recreation and leisure activities personnel, and any others in the community who work with persons with disabilities will find this text useful.

This text should stimulate the development of programs for the level and culture in which the individual reader is living. We hope to give you enough information that you can alter the appropriate processes for your own use. In some grander sense, we are hoping that this information will assist you in providing better programs for persons with disabilities. We do not encourage you to imitate, but to manipulate and mold these experiences to fit the needs of the particular system of which you are a part. We hope that in time, you can share your progress with us. We will try to follow this up with new information for other readers.

BOOK STRUCTURE

This text is intended to give the reader two views folded into each area. One is an overview of how the person with a disability can live their daily life, and the other is how their ability is accomplished or hindered in the world we live in. The authors represent different constituencies, countries, and parts of the lives we all live day in and day out.

Part I, Schools

This section is totally focused on that time frame in life where one makes the transition from school into adulthood life. For the person with a disability, this section specifically addresses how these individuals will cope with life after school, when the protective environment of the schools has left and the reality of the community and adulthood has arrived. For the person with a disability, this transition is complicated by the quick reduction of people who are always there to help, the loss of friends, and a society whose goals may or may not focus on the individual.

In chapter 1, Wehman and Noonan Walsh look at the status of American society and the structures that do and do not exist to assist the individual with disabilities in this transition. This chapter is followed by Garber, McInerney, and Osher (chap. 2), who review what has happened to many persons with disabilities and whether transition has been both cost effective and productive. In chapter 3, Young, Pedrosa, and Kavanaugh look at that very special site of the U.S. and Mexican border where emerging industries, changing environments, and clashes of culture affect the lives of persons with mental disabilities and their families as they try to cope and survive. Chapters 4 (Hitchings, Natelle & Ristow) and 5 (Ling) give the reader views of parent involvement and community involvement in two very different sites and countries. A midwestern view is presented from the United States of how parents are involved in this transition process, followed by an Australian view of community living, policies that have been passed, and their real affect on the lives of persons with disabilities.

Part II, Personal and Social Inclusion

The text moves to an in-depth look at what is happening in various communities and countries as persons with disabilities enter into them. Realistic looks are presented from the perspectives of persons with disabilities at the essence of their lives as life goes by day-to-day and how they cope.

Chapter 6 (MacNeil & Anderson) starts with a look at how and what is available for leisure time activities (what can and is being done, what are the possibilities of programming, including and attaining the power for planning activities). In chapter 7, Shaughnessy, Glover, Greene, and Choy address the issue of persons with disabilities becoming parents (specifically, people with mental retardation learning their rights and responsibilities of deciding to be a parent and how best to go about providing this information to them). Ramot and Gitelman (chap. 8) discuss the implementation of interventions in emerging societies for services for those with a disability. Specifically, they investigate how to access the models being used for community openness and how to interpret what is available to a different society, which may have different values and resources. In chapter 9, Corbett discusses strategies used in England for developing survival strategies for those with disabilities. Specific areas such as abuse, resource assistance, and support are discussed and described.

Part III, The Community

The essence of one's life ultimately ends up in the community in which one lives. For those with disabilities, this transition can be a very significant one, with its new experiences, challenges, and frustrations. Each community has it own state of preparedness for those with disabilities. Communities also have a public model and a realistic everyday model. The following authors review both levels of community so that the reader can see the various levels with which many people with disabilities must cope.

Herr (chap. 10) discusses Israeli immigration policy at two levels. The general view is that all have rights to the specific implementation of the policy and then the rights are tempered by those who deliver the services. Brown and Streumer (chap. 11) continue to discuss these same issues as they relate to employment. There are continuing differences between what is said and what is done on a daily basis. Each person with a disability must ultimately face what is done on a daily basis rather than believe what is the public policy. Rojewski (chap. 12) concludes this section with a comprehensive review of what has been done internationally in vocational preparation and discusses options that are available or that have been tried.

Part IV, Cross Cultural–Future

Many people would claim that we have made great strides around the world to welcome persons with disabilities into a full life. Of course it is uneven from country to country, region to region, and community to community. The next three chapters try to view what the future holds from a policy view, from the use of technology, and from the cultures that exist around the person with a disability.

Mitchell (chap. 13) uses his research in New Zealand to view how systems look at themselves and those who are part of the system. The research is also used as a means to predict how the system will move into the future. Siegel (chap. 14) looks at the advancements in technology and its affect on assisting the mentally retarded into society. Schalock and Kelly (chap. 15) view sociocultural factors in societies that influence vocational possibilities in the near and far term.

On finishing this text, the reader should have a beginning understanding of what is occurring in many different countries as persons with disabilities make the transition into society. Who is the most advanced? Who can we all learn from? Clearly the answer lies in learning from all and not being satisfied at the level we are at today.

—*Paul Retish*
—*Shunit Reiter*

PART I

Schools

CHAPTER I

Transition From School to Adulthood: A Look at the United States and Europe

Paul Wehman
Virginia Commonwealth University

Patricia Noonan Walsh
University College Dublin

Sam is 23 years of age; he graduated from the local special education program last year. He has a diagnosis of severe mental retardation with an IQ score of 27 and a secondary diagnosis of mild cerebral palsy, as well as a visual impairment. He has a long history of getting his own way by acting out when he gets upset. On occasion this behavior has been directed at teachers when they have attempted to intervene. Typically, however, his aggressive behavior is limited to temper tantrums.

Sam lives at home with his biological parents. They hope that he will be able to work soon. Until recently, his parents thought that his only alternative was a sheltered workshop or an activity center. Sam assists his family in household chores such as cleaning, laundry, and lawn work, and he participates in a Men's Club with his father and other retired men in his community.

After graduation from school, Sam was referred to the vocational rehabilitation program which arranged for him to receive a vocational evaluation. This testing indicated that Sam had a short attention span and performed poorly on routine, manipulative, and sorting tasks. Sam was able to follow simple directions when they were specific and when prior demonstration had occurred. However, he became uncooperative and noncompliant after working on a task for several minutes.

What will Sam and his family do now that his special education is completed? Who will help him get a job or more training? What hope can Sam have for his future? We will return to Sam and his situation and answer these questions a little bit later in this chapter.

These are the questions considered by thousands of youth with disabilities and their families as they move closer to the completion of their secondary-level education (Clark & Kolstoe, 1994; Enchelmaier, Kohler, & Rusch, 1994. The opportunities and challenges that await them in the adult community are very unclear and depend heavily upon local economies and job opportunities, residential and transportation services, and community awareness and support for persons with disabilities. For example, those individuals with severe cerebral palsy who live in one city may have tremendous opportunities at special travel accommodations and work opportunities. Yet only 75 miles away, in another town with less money or interest in helping people with disabilities, virtually no extra help may be available.

When they complete their secondary-level education program, young people like Sam leave the familiar education environment where they are legally entitled to a coordinated education plan called the IEP. They enter a multilayered adult service system with frequently unfamiliar and sometimes inconsistent or contradictory languages, policies, and practices. Sam and his family need guidance in understanding the opportunities and potential pitfalls involved in working with adult services, as well as preparatory experiences in participating in the adult community. The high school educator is a key resource person in helping the family to understand how to identify and utilize needed services and supports in the community. Educators can also facilitate the involvement of the adult community with the education program of a youth with a disability through arranging community-based training and work opportunities and by arranging referrals and joint conferences for families with adult service representatives.

These issues are true around the world. As young people with disabilities grow up they face new challenges of adulthood. While the terminology, training opportunities, and overall capacity varies greatly from country to country the same issue remains: What will happen to Sam when he grows up? In this chapter we will focus on the transition from school to adulthood as it is in most states, provinces, and countries, with a primary focus on the United States and European countries.

WHAT IS TRANSITION?

Experts in the fields of special education and rehabilitation recognize that the transition process must include the provision of quality services for all handicapped youth as they prepare to leave school. In fact, the federal Office of Special Education and Rehabilitative Services (OSERS) has made school-to-work transition a national priority and regularly provides special discretionary funds to educational and community agencies that are establishing model transition programs. What does the transition process encompass? Why is transition important? What transition models are involved?

Perhaps one of the most significant reasons that transition from school to adulthood has emerged as a major area of interest throughout the 1980s and well into the 1990s is that literally thousands of young people with disabilities are leaving special education with no jobs. There have been numerous studies looking at student outcomes after leaving school (e.g., Peraino, 1992). These have repeatedly shown that people with mild as well as severe disabilities are unable to consistently gain good quality employment with decent pay and fringe benefits. By most accounts over 50% of young adults with disabilities are unemployed when they leave school, with figures much higher with those with severe disabilities. Many professionals have begun to question the validity of the secondary / special education curriculum and the efforts at providing effective teaching interventions for these students (Edgar, 1987; Edgar & Polloway, 1994). There is a very serious concern that much of what happens in special education at the secondary level is not being very useful or functional in the context of ultimately gaining employment and making successful transitions into adulthood (Clark, 1994).

Transition for any student with a disability involves several key components, including: (a) an appropriate school program; (b) formalized plans involving parents and the entire array of community agencies that are responsible for providing services; and (c) multiple, quality options for gainful employment and meaningful postschool education and community living (Ivancic & Schepis, 1995).

Although the goal of our educational system is to help students become productive members of society as adults, few schools have guided students with disabilities into meaningful employment opportunities appropriate for their abilities. Because most students who are disabled do not benefit from systematic transition from school to work, approximately 50 to 75% of all adults with disabilities are unemployed (Louis Harris & Associates, 1994). Until recently, most parents of children with disabilities have rarely considered the possibility of a career for their children after graduation.

In the United States the mandatory special education law is called the Individuals with Disability Education Act (IDEA—1990). IDEA is specific about the responsibility of the local education agency about transition planning. In Section 300.18 the law states:

> The IEP for each student, beginning no later than age 16 (and at a younger age, if determined appropriate), must include a statement of transition services. . . . (Sec. 300.346)
>
> (a) As used in this part, "transition services" means a coordinated set of activities for a student, designed within an outcome-oriented process that promotes movement from school to post-school activities, including postsecondary education, vocational training, integrated employment (including supported employment), continuing and adult education, adult services, independent living, or community participation.
>
> (b) The coordinated set of activities described in paragraph (a) of this section must:

(1) Be based on the individual student's needs, taking into account the student's preferences and interests; and

(2) Include (i) instruction, (ii) community experiences, (iii) the development of employment and other post-school objectives, and (iv) if appropriate, acquisition of daily living skills and functional vocational evaluation. (Sec. 300.18)

Transition by young people with disabilities cannot be faced by the school systems alone. All forces within the community and family must work together to help increase the likelihood of successful adult adjustments. We must not lose sight of why we send students with disabilities to school: these students participate in school for the purpose of learning how to work independently, how to live in a community, and how to develop a quality of life which will insure happiness and satisfaction.

TRANSITION PLANNING

Transition from school to work is a process that focuses on the movement of students with disabilities from school into the world of work (Bullis, Bull, Johnson, & Peters, 1995). Facilitating a student's transition from a school program to the workplace requires movement through school instruction, planning for the transition process, and placement into meaningful, community-integrated employment. Currently, special education and vocational rehabilitation programs are required by legislation to cooperatively plan for the transition of students with disabilities into the work environment. Effective transition planning and implementation requires the participation, cooperation, and coordination of all local school and adult service agencies who provide services and supports to individuals with disabilities. A team effort increases the chances that all the necessary services and supports are made available to a student so as to assure a smooth transition into the labor force upon graduation. The rehabilitation counselor is a key player in this and must be an active participant in the transition team planning and implementation (Tooman, Revell, & Melia, 1988).

A rehabilitation counselor's role in transition programs varies according to the local needs and resources (Szymanski & King, 1989). Rehabilitation counselors can also be school-based and employed by a school district or cooperative of districts. However, most counselors are employed by state vocational rehabilitation agencies and often have limited time and resources to devote to coordination of transition services. Whether a counselor is school-based or state agency based, his or her activities may include career and psychosocial counseling consultation with special education and vocational education teachers, and coordination with school, family, and community efforts in career planning and implementation. Additionally job placement coordination of job support service, referral to and coordination with adult services, and planning and coordination with postsecondary programs is also done regularly (Wehman, 1995). Later in this chapter is an example of an actual student's plan.

The key components that should be included in a transition planning process are:

- functional, community-referenced secondary educational curriculum
- community-based service delivery
- interagency planning and service delivery efforts
- availability of an array of postsecondary options
- availability of ongoing community-based support services
- student, parent, and family involvement throughout the transition process

INTERAGENCY PLANNING AND SERVICE DELIVERY EFFORTS

An Interagency Transition Planning Team should be comprised of professionals from various disciplines who provide direct educational services or are targeted to provide adult services to transition-age students and the students' families. The team's major responsibility is to develop, implement, and monitor the individualized transition plan (ITP) for the student. The team should develop a plan that identifies the target outcomes in the areas of employment, community living, and recreation that the student and his or her family desire at the time of his or her graduation (Wehman, 1995). The plan should identify the supports necessary to achieve and maintain these outcomes and who is responsible for each step.

The ITP addresses goals in a number of postsecondary areas. These goals are not achieved while the student is in their secondary program. The ITP can serve to focus educational services on the development and practice of skills that will enhance the opportunity for the student to achieve these goals upon completion of their secondary level program. The key elements of a plan that should be considered are:

- Does formal transition planning begin for students when they reach the age of sixteen?
- Are the appropriate school and adult service personnel involved?
- Has a transition planning meeting been held? And has an individualized transition plan been developed?
- Does the transition plan cover the appropriate target areas such as employment, postsecondary education, independent living services, financial and income needs, recreation and leisure needs, medical and therapeutic needs, social and recreational needs, transportation needs, and advocacy and legal needs?

- Does the plan reflect a true vision of the potential of the student or is it merely a plan that offers only what the service delivery system currently provides?
- Is the plan updated annually at a minimum?
- Are exit meetings held to finalize plans for the transition from school to employment?
- Are appropriate elements of the transition plan included in the IEP?

WHAT HAPPENS AFTER SCHOOL?

Employment is a major element in the lives of people with or without handicaps. The type of work a person does, the amount of money they earn, and career advancement opportunities directly affect how individuals look at themselves (Unger, 1995; Wehman & Moon, 1988). What is most important is to develop multiple employment choices for individuals with disabilities that reflect the array of job opportunities available to nondisabled individuals in the same community. For example, the types of jobs and supports that need to be developed for those jobs are crucial to an effective transition plan for students with severe disabilities. Consider some of the issues below:

- Into what types of jobs are people being placed? Are these jobs reflective of the array of jobs available in the community? Are placements occurring only in entry level positions?
- Do the jobs people are working provide a "livable wage" with benefits?
- Are people working in community-integrated jobs?
- Have the provision of training and ongoing support services been identified prior to placement?
- Once a placement has been initiated, has the fading process been implemented appropriately?
- Are all parties involved in the placement satisfied with the current outcome and level of support?
- Have appropriate arrangements been made for the transfer of case management activities to a long term support agency (if one exists)?

Career/Vocational Education

Career and job choices are difficult for all individuals. Frequently, students with disabilities have had little or no exposure to vocational options available within the community, making it difficult for them to choose what type of job they want at graduation, or what they want to do as a career. The educational team (and especially the rehabilitation counselor) should begin involvement in career/

vocational counseling with students by the time they reach 16 years old. They should arrange to meet with the student, his or her family, and school personnel to discuss the employment opportunities available in the community. The counselor should act as a consultant to the teachers and other school personnel involved in the development of individual education plans to ensure that students are exposed to a variety of vocational opportunities. Concerted efforts on the part of all involved can provide the student with an background that will enable him or her to make job/career choices as graduation nears.

At times, particularly in heavily populated urban areas, the size of a special education program makes it prohibitive for the available vocational rehabilitation counselor to meet with all students 16 years of age and older. The counselor might work with the school program to prioritize services to those students most in need of the career/vocational counseling. The counselor should assume that those students with the more challenging disabling conditions in terms of employment preparation and eventual job placement will be included in the group receiving services.

Case Management

Traditionally, rehabilitation counselors working with a public agency have assumed a primary responsibility related to case management (Neal & Bader, 1991). As a member of a transition planning team, the counselor should also ensure dissemination of accurate information to parents and educators. For example, here are some typical responsibilities of a case manager:

- *Develop* vendorship and purchase of service agreements
- *Establish* local agreements with key agencies
- *Participate* in local interagency transition planning
- *Provide* inservice training to school personnel and parents on the federal and state vocational rehabilitation criteria for eligibility and provision of services
- *Attend* Individual Transition Planning meetings
- *Serve* as a member of the transition team throughout the secondary years
- *Gather* and interpret vocational assessment information
- *Coordinate* and *monitor* supported employment placement of post-secondary students
- *Identify* referral needs and ensure referrals are made to the appropriate agencies and or services

Transition planning involves many different members of the educational team and the community as well as the choice of students and family members. This process is as important as the student's plan for life after school.

Community-Based Instruction with Students

Many youths with a disability and their families experience a sense of isolation from the community (O'Brien & O'Brien, 1992; O'Connell, 1992). A primary example of this isolation is the limited participation of youths with a disability in work and work-related activities. By encouraging and supporting middle- and secondary-age youth with disabilities to obtain ID cards, develop and maintain resumes, and to seek out work opportunities, the school program can expand the student involvement in the community, knowledge of work requirements, and awareness of individual interests. These activities provide a firm base of information for the transition committees to use in assisting the individual student to plan for postsecondary interests and needs.

A formalized approach to expanding the community awareness and participation of a secondary-age youth with a disability is the incorporation of community-based instruction and supported employment into the school activities (Moon & Inge, 1993). Community-based instruction is defined by Wehman as involving "teachers and other education personnel teaching educational objectives in natural environments, such as work sites, shopping malls, and restaurants" (1992, p. 170). Training experiences in the community help students with disabilities determine job preferences and develop a work history. The focus of community experiences can also move from training to actual employment as the student, for example, nears completion of secondary education.

When designing a vocational training program, it is important to analyze the community and identify jobs that are appropriate for students with severe disabilities. Training experiences should provide students with the opportunity to become a part of the work culture and train alongside regular employees. Finally, a training program should be designed that reflects an increase in the number of hours spent in the community as students near graduation. In fact, it is ideal for a student to obtain employment by the end of each school year. The result is a "work résumé" that demonstrates inclusion in a variety of jobs within a number of different work settings. The information in Table 1.1 is offered as a guide to teachers for setting up community-based training sites.

VOCATIONAL REHABILITATION IN THE U.S.

The federal legislative history of vocational rehabilitation dates back to 1918. The initial focus was on assisting World War I veterans with disabilities obtain employment. During the last 75 years, the federal legislation has expanded the scope of the rehabilitation program substantially to include services to persons with mental retardation or psychiatric disabilities, nondiscrimination of persons with disabilities, and the use of independent living program.

The purpose of the current federal Rehabilitation Act, most recently reauthorized as the Rehabilitation Act Amendments of 1992, is to empower individuals with disabilities to maximize employment, economic self-sufficiency, independence, and inclusion and integration into society (Public Law 102-569, 1992). The congressional intent for the rehabilitation program is to help people with disabilities get jobs and become adjusted to their communities. Every state and local community in the United States has a vocational rehabilitation program with counselors who can help people with disabilities and their families. The most recent update to the Rehabilitation Act, the Rehabilitation Act Amendments of 1992 (Public Law 102-569), combines with the Individuals with Disabilities Education Act (IDEA) and the Americans with Disabilities Act (ADA) to put in place a consistent set of legislation based on the following public policy:

> Disability is a natural part of human experience and in no way diminishes the right of individuals to—(A) live independently; (B) enjoy self-determination; (C) make choices; (D) contribute to society; (E) pursue meaningful careers; and (F) enjoy full inclusion and integration in the economic, political, social, cultural, and educational mainstream of American society. (Public Law 102-569, 1992)

The Rehabilitation Act Amendments of 1992 are the main source of funds through which employers and persons with disabilities can find assistance and expertise in locating employment. Every state in the United States has such a program, which can be found in the local telephone directory.

Relationship of the Rehabilitation Act to School Programs and Youth with Disabilities

The Rehabilitation Act Amendments of 1992 emphasize the provision of support and services through the rehabilitation system for high school–aged students with disabilities exiting or preparing to exit school programs. The Rehabilitation Act Amendments contain a definition of transition services (discussed later) that matches the definition contained in the IDEA. Transition is the process of planning for movement from high school to the world of work and other aspects of adult life (e.g., Wehman, 1992). The young man, Sam, who was referred to at the beginning of the chapter, is an example of a student who needs transition services. The transition services as defined in the Rehabilitation Act Amendments of 1992 are:

1. A coordinated set of activities for a student, designed within an outcome-oriented process, that promotes movement from school to post-school activities, including postsecondary education, vocational training, integrated employment (including supported employment), continuing and adult education, adult services, independent living, or community participation.

2. The coordinated set of activities shall be based upon the individual student's needs, taking into account the student's preferences and interests,

TABLE 1.1

Designing and Implementing a Community-Based Instructional Program

Steps	Activities
I. Conduct a job market analysis to identify potential jobs in the community that would be appropriate for students with severe disabilities.	1. Survey the telephone yellow pages. 2. Read the classified section of the newspaper. 3. Contact local business organizations—i.e., Chamber of Commerce. 4. Survey school graduates to determine jobs held by individuals with disabilities in the community.
II. Identify businesses with the targeted jobs.	1. Establish a school policy for contacting businesses. 2. Identify individual(s) responsible for business contacts. 3. Determine school insurance coverage and liability issues. 4. Develop a list of employers to approach. 5. Schedule a time to write letters, telephone and visit employers. 6. Compile a file for each business contacted.

III. Contact the Personnel Director or Employer.	1. By letter and/or telephone:
	  a. Briefly describe the school's community-based program.
	  b. Identify jobs that may be appropriate for training.
	  c. Schedule a time to visit and explain the program further.
	2. Visit in person:
	  a. Describe the purpose of community-based instruction.
	  b. Discuss the employer, teacher, and student responsibilities on the job site.
	  c. Discuss the school's insurance and liability policies.
	  d. Target tasks and time periods for training.
	  e. Schedule a visit to observe the identified tasks to develop job duty and task analyses.
	  f. Send a thank-you note.

IV. Select and analyze appropriate jobs for community-based training.	1. Visit the job site location. 2. Discuss the identified jobs with the site supervisor. 3. Discuss the job site rules and regulations.

(Continued)

TABLE 1.1 (Continued)

Steps	Activities
	4. Observe the coworkers performing the job duties.
	5. Select the tasks best suited for students with severe disabilities.
	6. Develop a job duty schedule and task analyses for the activities selected.
	7. Identify available times with the employer or department supervisor for training.
	8. Request at least 1–2 hour blocks of time for each site identified.
	9. Agree on a start date.
V. Schedule community-based training.	1. Identify students to receive vocational training.
	2. Hold IEP/ITP meetings for students.
	a. Identify student training needs.
	b. Discuss purpose of community-based vocational training with transition team members.
	c. Write vocational goals/objectives.
	3. Match students to available sites.
	4. Sign community-based training agreements (student, parents, employer, school representative).
	5. Develop a daily schedule.
	6. Develop a transportation schedule.
	7. Send a copy of the schedule to the school principal, special education supervisor, parents, employers, etc.
	8. Provide parents with information on individual insurance coverage for liability.
VI. Design individual systematic instruction programs.	1. Modify job duty schedules and task analyses based on student characteristics.
	2. Select a data collection procedure.
	3. Take a baseline of student performance on all tasks to be taught.
	4. Select an instructional procedure.
	5. Select a reinforcer.
	6. Implement the training program.
	7. Take probe data on student performance.
	8. Routinely review student data and modify program format as needed.
	9. Review student goals and objectives for training and update as needed.

and shall include instruction, community experiences, the development of employment and other postschool adult living objectives, and, when appropriate, acquisition of daily living skills and functional vocational evaluation.

This definition is a balanced statement of how the transition process is embedded in the Rehabilitation Act Amendments. As the reader can see it is similar to and coordinated with the IDEA definition of what the schools transition responsibilities are. Why is this important to students like Sam? The reason is simple: parents and professionals alike can draw on the resources provided by this law to help focus on Sam's transition from school to adulthood needs.

Part I of this definition focuses on services occurring after the individual exits the school program. These services reflect a representative sample of the wide array of postschool activities that might be used by individuals with a disability entering the adult community. At times these services are used in sequence, such as postsecondary education followed by employment. Services might also be used simultaneously, such as supported employment (discussed later) along with other adult services and community living supports. Part II of the definition of transition services focuses on activities that may occur during the school program to support the preparation and planning for transition. This section emphasizes relating the school program to the community and the incorporation of postschool employment and daily living objectives into classroom activities and planning.

THE VOCATIONAL REHABILITATION COUNSELOR AND THE SCHOOL PROGRAM

The goal of the cooperative relationship between the vocational rehabilitation program and the education system is for there be no gap in services as youth with disabilities make the transition from school into their postsecondary activities. The number of persons with disabilities served at any one time by a vocational rehabilitation counselor varies nationally, however, and it is not unusual for an individual counselor to have responsibility for assisting 100 to 200 people at various stages of the vocational rehabilitation process. Even those vocational rehabilitation counselors who spend the majority of their time working with youth with disabilities usually carry large caseloads. Vocational rehabilitation counselors cannot possibly attend every IEP meeting for every student with a disability age 14 and older and still effectively respond to the multiple and diverse needs of the full range of persons for whom they coordinate services.

The vocational rehabilitation counselor helps a client plan for and secure appropriate employment. This ideally should occur during the transition period from school to adulthood. Some students secure employment during their exiting school year, and the vocational rehabilitation counselor helps maintain and support them in their work and community adjustment. Other students pursue postsecondary training/education in preparation for employment, and the counselor can potentially assist in planning and securing postsecondary activities leading to employment. Finally, some will seek employment directly upon exiting their school program. They will need timely, well-planned job development and job placement assistance to bridge the gap between school and work.

The challenge therefore for the vocational rehabilitation counselor, the youth with a disability, and the school program is to design student specific education, transition, and employment plans for a population whose individual interests and needs vary considerably. The vocational rehabilitation counselor can provide and coordinate a variety of services and supports including: job and career oriented assessments, counseling, and guidance; sponsorship of postsecondary training; job development, analysis, placement, and restructuring; use of rehabilitation technology to assist, for example, in making job site accommodations; and identification and management of support services.

SUPPORTED EMPLOYMENT: A NEW WAY OF HELPING YOUTH WITH SEVERE DISABILITIES

An approach that was implemented in the early 1980s in the U.S. for people with severe disabilities that has become very popular is called *supported employment*. This approach was developed as an alternative to segregated adult day programs but is also being used in school systems for transition-age students. It has spread throughout Europe (see next section) as well as other parts of the world. With supported employment, a person with a disability is placed into a community-based competitive job with the help of an individual usually called a job coach or an employment specialist. This approach was developed in order to help people who were thought to have disabilities too extensive for them to work (Wehman & Moon, 1988). Job coaches can be teachers, counselors, or people from other disciplines. They work extensively with clients and their families to determine the individual preferences for various types of work, the effect of employment on each individual's overall financial situation (including financial benefits and health care), and each person's expectations of the program. Because the job coach provides direct instruction to the individual with a disability at the actual work site, clients may elect to work in jobs that they are initially unable to perform. The job coach is the most integral as key aspect in making this approach work.

Job site training focuses on direct training on job duties to enable the supported employee to meet the performance standards of the employer. In addition to systematic instruction, the job coach may restructure the work environment or prescriptively modify the job duties of a given position. The client can be assisted in adapting to the social environment of the work setting, including appropriate interactions with coworkers and supervisors. In many instances the job coach will remain at the job site for all of the individual's work time for several weeks.

In contrast to alternative placement approaches, supported employment services do not terminate once an individual has demonstrated the ability to perform all job duties to the standards and expectations of the employer. Ongoing support services are provided as long as the individual is employed. This has been a positive development for young people with disabilities who are starting their first jobs. The intent of the support services is to identify and remediate any problems experienced by the client before they jeopardize the individual's employment. Support may frequently be provided to address difficulties the client encounters outside the work settings that may ultimately affect job performance, such as interference with benefits, changes in the individual's residential setting, or transportation problems.

Larry: Entering Supported Employment from School

Larry is naturally suited for his job as a dining room attendant. He has worked at a local hotel in Richmond, Virginia for the past 2 years. Larry's friendly manner, outgoing personality, and seriousness about his job responsibilities have contributed to his successful employment. Larry is 20 years old. His primary disability is mental retardation with secondary disabilities including low vision in his left eye, a severe hearing impairment, and a speech-language impairment. Larry attended a segregated school for students with multiple disabilities. Upon graduation he sought employment through traditional job training options in the community. These experiences proved unsuccessful because of the complexities of his dual sensory disability. He needed the specialized services provided in supported employment including assessment, job matching, intensive job site training, consistent fading strategies, and follow-along support.

The dining room attendant position was targeted because Larry expressed the desire to work in a fast-food restaurant. His duties include maintaining a clean dining room, replenishing the condiments and cold bar, and checking the restrooms for cleanliness. When additional job training is needed, Larry's job coach provides these services. Larry has become a valued employee.

Larry has a tremendous family support system and could live at home. However, supported employment has given him a new sense of independence and he is now living in his own apartment.

INDEPENDENT LIVING

As important as employment is for young people with disabilities, there are other parts of an individual's life as well. As was noted earlier, there are many types of transitions that we all go through as we move from adolescence into adulthood, such as independence in mobility, developing friendships, choosing recreation options, and planning for the future (Mount & Zwernik, 1988; Wehman, 1992).

This section concerns community living, transportation, and leisure, three areas of critical importance in the transition process for young people with disabilities. It should be noted that the vocational rehabilitation counselor, the case manager, and other adult service personnel will need to play an active role in helping the student to arrange any of these options as well as employment opportunities.

Community Living

When students grow up and leave school, one of the first questions that they normally ask is "Where am I going to live?" — their parents are often asking them the same question. It is perfectly normal to live at home through school and through the college years as well, but as one enters adulthood there is a need for independence in living arrangements.

There are many different living alternatives as students make the transition out of school and into adulthood. At one time in the not too distant past, individuals with severe disabilities lived in state institutions that had as many as several hundred residents living at the facility. Those students who stayed in the community would continue to live with their mother and father until their parents grew old and passed away. At that time they would be sent to a nursing home. Within the past decade there has been an emergence of more group homes, which would house as many as 8 to 12 disabled individuals in a house within a regular neighborhood. Within this arrangement, there would be different shifts of live-in residential counselors that would provide around-the-clock supervision. The group home is probably the most prevalent nonresidential option that is available in the United States today for people with significant levels of disability.

Within the last 5 to 6 years, however, there has been a dramatic upswing in the use of another residential alternative, which is called *supported living*. With this arrangement, individuals with disabilities are helped to find apartments or other types of housing that would house two or three people and sometimes only one. In much the same way as the supported employment model is used, counselors or case managers help to provide support on a regular basis through visits, providing only the amount of supervisory help that is absolutely necessary. This is, of course, a highly attractive option that is predicated on a reasonable degree of domestic skill competence on the part of the student when they leave school.

It is interesting to note the degree of progress that has occurred in the types of models and philosophies associated with the different models over the past 30 years. During the 1960s virtually all people with any significant disabilities were housed in large institutions or residential facilities, usually at the suggestion of the family pediatrician. As we moved into the 1970s, when writers such as Wolfensberger (1972) wrote about deinstitutionalization, there was an emergence of large group homes in the community and what are also known as Intermediate Care Facilities (or ICF-MRs) that, in a sense, were small institutions with many as 75 to 100 people living in a facility. By the late 1970s and first half of the 1980s, there was a clear move to rapidly downsize institutions and even group homes to smaller group homes; this thinking has lead to the concept of supported living (Wagner, Long, Reynolds, & Taylor, 1995).

The key element to community living arrangements, both philosophically as well as from a programmatic implementation standpoint, is assessing the amount of help or support that a person with a disability needs. This is a radical departure from the thinking of 10 to 20 years ago, when most programs were structured to "take care of" or to "fix the problem" of people with disabilities. Therefore, large scale shuttling of individuals into large facilities in rural or remote areas, where most institutions were based, was viewed as the most expeditious way to handle this problem. However, as it became increasingly clear through an abundance of research literature that individuals with significant disabilities could be taught many more independent living skills and were able to demonstrate greater overall competence, the notion of segregating them into a large institution area was viewed increasingly as highly inappropriate. Subsequently, the philosophical directions moved toward providing the necessary array of supports to help the individual attain their community living preferences.

Transportation and Community Mobility

Community mobility refers to movement from one place to another within a particular setting, as well as the ability to travel between two community locations. Transportation is critically important to all individuals, as the inability to get from one area to another leads to tremendous dependence on others. In the Americans with Disabilities Act, Title III is fully devoted to the issues of transportation accessibility and mobility. The pioneers who lead to the passage of the Americans with Disabilities Act realized that the ability of an individual to participate independently or semi-independently in work and community life is heavily dependent upon mobility. Therefore, transportation is crucial to making transition from school to adulthood a viable possibility. It is equally crucial in the preparation for community living of many school-aged young people with a disability. As important as transportation is, this is still one of the most difficult services to obtain on a consistent basis.

For example, it is not uncommon to hear a school principal deny a special education teacher use of the school bus for community-based training in shopping skills because "we just can't afford field trips." The importance of teaching skills to some students in community settings in which it will be used, such as teaching in restaurants or grocery stores, is sometimes lost through well-meant but mis-placed overprotectiveness.

The availability of transportation is a key factor in the attainment and mainte-nance of employment by youths with fiscal disabilities. Without it, employment, community-based training, and access to many of the normal services available in the community will not be possible, and those affected will become isolated and shut in.

Leisure Skill Alternatives

Educators increasingly have recognized the importance of leisure in the develop-ment and socialization of all people. Individuals with disabilities are no excep-tion. It has been suggested that active participation in planned leisure activities within the community will result in positive gains in the following areas:

1. Health and physical fitness
2. Mobility
3. Language
4. Social skills
5. Self-fulfillment or self-image.
   (Moon, 1994; Schleien & Ray, 1988; Wehman & Schleien, 1982)

Many people with disabilities have substantial amounts of time are available for leisure activities. Constructive use of this time may provide educational ex-perience, as that maximizes chances for adjustment within community setting. Although participation in recreational activities should be voluntary, few indi-viduals with significant disabilities are self-directed or even aware of what their options in leisure might be. Therefore, educators must work closely with com-munity recreation specialist to plan specific goals and instructional experiences that can help enhance the transition from school to adulthood.

THE EUROPEAN EXPERIENCE: MOVING INTO REAL JOBS

Traditionally, men and women with intellectual disability (mental handicap) in more economically developed countries have been offered sheltered work once they reach adulthood. This is true in North America, Europe, Asia, and Australia as well as other parts of the world. Sheltered workshops may be attached to in-stitutions such as hospitals or they may stand alone in cities and towns. The hall-marks of this dominant form of employment are:

- Groups of adults with intellectual disability congregate together
- They receive a token payment unrelated to productivity or experience
- Contract with nondisabled peers is minimal

- Employment lasts many years, perhaps a lifetime
- Workers are usually screened on admission: those who do not meet medical or adaptive criteria may be allocated to another type of day activity

In Ireland, to take one example, sheltered work—more properly called "long-term vocational training"—is available throughout the country, managed by various voluntary, religious, and statutory bodies (McConkey & Murphy, 1988). Indeed, the numerous cohort of young adults in Ireland and the dearth of adequately funded training programs have swelled waiting lists for vocational training centers. Some centers produce and market their own products, such as pottery. But often the sheltered workers carry out assembly jobs for outside firms on a contractual basis. In Germany, by contrast, such workshops are more formally established and regulated as a parallel, self-sustaining system of production and income transfer (Samoy, 1992).

What is wrong, one may ask, with such a permanent, secure, and familiar workplace? Surely this is the universal aspiration of adults with intellectual disability and their families? Many sheltered workplaces appear benign, and yet appearances may deceive us into accepting a restrictive practice of "dead-end activities" as the norm (Bonanno, 1990, p. 13). Those providing employment services must now ask what they offer to the individual with intellectual disability (mental handicap). Will the individual's current position lead to a working life marked by choices, satisfaction, career development, payment for the job done, and companionship with coworkers with varying abilities? These are remorseless questions. They will not go away merely because they cause discomfort.

Current Alternatives

A number of employment initiatives and studies have been carried out that examine various models of employment that have been applied on behalf of adults with intellectual disability (mental handicap) during the past ten to fifteen years. What can we learn from the available evidence?

One alternative employment opportunity already noted in an earlier section is still young, but thriving nonetheless in Europe. This is supported employment, which we define as "real work in an integrated setting with on-going support" (National Development Team, 1992).

This approach differs both from sheltered employment and open employment, in which no ongoing supports are provided. It is, rather, a flexible response to the perennial barriers that have prevented the participation of men and women with intellectual and other disabilities—the very long-term unemployed—in the labor force. Fueled by the initial success in the 1970s and early 1980s of applications of systematic teaching methods among adults with intellectual disability (mental handicap) in work settings, and also by the compelling surge toward normalization, many professionals began to question the very nature of existing vocational services (Kregel & Wehman, 1989). The new alternatives, by contrast, promoted real work—that is, work that someone else would have to do if the person with intellectual disability did not do it—real wages, and real workplace with coworkers, not all of whom have disabilities.

Supported employment may be provided in different forms, although the first —individual placement—is perhaps best-known; the individual worker is first

1. placed in job suited to his/her preferences;
2. trained in the needed skills on-site by a job coach; and then
3. maintained in the job through a mix of special and natural supports (Walsh, Rafferty, & Lynch, 1991).

There is no "pre-work" or preparatory period. Nor is any individual excluded from work on the basis of a priori assumptions of ability. Four models currently applied are:

1. Individual placement—single worker, one site
2. Cluster models—two or three persons, one site
3. Work crew—usually mobile, on contract
4. Small business—mixed workforce, one enterprise

In the United States, professionals and advocates who were convinced of the efficacy of supported employment helped to bring about the federal initiatives of 1984 and 1986, in which substantial funding was allocated to system change grants in order to change radically the vocational rehabilitation system at state level in 27 of the 50 states (Kregel & Wehman, 1989). More recently, Sale, Revell, West, and Kregel, (1992) reported that expenditure on supported employment grew by approximately 19% from 1989 to 1990. They concluded that many states in the United States are now reallocating the funds previously reserved for tradi-tional case services to supported employment programs. It seems, from these re-ports, that money is following rhetoric.

Shafer, Wehman, Kregel, & West (1990) have assessed the impact of federal initiatives and found that different options within the supported employment model are being developed. More diversity is the outcome—but as some cost: it seems that supported employees working within options other than individual placement are less likely to work for twenty hours or more weekly. These au-thors also found evidence or more creativity, and more innovation among pro-viders working outside of traditional vocational facilities—a notable finding.

SUPPORTED EMPLOYMENT OUTCOMES

Proponents of this model cite evidence to support their claims that successful supported employment can achieve two worthy objectives: it can (a) increase his/her income, a concrete outcome measure; and, further, it can (b) enhance the process through which an individual achieves integration into society.

Incomes

The evidence for improved levels of income is striking. In one study, Thompson, Powers, and Houchard (1992) examined the wage effects of supported employment. They concluded that wages did increase after individuals with developmental disabilities entered supported employment, and that the individual placement model had the largest effect on wages; by contrast, mobile work crews gained little. Thompson et al. (1992) cited the findings of the national survey of employment among 85,000 persons with developmental disabilities that was undertaken by Kiernan, McGaughey, and Schalock (1986): Mean quarterly wages for persons in sheltered workshops amounted to $402.75, compared with $786.00 for those in supported employment. The mean hour wages were, respectively, $1.31 and $2.59.

Integration

There is also evidence to suggest that successful supported employment can achieve a second objective: It can promote the social as well as the vocational integration of workers with intellectual and other disabilities. Rusch, Johnson, and Hughes (1990) examined the quality of the involvement of $N = 264$ supported employees with their coworkers who did not have disabilities. They conducted that the levels of contact and socializing observed were related less to the individual worker's disability than to the type of work placement. Far more involvement was observed in individual or clustered placements—that is, when one or only a few persons worked in an integrated workplace. Those in work crews or small business settings had relatively lower levels of contact. Rusch, et al. (1990) commented that "[W]ithout the opportunity to interact with nondisabled coworkers in the workplace, it is unlikely that employees with disabilities can participate as equal members of the workforce."

What of the other members of the workforce, the people who work alongside supported employees who have intellectual disability (mental handicap)? Shafer, Rice, Metzler, & Haring (1989) surveyed $N = 212$ American coworkers. They found that regular social contact enhanced acceptance (as measured by reported comfort) on the part of the coworkers; such contact does not appear to affect the perceived competence of the supported employees. These authors conclude that employment specialists should plan ways of promoting social contacts between workers both with and without disabilities in the workplace and even after the working day, and also improve the vocational competence of supported employees.

Other Outcomes

A related outcome of successful supported employment is the provision of choices to the men and women who obtain it—men and women who may have had little opportunity to make meaningful choices in their lives. West and Parent (1992) comment that traditional employment services were designed for stereotypes, not individuals. Many of us here today recall decisions that were made about young adults 18 or 20 years old in their absence—perhaps whether to admit or to exclude them from a sheltered workshop—"yes/no" decisions that would have lasting impact. These authors describe, by contrast, the approaches that successful supported employment providers may take in ensuring that jobs and workers are in harmony:

- interview the consumer, family, advocates;
- observe the individual at work;
- review records;
- visit the work site, ask questions, communicate;
- design situational assessments, trial work periods (West and Parent, 1992).

INNOVATIONS – CASE STUDIES

It is often said that the evidence from large-scale surveys and the very language of supported employment reflects North American traditions. Does this imply that supported employment is culture-bound? By no means: our colleagues around Europe have been engaged in a number of high-quality demonstration projects. With their cooperation, I am able to present a sample of these innovative activities to you today.

United Kingdom

In the United Kingdom, the National Development Team (1992) has published a report, "Supported Employment for People with Learning Disabilities." They concluded that supported employment has now reached a growth rate similar to that in the United States. The first part of the report presents the results of a survey of some 79 service agencies in England, Scotland, and Wales. A total of 1,600 client-workers within the supported employment were identified at the end of 1991. Based on the data available, the National Development Team reported that "... the running costs of most supported employment services were comparable with those of more traditional services."

One example from the United Kingdom helps to illustrate the diverse form that supported employment options may take: Deb Steele ("Excell," London). It is striking that the service that Steele and her colleagues have established in the heart of London advertises itself as a mainstream or "High Street" agency serving local employees by providing a high-quality employment service specializing in offering local employers access to qualified, trained local people. Some of the local people who obtain employment in this way are people with intellectual or other disabilities. In the "Excell" enterprise, the focus is on the quality and reliability of the product delivered—in this case, successful employment placements sustained through skilled job coaching.

The Netherlands

In the Netherlands, Rob Bastiaansen and his colleagues at Stichting VSO Arbeidstrajekt, Rotterdam, have joined with employers, service agencies, government departments, and young job-seekers themselves to develop supported employment options. With additional support from the FORCE initiative of the European Commission, the Rotterdam team have worked closely with local employers in order to identify what information is most helpful to them, what supports are most appropriate, and what training materials are most effective for them and their other employees. The hallmarks of this project are the consistently high quality of its professional dealings with all relevant parties, and the priority placed on rigorous, university-affiliated evaluation of the supported employment process and outcomes.

Portugal

In Portugal, individuals in Lisbon, Setubal, and Peniche have promoted the Agora project, another Horizon-funded transnational initiative. Together with their partners in Northern Ireland and the Netherlands, the Agora project team has applied the individual placement model of supported employment. Job coaches work closely with the employers and coworkers to ensure placement. Job training is provided on-site when it is required.

Ireland

In Ireland, with a population of 3.6 million, the efficacy of supported employment has been demonstrated in at least three quite distinct groups of people with intellectual disability (mental handicap).

Open Road was an innovative project funded by the European Social Fund from 1988 to 1991. As documented in the *Final Report* (1993) of this project, men and women with moderate or severe levels of intellectual disability who had no previous vocational experience found real, part-time work with the support of job coaches or coworkers. A striking feature of this project was its impact on the adaptive behavior of the participants: their scores in the range of social, communicative, and practical daily activities increased significantly during the life of the project (Open Road, 1993, section 4).

A second project, *Challenge,* is currently active within the *Horizon* initiative. Partners in Ireland, the United Kingdom, and Spain are successfully introducing men and women with severe intellectual, physical, and multiple disabilities to the wold of work. To date, 12 of the 15 participants in Ireland have regular, part-time employment with the support of job coaches and coworkers (Project Challenge, 1993).

A third project promoted by Ireland, *Connect,* has recently started its activities: it aims to provide the training and re-training required by men and women who have a mild or moderate level of intellectual disability (mental handicap) and who have worked for some time in traditional, sheltered settings. This project also benefits from the support offered through the Horizon transnational initiative funded from the European Commission.

Developing Countries

Fresh employment alternatives are not confined to the European community, no more than to North America. The monastic fathers in Europe used to say: "To work is to pray." But for some people with intellectual disability (mental handicap), to work is to live. In the developing countries, the crucial factor for adults is their own livelihood and that of the families who sustain them in the community. The priority for service providers in these countries is straightforward: to provide the family of the person with intellectual disability (mental handicap) with what is required as a livelihood—perhaps a house, or land, or a financial loan, or job training for the family breadwinner. For in these countries—Guyana, Sri Lanka, or the Philippines, for example—only family income can ensure that the person with intellectual disability (mental handicap) can be supported and cared for (R. McConkey, personal communication, October 17, 1993).

What employment opportunities present themselves to people with intellectual disability in developing countries? These must of course fit the local economy. Cottage industries—sewing, laundry services, stitching bags, or producing craft items—may be carried out at home, among family and neighbors. Some men and women may be sustained in their own small businesses in this way. Others may work with others in cooperatives, as in the Philippines, where persons with complementary abilities join forces. To take an example, some workers with intellectual disability might work alongside those with physical or sensorial disability, their respective strengths interlocking in common enterprise. Models of supported employment also lend themselves to the economies of developing countries. But there, as in the European community or North America, the same caution prevails on the continued desirability of large, congregate centers: too often, these shelters become costly, rigid structures with no exit.

Instead, policymakers and providers in the developing world are turning toward models of education that prepare men and women with intellectual and other disabilities for a livelihood even from their childhood. The policy of

UNESCO states that special education should be individual-centered, oriented to the local environment and aimed at productive work (McConkey, personal communication, 1993). "Livelihood earning" starts at an early age. The person with intellectual disability in the developing world must be perceived as a contributor to the family and—if the family is not there to care—then to the local community. Specially devised video training packages and other materials have been prepared to meet the needs of those helping to support people with intellectual disability and their families in the developing world (McConkey, Bradley, & Holloway, 1993; "Training for Work," Cheshire Foundation, International—available in Penang, Malaysia, or from the first author, McConkey).

Labor Force Issues

It may be seen that the reports of promising developments are widespread. The initiatives described here represent good practice on the part of those involved with the fortunes of people with intellectual disability (mental handicap) who are also, it must be recalled, citizens of their countries and members of the international community. We have robust evidence to back our claim that a supply of motivated, trained, and supported employees is available from within the ranks of persons with intellectual or other disabilities. But our colleagues in the International Labor Organization and in the private and public sectors have additional concerns about a much wider constituency. What about the current demand for labor?

Workforce

The workforce is undergoing profound structural changes. Trends toward its "feminization" (Walsh, 1993; Yelin, 1991) are apparent. A contributory factor has been the decline in the jobs and industries traditionally dominated by men—the coal-mining industry, to take one example. As Yelin (1991) has commented about trends in the United States,

> the overall labor-force participation rate—regardless of gender, age or disability status—increased 10 percent over the last two decades because the increase among young women overshadowed the decreases experienced by older men. Likewise, this overall increase masks substantial increases among persons without a disability (12 percent) and a worsening employment picture for those with disabilities (the labor-force participation rate fell by 4 percent among all working-aged persons with a disability, dropping even more, as noted above, among some subgroups). Thus, on balance, the person with a disability fared worse in the labor market at the end of the period than at the beginning, even though the labor force expanded both absolutely and relatively during this time. (pp. 134–135)

In Ireland, the number of women at work rose by 41% between 1971 and 1992, while there is a marked decline in labor force participation among older men (Walsh, 1993). These and other trends shape the context in which any initiatives on behalf of people with intellectual disability (mental handicap) must be implemented. Although we tend to act locally, we must nonetheless think globally.

Other Economic Trends

No one from the European community can ignore the impact of recessionary trends on overall levels of unemployment. Trends in employment are not uniform: these vary from sector to sector and region to region, and must be documented carefully. Ireland, to take one example, has a relatively high rate of unemployment. The numbers employed in agriculture have declined sharply, while those employed in retail distribution and financial services have risen (Walsh, 1993). In addition, tightened fiscal policies in Ireland and other countries also have increased the costs associated with placing people with disabilities in employment and supporting them in the long term.

High unemployment and high costs impact the availability of employment to persons with intellectual and other disabilities. Rising supply costs—for example, the costs incurred by employers attempting to accommodate to the recent American's with Disabilities Act in the United States—must be addressed. As Chirikos has suggested (1991), the burden of higher costs and other redistributive issues in generating employment may have to be shared by employers and employees alike. Chirikos identifies three crucial research needs: we must know more about how much it costs to accommodate persons with disabilities in the workplace; we need to know more about the labor supply in general—for example, the mix and severity of disabilities—and we need more information to say whether employment for persons with disabilities could be increased if costs were shared.

FURTHER WORK TO BE DONE

The findings available to us point to fruitful lines of action research. We suggest that the following research questions demand our urgent attention:

1. What are the short- and long-term costs of supporting people with intellectual disability (mental handicap) in integrated employment, and ow can we meet these costs?

2. A related question regards the interface of employment income and subsidies with national systems of benefits, allowances, and entitlements: what steps can we take to help rationalize these very diverse systems so that they sustain people with disabilities optimally? From my own experience and that of my col-

leagues in the League, I can assure you that this will not be a straightforward task.

3. As the National Development Team (1992) in the United Kingdom has suggested, we must address the evaluation of long-term outcomes of supported employment. Only the careful collection and analysis of data can help to determine whether this model, in all of its forms, truly benefits employees with disabilities. We often hear voices raised with doubts about supported employment: "Only some can benefit," or "It is really just part-time work," or "It is only for Americans," or "In that project, the people selected were the most able / the least able," or "Our parents, or staff, or clients, prefer their familiar workshop," and so forth. These responses to radical change are to be expected: many are driven by a genuine concern about the well-being and acceptance of people with intellectual disability (mental handicap) in a world of hard times. It is important to provide timely, reliable, data about this employment option or any other.

One strategy might be to coordinate the findings from Horizon and other initiatives. We might also join with new structures such as the European Union on Supported Employment in developing friendly, transferrable, evaluative tools so that employment outcomes may be compared among different countries and over time. Most important is the involvement of people with disabilities themselves in the work of evaluating their own employment experiences and preferences. There is much work to be done here.

Systemic Change

Finally, it is apparent that radical changes will be required if we wish to develop alternatives to the well-entrenched sheltered tradition of employment. Beare, Severson, Lynch, and Schneider (1992) described the conversion of a small service agency in the western part of the United States to the community-based employment. The crucial factor was the philosophical change brought about at executive and board level, followed by the commitment of staff and support of parents. Were there difficulties? Certainly: the authors reported occasional job dissatisfaction, coworker dissatisfaction, and the challenges posed by providing transport across rural area, among others. Other barriers were the prevailing financial systems and the "developmental thinking" of staff who believed that clients deserved care, not jobs. And yet this small service agency successfully change its mission from the top down and securing supported employment of good quality for most of the adults referred to it (Beare, et al., 1992).

What can we do to turn our respective agencies around? This will be a painful step, as we must turn ourselves around in the process (Kregel & Wehman, 1989). The outcomes of systematic change will certainly provide a worthy topic for a future researchers and practitioners.

SUMMARY

The transition process necessary for students with a disability to move effectively from school to work has two primary points of emphasis. First, attention must be focused on the students' in-school activities involving both preparation and planning for living and working in the community. Objectives focused on working competitively and living in an independent, integrated fashion in the community should be emphasized in the student's educational program. Educators must be familiar with resources in the community that will be utilized as the student enters the adult community, and these resources should be brought into the school to assist in the planning of transition oriented activities. Second, attention must be focused also on the postschool objectives and services that will provide and maintain the supports necessary for the individuals with a disability to make a successful transition from school to work. These services might support a period of postsecondary education/training or possibly direct movement into employment. The likelihood that these postschool services will be available and provided in a timely and responsive manner are enhanced substantially if they are identified and arranged prior to the completion of the student's school program.

REFERENCES

Americans with Disabilities Act of 1990, 42 U.S.C., §12101 *et seq.*

Beare, P. L., Severson, S. J., Lynch, E. C., & Schneider, D. (1992). Small agency conversion to community-based employment: Overcoming the barriers. *Journal of the Association for Persons with Severe Handicaps 17*(3), 170–178.

Bonanno, B. (1990). *Work Opportunities for People with Mental Handicap.* Brussels: ILSMH.

Bullis, M., Bull, B., Johnson, B., & Peters, D. (1995). The school-to-community transition experiences of hearing young adults and young adults who are deaf. *Journal of Special Education, 28*(4), 405–423.

Chirikos, T. N. (1991). The economics of employment. *Milbank Quarterly 69*(Suppl. 1/2), 150–179.

Clark, G. (1994). Is a functional curriculum approach compatible with an inclusive educational model. *Teaching Exceptional Children, 26*(2), 36–39.

Clark, G., & Kolstoe, O. (1994). *Career education and transition.* Boston: Allyn and Bacon.

Edgar, E. (1987). Secondary special education: Is much of it justifiable? *Exceptional Children, 53*, 555–561.

Edgar, E. & Polloway, E. (1994). Education for adolescence with disabilities: Curriculum placement issues. *Journal of Special Education, 27*(4), 438–452.

Enchelmaier, J., Kohler, P., & Rusch, F. (1994). Employment outcomes and activities for youth in transition. *Career Development for Exceptional Individuals, 17*(1), 1–16.

Individuals with Disabilities Education Act of 1990, Pub. L. No. 101-476, Title 20, U.S.C. 1400–1485 (1990). *U.S. Statutes at Large, 104*, 1103–1151.

Ivancic, M. T., & Schepis, M. M. (1995). Teaching key use to persons with severe disabilities in congregate living settings. *Research in Developmental Disabilities, 16*(5), 415–423.

Kiernan, W. E., McGaughey, M. J., & Schalock, R. C. (1986). *National employment survey for adults with developmental disabilities.* Boston, MA: Children's Hospital, Developmental Evaluation Clinic.

Kregel, J., & Wehman, P., (1989). Supported employment: Promises deferred for persons with severe disabilities. *Journal of the Association for Persons with Severe Handicaps 14*(4), 293–303.

Louis Harris and Associates. (1994). *Survey for the international center for the disabled. The ICD survey II: Employing disabled Americans.* Washington, DC: National Organization on Disability.

McConkey, R., Bradley, S., & Holloway, S. R. (1993). *Training for Work.* Glasgow, Scotland: Cheshire Foundation, International.

McConkey, R., & Murphy, R. (1988). A national survey of centers and workshops for adult persons with mental handicaps. In R. McConkey & C. Conliffe (Eds)., *The person with mental handicap.* Dublin: St. Michael's House Research Trust; Belfast: Institute for Counselling and Personal Development.

Moon, M. S. (1994). *Making social and community recreation fun for everyone.* Baltimore: Paul H. Brookes.

Moon, M. S., & Inge, K. (1993). Vocational preparation and transition. In M. E. Snell (Ed.), *Instruction of students with severe disabilities* (4th ed., pp. 556–587). New York: Merrill.

Mount, M., & Zwernik, J. (1988). *Personal futures planning.* Minneapolis: Metropolitan Planning Council, Minnesota Developmental Disabilities Council.

National Development Team. (1992). *Supported Employment for People with Learning Disabilities.* Manchester: Hester Adrian Research Centre.

Neal, S., & Bader, B. (1991). Case management. In P. McLaughlin & P. Wehman (Eds.), *Mental Retardation and Developmental Disabilities* (pp. 172–183). Austin, TX: PRO-ED.

O'Brien, J., & O'Brien, C. (1992). Members of each other: Perspectives on social support for people with severe disabilities. In J. Nisbet (Ed.), *Natural supports in school, at work, and in the community for people with severe disabilities* (pp. 217–231). Baltimore: Paul H. Brookes.

O'Connell, M. (1992). *Community building in Logan Square: How a community grew stronger with contributions of people with disabilities.* Evanston, IL: Northwestern University Center for Urban Affairs and Policy Research.

Open Road. (1993). *Final Report.* Dublin: St. Michael's House Research.

Parent, W. (1991). Situation assessment and vocational evaluation. In S. Griffin and G. Revell (Eds.), *Rehabilitation counselor desktop guide to supported employment* (pp. 117–131). Richmond, VA: Virginia Commonwealth University.

Peraino, J. M. (1992). Post-21 follow-up studies: How do special education graduates fare? In P. Wehman (Ed.), *Life beyond the classroom: Transition strategies for young people with disabilities* (pp. 27–70). Baltimore: Paul H. Brookes.

Project Challenge. (1993). *Interim Report.* Newbridge, Co. Kildare, Ireland: KARE.

Rehabilitation Act Amendments of 1992, 20 U.S.C. §1400, *et seq.*

Rusch, F., Johnson, J. R., and Hughes, C. (1990). Analysis of co-worker involvement in relation to level of disability versus placement approach among supported employees. *Journal of the Association for Persons with Severe Handicaps 15*(1), 32–39.

Sale, P., Revell, W. G., West, M., & Kregel, J. (1992). Achievements and challenges II: An analysis of 1990 Supported Employment expenditure. *Journal of the Association for Persons with Severe Handicaps 17*(24), 236–246.

Samoy, E. (1992). *Sheltered Employment in the European Community.* Leuven: Hoger Instituut voor de Arbeid.

Schleien, S., & Ray, T. (1988). *Community recreation programs.* Baltimore: Paul H. Brookes.

Shafer, M. S., Rice, M. L., Metzler, H. M. D., & Haring, M. (1989). A survey of nondisabled employees' attitudes towards supported employees with mental retardation. *Journal of the Association for Persons with Severe Handicaps 14*(2), 136–146.

Shafer, M., Wehman, P., Kregel, J. & West, M. (1990). National Supported Employment Initiative: A preliminary analysis. *American Journal on Mental Retardation 95*(3), 316–27.

Szymanski, E. M., & King, J. (1989). Rehabilitation counseling in transition: Planning and preparation. *Career Development for Exceptional Individuals, 12*(1), 3–10.

Thompson, L., Powers, G., & Houchard, B. (1992). The wage effects of supported employment. *Journal of the Association for Persons with Severe Handicaps, 17*(2), 8794.

Tooman, M., Revell, G., & Melia, R. (1988). The role of the rehabilitation counselor in the provision of transition and supported employment programs. In S. E. Rubin & N. M. Rubin (Eds.), *Contemporary challenges to the rehabilitation counseling profession* (pp. 126–141). Baltimore: Paul H. Brookes.

Unger, K. V. (1995). Unfinished business: Providing vocational services to transition-aged youth with serious emotional disturbance. *Journal of Vocational Rehabilitation, 5*(2), 159–165.

Wagner, B. R., Long, D. F., Reynolds, M. L., & Taylor, J. R. (1995). Voluntary transformation from an institutionally based to a community-based service system. *Mental Retardation, 33*(5), 317–321.

Walsh, B. M. (1993). Labour force participation and the growth of women's employment. Ireland 1971–1991. *The Economic and Social Review 24*(4), 369–400.

Walsh, P. N., Rafferty, M., & Lynch, C. (1991). The OPEN ROAD project: Real jobs for people with mental handicap. *The International Journal of Rehabilitation Research 14*, 155–161.

Wehman, P. (1992). *Life Beyond the Classroom: Transition strategies for young people with disabilities.* Baltimore: Paul H. Brookes.

Wehman, P. (1995). *Individual transition plans: A teachers curriculum guide to planning transition.* Austin, TX: PRO-ED.

Wehman, P., & Moon, M. S. (1988). *Vocational rehabilitation and supported employment.* Baltimore: Paul H. Brookes.

Wehman, P., & Schleien, S. (1982). *Leisure programs for handicapped persons.* Austin, TX: PRO-ED.

West, M. D., & Parent, W. (1992). Consumer choice and empowerment in Supported Employment services: Issues and strategies. *Journal of the Association for Persons with Severe Handicaps 17*(1), 47–52.

Wolfensberger, W. (1972). *Principles of normalization.* Toronto: National Institute on Mental Retardation.

Yelin, E. H. (1991). The recent history and immediate future of employment among persons with disabilities. *Milbank Quarterly 69*(Supp. 1/2), 129–149.

A Preventive Education Model for School Restructuring: Creating Parent–Student–Teacher Partnerships to Prevent Postschool Maladjustment

HOWARD L. GARBER
Milwaukee Center for Independence
Milwaukee, Wisconsin

MAURICE MCINERNEY
DAVID OSHER
American Institutes for Research
Washington, DC

This chapter describes a preventive education model for school restructuring. The purpose of the model is to anticipate and prevent problems of postsecondary school transition among youth with disabilities.

School-to-work transition includes the time span before and immediately following the completion or dropping out of high school (Wagner et al., 1991; Will, 1984). Adolescents and young adults experience transition in different ways. Some do so as they begin the process of finishing their education, leaving their family home—often for the first time—finding a stable job, and establishing an independent life in the community (Affleck, Edgar, Levine, & Kortering, 1990). Others do so as they move from school to school, drop out, and confront a hostile job market and an unfriendly and often inaccessible social service system (Clark & Foster-Johnson, 1994; Wagner, Blackborby, Cameto, Hebbeler, & Newman, 1993). In either case, transition is typically a challenging time for many youth with disabilities as well as their nondisabled peers (Ginzberg & Vojta, 1981). As a result, Richardson, Koller, and Katz (1988), among others, emphasize that all adolescents and young adults need to develop the personal competence required for successful transition into the local community.

Youth with disabilities are, unfortunately, among those who are most likely to experience problems of postschool maladjustment (U.S. Department of Education, 1992). Over 38% of adolescents with disabilities drop out of school (Wagner, et al., 1993). In addition, adolescents and young adults with disabilities are less likely than their nondisabled peers to live independently (Wagner, D'Amico, Marder, Newman, & Blackborby, 1992) and are more likely to be unemployed for extended periods or to be employed at low paying, part-time jobs after high school (Schalock & Lilley, 1986; Wagner et al., 1993). Furthermore, these youth are likely to depend on extended financial and social support from their family and friends (Kiernan & Brinkman, 1988) or the public welfare system (Mithaug, Horiuchi, & Fanning, 1985).

These problems are particularly pronounced among three groups of students: students from economically disadvantaged backgrounds, students whose linguistic and cultural background is not part of the social mainstream, and students of color (Wagner et al., 1991). Many of these students are overrepresented among students with disabilities (Wagner et al., 1993) and among those students who are placed in more restrictive placements (Chinn & Hughes, 1987; Edelman, 1987). At the same time, the National Longitudinal Transition Study (1991) found that some of these students (particularly those with emotional and behavioral disorders) are underrepresented among those students with disabilities who do receive such needed transition services as counseling and vocational educational training.

African American students with disabilities provide a case in point. When the National Longitudinal Transition Study of Special Education Students controlled for other differences, it found that African American students with disabilities were significantly less likely than their White counterparts to find a competitive job or earn competitive wages, and significantly less likely to be living independently and fully participating in the community (Wagner et al., 1993).

This chapter considers issues of preventive education and school restructuring in identifying and serving youth with disabilities. We describe a three-factor (parent-student-teacher) risk model of preventive education that can address the needs and build upon the strengths of different students, schools, communities, and cultural groups. The model reflects our understanding of those factors that deleteriously affect children's development. If implemented in a culturally competent manner, this model offers a promising approach to restructuring traditional approaches to education in this country.

PREVENTIVE EDUCATION GOALS
FOR SCHOOL RESTRUCTURING

Preventive education is a model by which local communities can restructure their schools by creating cooperative partnerships that empower parents, students, and teachers:

- *Parent empowerment* means that parents and other family caregivers should be enabled and encouraged to accept shared responsibility with the school to help their adolescent offspring become independent young adults
- *Student empowerment* means that adolescents and young adults should be enabled to develop the knowledge and problem-solving skills that are required for success in our increasingly technological society
- *Teacher empowerment* means that classroom teachers and other local school staff should be given adequate resources and then held accountable for preparing their students for successful school-to-work transitions

The model involves establishing an information system that effectively moves the point of referral for postschool transition problems back in time to the high school (and even the junior high school) period where these problems originated.

Under a preventive education model, both students with disabilities and their families participate in an individualized program of transition services. The intent of this intervention is to preventively teach and facilitate the development of the skills required for postschool success before — not after — students leave high school and begin the transition process. In addition, local secondary schools — at both the high school and middle school level — reorganize their delivery systems to establish communication systems necessary to implement preventive education strategies. The result of this restructuring is likely to be more effective services for individual youth and their families, fewer dropouts, and a more efficient use of educational resources available to the local school district.

Previous School Restructuring Initiatives

There have been at least three distinct waves of school restructuring initiatives over the last 25 years. The first wave, which began in the late 1960s and early 1970s, emphasized improving educational outcomes by disseminating information about effective educational practices (Emrick & Peterson, 1978). For example, the U.S. Department of Education's National Diffusion Network disseminated information about locally developed curricula and programs with a proven track record of success (Miles, 1980). Such authors as Louis and Rosenblum (1981) suggest that the National Diffusion Network model can benefit students when schools are provided high quality information, appropriate technical assistance, and a small amount of funds to implement recommended changes. However, a consistent body of research and analysis suggests that local commitment by school-based practitioners is necessary if effective practices are to be implemented (or adapted) effectively (Fullan, 1990; Osher & Kane, 1993).

The second wave of reform was sparked by the publication of *A Nation at Risk* (Boyer, 1983), a highly critical evaluation of the quality of education in the country's public schools. Second wave reformers emphasized a "top-down" approach in which school administrators, often at the federal or state level, mandated specific curricular changes in local school buildings and classrooms (Goodlad, 1984). These mandates included calls for increased graduation requirements, a longer school day, higher standards for teachers, and more testing for students. Such authors as McLaughlin (1990) point out that the impact of these reforms has been mitigated, in part, because legislative mandates alone are typically insufficient to create systemic changes in complex, social institutions such as our public schools.

The third wave of school restructuring began in the late 1980s, in part due to dissatisfaction with second wave reform initiatives (Cuban, 1990). This period was characterized by a "bottom-up" approach to school restructuring (Elmore & McLaughlin, 1988). Changes suggested during this period included interdisciplinary collaboration, the development of approaches to actively engage families in the development and evaluation of interventions, and the decentralization of control from the state and school district level to the community and school. For example, school-based site management teams were established to evaluate local programs and make local decisions about how and when to improve their educational practices. In addition, there was increased staff development, training, and support to ensure that recommended restructuring initiatives were implemented as intended or adapted effectively and to enable teachers to work more effectively with students from diverse cultural and socioeconomic backgrounds (Fullan & Miles, 1992; Louis & Smith, 1991).

Cultural Context for School Restructuring

During the past decade, researchers and practitioners in mental health, social welfare, and education developed a conceptualization of cultural competency. When implemented effectively, culturally competent approaches can enable professionals and organizations to work more effectively with students from diverse cultural and socioeconomic backgrounds (Isaacs & Benjamin, 1991; U.S. Department of Education, 1994). Culturally competent approaches (American Humane Association, 1992; Cross, Bazron, Dennis, & Isaacs, 1989; Focal Point, 1994; Orlandi, 1992) respect individual differences and appreciate the differences and similarities within, among, and between cultures and individuals. Because these approaches recognize the cultural grounding of the teachers' (or other service providers') views, behaviors, and methods, they reduce the risk that already marginalized students and families (whether due to poverty, culture, language, race, religion, or even disability) will: (a) be "blamed" for their differences (Darling, 1979; Ryan, 1971), (b) receive inappropriate services and lowered expectations (Federal Resource Center for Special Education, 1993; Hilliard, 1989; Richardson & Colfer, 1990), and (c) again be subjected to what Asa Hilliard referred to as "a protocol of interactive behaviors" (1989, p. 68) in which teachers expect less, give less support, and are more critical of students for whom they have lower expectations (Meier & Brown, 1994; Page, 1991). While minimizing the negative impact of self-fulfilling prophecies, culturally competent approaches also minimize the risk that students and their families will reject or undermine transition plans because they do not understand them or find them to be intrusive or culturally inappropriate (Bower, Thompson, & Fullilove, 1990; Harry, 1992).

Preventive Education Approach to Restructuring Public Schools

Our preventive education model incorporates selected features of each of these previous school restructuring initiatives. For example, preventive education emphasizes locally developed curricula (i.e., first wave reform), increased accountability (i.e., second wave reform), and family-school collaboration and ongoing staff training and technical assistance (i.e., third wave reform). The intent of these reform initiatives is to reorganize local delivery systems in ways that will help improve postschool transition outcomes for students with disabilities and their families.

Table 2.1 contains a list of preventive education goals and strategies for school restructuring. These goals are organized within three categories: parent empowerment, student empowerment, and school empowerment. Selected strategies to help achieve the successful implementation of each goal are also identified. These goals and strategies are described in greater detail below.

Parent Empowerment

The importance of family involvement in children's schooling has long been recognized. For example, families influence both adverse and positive developmental outcomes for children with disabilities (Garber & McInerney, 1982; Upshur, 1991). Similarly, family influences have been shown to either facilitate or impede the intellectual and affective development of normal (Majoribanks, 1976), disadvantaged (Rutter & Madge, 1976) and at-risk children (Werner & Smith, 1977).

Surprisingly, given the importance of families, parents have been given little substantive involvement in most school reform efforts to date. The most publicized role involves "choice" initiatives, where parents are provided school vouchers and allowed a choice about where their children are educated. However, as Smith and O'Day (1990) point out, the school choice movement presumes incorrectly that most parents are dissatisfied with their children's neighborhood school and are motivated to take the time to choose another school—especially if that school requires extensive travel from the family home. Instead, choice seems likely to benefit well-educated, middle- and upper-middle-class parents. These individuals have both the time to obtain information about the range of available choices as well as the resources to adequately evaluate which option is best for their children.

A preventive education model emphasizes parent empowerment—rather than for what most families is a forced "choice" between unwanted options. As indicated in Table 2.1, there are perhaps five key strategies to empowering parents to become active supporters and accept shared responsibility for their children's education. First, school policies and procedures are modified to encourage and support active parent participation. Second, parents are provided full and accessible information in a family-friendly, linguistically accessible, and culturally appropriate manner about how to develop and implement appropriate transition

TABLE 2.1
Preventive Education Goals and Strategies for School Restructuring

	Parent Empowerment
Goal	Parents should participate in the development of transition goals and accept shared responsibility with the school to help adolescents become independent young adults.
Strategies	Parents are enabled to participate in transition planning and implementation in a respectful and family-friendly manner. Parents are provided with information about appropriate transition goals and objectives in a culturally competent and linguistically appropriate manner. Parents actively participate in the development of goals and objectives and in the monitoring of their implementation. Parents receive support and advice about how to help prepare their children for transition success. Parents are referred to available local services for more intensive treatment or support, as needed and appropriate.
	Student Empowerment
Goal	Students should develop the critical thinking skills that are required for success in our increasingly technological society.
Strategies	Students are provided with an opportunity to develop appropriate work habits and other prevocational skills needed on local job sites. Students are provided with an opportunity to learn how to solve common social problems at home, in school, and in the community. Students are provided structured opportunities to explore possible career paths after high school. Students actively participate in the development of transition goals and plans and in the assessment of their implementation.
	Teacher Empowerment
Goal	Teachers should be held accountable for preparing their students for successful school-to-work transitions and are provided with the training and support that will enable them to do so.
Strategies	Teachers participate in site-based management teams that work with families and students to identify local goals and objectives for transition. Teachers implement an interdisciplinary curriculum to teach requisite transition skills. Teachers receive needed training and support to ensure their professional growth as transition specialists.

goals, objectives, and options for their adolescent children. Third, parents actively participate in the development of goals and objectives and the monitoring of their implementation. Fourth, parents receive support and advice about how to help prepare their children for transition success. Fifth, parents are referred to available local services for more intensive support or treatment.

As Clarke (1980) points out, the recognized importance of family support belies the fact that family factors are largely outside the realm of the existing educational delivery system. Thus, under a preventive education model, parents provide a previously untapped source of support for their children's growth, achievement, and postschool success. The active involvement of families provides many benefits in increasingly diverse and mobile societies. First, it can produce enthusiasm from parents whom educators have hitherto been unable to reach (Edwards, 1993; Levin, 1993). Second, it enables educators to develop culturally responsive models that build on student and family strengths (Osher & Osher, 1994). Finally, it contributes to the harnessing and sustaining of natural supports that will be available to the student after he or she leaves school (Eber, 1994; Seligman, 1991).

Student Empowerment

The need for student empowerment can be seen in terms of the large numbers of former students who fail to make adequate postschool transitions (Wagner, 1993). For example, the U.S. Commission on Civil Rights (1983) reported that over 250,000 youth with disabilities exit school each year but fail to find a job and secure an independent home life. Moreover, these data underestimate the actual number of youth who experience transition difficulty due to learning and behavioral problems. Nationally, nearly 1.7 million youth exit high school annually with at best minimal literacy, many without a diploma, and lacking the critical thinking skills and work habits expected of a technologically sophisticated work force (Porter, Archbald, & Tyree, 1991). We call this group *youth at risk*.

Many youth at risk present a developmental history of learning and behavioral problems prior to their school exit. Some youth develop antagonistic styles of learning that are transferred from their families (Hess, 1970; Ogbu, 1992) as early as preschool (Garber, 1988). Many youth at risk typically have poor work habits throughout their school careers. These youth often exhibit increased antisocial behavior as elementary and middle school students, due to both frustration and inability to succeed in school (Gresham, 1981; Osher & Osher, 1994) and the inhospitable climate they face in school (Cummins, 1986b; Page, 1991). In addition, these youth often emulate poor vocational role models at home (Garber & McInerney, 1991) or react negatively to what they perceive as a lack of future economic and educational opportunities (Ogbu, 1978; Taylor, 1990). Furthermore, these students often are unable to access local employers and obtain job references that are stepping stones to postschool employment (Hasazi, Gordon, & Roe, 1985).

It is possible to design alternative school curricula that address these developmental characteristics of youth at risk. If these curricula are to be effective, however, they must be developed and implemented in a manner that (1) actively engages students and (2) takes into account what John Ogbu describes as the "social pressures discouraging involuntary minority students from adopting the standard attitudes and behavior practices that enhance school learning" (1992, p. 10). This requires listening to students (Delpit, 1988; Franklin, 1992) and addressing the social and cultural tensions that structure the relationships between socially marginalized students and their teachers (Dryfoos, 1990; Williams & Kornblum, 1994). Once we do so, it becomes possible to implement culturally responsive curricula that address the emotional and cultural needs of these students (Cummins, 1986a; Smey-Richman, 1991).

Table 2.1 contains illustrations of these preventive education strategies. For example, evidence that students have poor work habits can lead to pre-employment practica. These practica can be linked to collaborative feedback sessions that acknowledge different cultural styles but enable students to actively adapt to culturally acceptable approaches, follow directions, work independently on local job sites, and integrate these changes into their community life. Similarly, students with poor or inappropriate social skills can develop these skills, and discover techniques they can employ to solve common social problems at home, in the school, and in the community. This can be done through counseling that respects the student and his or her culture, and by providing students with an opportunity for culturally competent counseling and role playing, and to examine and critically reflect upon the problems they encounter and the choices they make. Furthermore, students who lack vocational role models can be provided structured opportunities to explore possible future career paths during high school. Finally, many students will have to advocate for, access, design, and evaluate support services after leaving school (e.g., assistive technology for individuals with sensory or physical disabilities and "invisible" consumer-directed "wrap-around supports" for individuals with cognitive and emotional disabilities.) These students can learn to do so while in school by participating in the development of transition goals and plans and in the assessment of their implementation.

We believe that the key to empowering students at risk lies in appreciating both the developmental history and ecological logic of these students' learning and behavioral problems (Brofenbrenner, 1979; Greenwood et al., 1992). Traditional school curricula are typically not coordinated across grades, and children's achievement is often uneven across different curricular areas. At the same time, the cultures of many schools are inhospitable to the emotional needs and learning styles of many of these students (Office of Educational Research and Improvement, 1993; Pine & Hilliard, 1990). Alternatively, under a preventive education model, schools reorganize their delivery system to preventively anticipate and prevent long-term problems in adjustment during and after high school. The results are two-fold. Fewer students drop out, and more students are enabled to develop needed transition skills before they begin the process of postschool transition.

Teacher Empowerment

Teachers are often frustrated by our large, complex, and regimented systems of public education. Public school resources are often fixed (Kakalik, 1981), yet costs are rising (Parrish, 1994). Furthermore, teachers are asked to shoulder even more responsibility for mitigating such social problems as teenage pregnancy and drug addiction (McInerney, Kane, & Pelavin, 1992).

Such authors as Smylie (1995) suggest that public school teachers would benefit from a systems change in which educational authority is decentralized. As indicated in Table 2.1, under a preventive education model, teachers participate in site-based management teams to identify transition goals and objectives. However, our previous experience with school reform suggests that decentralization alone is not sufficient to empower teachers to improve educational outcomes for their students (Smith & O'Day, 1990).

Information in Table 2.1 identified two additional strategies that we believe should accompany site-based management initiatives. First, alternative education programs and curricula are needed; employer surveys are one source of information for developing new instructional sequences under a preventive education model. For example, employers report that the skills needed for postschool jobs include (a) appropriate reading and communication skills, (b) problem solving ability, and (c) positive work habits (Johnston & Packer, 1987). Teachers can implement an interdisciplinary curriculum to teach prerequisite transition skills in these areas.

Second, there are accompanying needs to provide ongoing training and support to teachers that will enable them to implement interdisciplinary, collaborative efforts that address the individualized needs of culturally and linguistically diverse learners. Traditionally, this involved preservice training that culminated in awarding new graduate degrees and accreditation as transition specialists (Holmes Group, 1986). However, developing university degree programs would not necessarily address continuing problems regarding teachers' lack of "content knowledge" about required transition skills (Smith & O'Day, 1988), experience in collaborating across disciplines or working with family members in a culturally competent manner (Osher & Osher, 1994).

As suggested in Table 2.1, teachers can be enabled to develop, implement, and evaluate new transition curricula. Such training can perhaps best be accomplished through field-based training and on-site technical assistance that enables all school staff who are involved in transition preparation to try out, reflect on, and adapt new approaches (Gersten & Woodward, 1992; Louis & Miles, 1990).

To date, local public schools have been largely unsuccessful in translating information about needed job skills into curricular sequences to better prepare students for the demands of employment and independent life in the community. The preventive education model we are proposing requires systemic changes in how educational resources are allocated and how teachers conceptualize and conduct their daily responsibilities in the classroom. Teachers need to be empowered with site-based management, alternative curricula, and ongoing training and support so that increased teachers' accountability for their students' transition success is a realistic, attainable goal.

CREATING PARENT, STUDENT, AND TEACHER PARTNERSHIPS TO PREVENT POSTSCHOOL MALADJUSTMENT

Our overriding recommendation to restructure schools is to create culturally competent, parent-student-teacher partnerships that build upon the strengths and respond to the needs of families, students, and schools. These partnerships would help local schools and families to anticipate and prevent learning and behavioral problems that contribute to postschool maladjustment. This section of the chapter contains research evidence that demonstrates the importance of parent-student-teacher partnerships. We also offer several practical suggestions about the creation of effective partnerships at the local school level.

STORRY Research Program

Our preventive education model for school restructuring is based on Sequencing the Transition of at Risk and Retarded Youth (STORRY). STORRY was a longitudinal program of research, training, and technical assistance conducted at the University of Wisconsin–Madison. The STORRY model of preventive education was replicated in several local school districts throughout the state of Wisconsin (Garber & McInerney, 1989).

Table 2.2 summarizes results from various STORRY treatment activities. Prescribed treatments are organized with respect to their primary activity and purpose. There are three broad categories of preventive intervention: (a) school-to-family outreach, (b) transition plan case management, and (c) pre-employment experience and education. For each category, the setting, change agents, and target problem behaviors are identified. Relevant subject characteristics and observed results are detailed for particular interventions. In addition, the impact of these preventive interventions on local service delivery systems is described.

Individual research studies examined different combinations of preventive interventions. Preventive strategies were employed at home, at school, and in the community on local job sites. Local public school districts provided the primary communication and coordination linkages that were required to initiate these intervention programs.

Treated youth varied with respect to chronological age (i.e., 12–18 years) and

TABLE 2.2

Results of Preventive Rehabilitation Treatments

Preventive Activities/Purpose	Setting Change Agents	Problem Behaviors	Treatment	Preventive Subjects	Strategies Results	Local Impact
School-to-Family Outreach Provides training to parents to develop support competency and to help them act as more effective partners to enhance the impact of prescribed treatments.	*At home* Parents Grandparents Siblings	Inappropriate role models Social isolation from community activities Frequent family crises Family not future goal oriented	Job Information Exchange Parent Support Groups Individual Education Plan and Individual Transition Plan Communication	25 at-risk 12th graders and their families 81 high school students with mental retardation and their families	Competitive jobs at self-sufficient wages were secured within one year postschool Adaptive behaviors increased prior to high school exit Social and prevocational skills increased prior to high school entrance	Preventive rehabilitation strategies are able to anticipate and treat predicted problems of community adjustment and thereby reduce the likelihood of demand for referral to local agencies Increased family ability to support rehabilitation objectives helps maintain and generalize the benefits of prescribed treatment for transition process
Transition Plan Case Management Provides transition coordinator to both prescribe and evaluate sociovocational instruction and counseling during and immediately after high school	*At School* Teachers Counselors Classmates	Frequent unexcused absences Cannot resolve complex social problems Disruptive antisocial behaviors Repeated academic failures	Drop-out Prevention Social Problem Solving Training Study Skills Tutorial	15 high school drop-outs enrolled in a G.E.D. completion program 20 at-risk 9th and 10th grade students 33 at-risk middle school and 36 at-risk high school students	Drop-out rates were halved at the target high school Social skill gains were maintained across school years Grade point average and class rank increased by the end of the school year	Preemployment placements and outreach to consortiums of local employers increase opportunities to hire workers with handicaps and provide job stability Improved interagency cooperation eliminates service gaps and increases the cost savings benefits of total community integration

(Continued)

TABLE 2.2 (Continued)

Preventive Activities/Purpose	Setting Change Agents	Problem Behaviors	Treatment	Preventive Subjects	Strategies Results	Local Impact
Preemployment Experience and Education Derives sequences for sociovocational training curricula that emphasize skills to support transition	At work Job Coach Employers Peers	Poor work habits Disrespectful attitudes Unrealistic career goals Low personal ambition	Vocational Education Practice Career Awareness and Job Search Skills Early Screening and Identification	30 high school students with special needs 75 and at-risk high school students with special needs 115 regular and special education 8th grade students	Competitive local jobs were maintained 1-3 years after high school Self-concept and general knowledge increased prior to high school exit Referrals to work experience program included at-risk youth who were not previously identified	

severity of disabling condition. Skill comparisons between treated and non-treated subjects were provided for each study. Repeated assessments were used to evaluate the responsiveness of individual students to the intervention program. The performance of untreated students was the referent to evaluate skill gains observed for treated subjects.

Before high school entrance, treated youth improved their academic grade point average and demonstrated increased social and prevocational skills in such areas as personal attitudes, behavior management, and general knowledge. These students were also screened more appropriately and referred to high school alternative learning programs.

During high school, treated youth continued to demonstrate increased social and prevocational skills. Skill gains were observed for different groups of students across successive school years. For example, there was a significant increase in adaptive behavior among a treated group of adolescents with mental retardation. In addition, treated students were highly successful in completing requirements for their high school diploma.

After high school, treated youth were most successful in transitioning into their respective local communities. These students demonstrated competence in looking for and securing local jobs. Their wages were competitive and sufficient to sustain an independent lifestyle. In addition, job stability was maintained, in some cases, up to three years after high school exit.

Practical Strategies to Implement Preventive Education

Our previous work on STORRY suggests that it is possible to identify risk characteristics that predict the likelihood that youth with disabilities will experience postschool problems. Under a preventive education model, local schools use this information to work with parents and students to design specific intervention plans that empower parents, students, and teachers to create partnerships and work cooperatively to prepare students for successful school-to-work transitions. Field-tested strategies that illustrate how to create these parent-student-teacher partnerships are presented later in this chapter.

Parent Empowerment Strategies

As indicated in Table 2.3, the long-term goal of parent empowerment strategies is to enable parents to actively participate in developing and implementing prevention plans and, when necessary, to gradually transform a family's high-risk characteristics into low-risk characteristics that support transition-related objectives. For example, planning meetings can be scheduled and conducted in a manner that encourages parental participation, solicits parental expertise, and invests parents in transition plans (Osher & Osher, 1994). Similarly, parents who initially provided inappropriate vocational role models can develop strategies to encourage their children's prevocational exploration of different possible career paths.

TABLE 2.3

Examples of Parent Empowerment Strategies for School Restructuring

Parent Empowerment Strategies	High-Risk Characteristics	Low-Risk Characteristics
Parents are enabled to participate in transition planning and implementation in a respectful and family-friendly manner.	Parents are alienated from the school or its staff because of previous experiences or because of a lack of fit between family culture and structure and school culture and structure.	Parents are enabled to participate in transition planning by addressing the lack of fit between family and school culture (cultural competency) and structure (family-friendly approaches).
	Parents are unable to communicate their needs and strengths (and those of the student) to school-based professionals.	Parents actively participate in planning that addresses the individual needs and strengths of the student and family.
Parents are provided with information about appropriate transition goals and objectives in a culturally competent and linguistically appropriate manner.	Parents lack information about appropriate postschool goals for their adolescent children.	Parents are advised about possible postschool options for their children after high school.
	The family home has few — if any — transition-related brochures or other written materials (e.g., job notices or application forms).	Parents are provided with transition-related materials.
	The family cannot understand the information that is provided.	Parents are provided with information and materials in a manner and language that is appropriate to them.
Parents actively participate in the development of goals and objectives and the monitoring of their implementation.	Parents do not buy-in to transition goals and implementation.	Parents buy-in to transition goals and implementation.
	Parents do not monitor the implementation of transition plan.	Parents monitor the implementation of transition plan.

(Continued)

TABLE 2.3 (*Continued*)

Parent Empowerment Strategies	High-Risk Characteristics	Low-Risk Characteristics
Parents receive support and advice about how to help prepare their children for transition success.	Families live alone and are generally isolated from their extended family, friends, and neighbors.	Families have direct access to support groups through a network of parents with adolescent children.
	Parents employ authoritarian, coercive styles of child-rearing with their adolescent children.	Groups of parents "brainstorm" how to enforce consistent standards of behavior at home. If needed and desired, parents receive support to implement these approaches.
	Daily family life is disorganized and the responsibilities of family members are ill-defined and fragmented.	Parents learn from other parents how to establish daily schedules and assign responsibilities for completing routine chores and, if desired, receive support to implement these approaches.
Parents are referred to available local services for more intensive treatment, as needed and appropriate.	Parents are generally passive, have a poor self-image, and lack self-confidence.	Parents receive therapeutic counseling or are enabled to experience more control in their lives (e.g., by helping shape effective transition plans.)
	Adult family members are often unemployed or underemployed for extended periods of time.	If they desire, adult family members are provided local job training and placement services.
	Family life is disrupted by repeated financial crises and related interpersonal conflicts.	If they desire, families are referred to local agencies that provide basic necessities (i.e., food, clothing, and shelter).

Finally, parents who initially employed authoritarian styles of child-rearing can be provided with tools and support that can enable them to implement alternative management strategies that reinforce consistent standards of behavior.

Families differ in their structure, culture, resources, and values. School-based outreach to empower parents may be provided in different forms to accommodate the individual needs and build upon the strengths of different families. We used three methods in STORRY:

• *Information brokerage.* Parents were provided with information about appropriate activities at home that would reinforce instructional objectives at school. In addition, parents received information about services that were available in the local community. This information was communicated either verbally or in a parent newsletter;

• *Parent support groups.* Parents were encouraged to participate in monthly meetings at family homes or at school. Parents used these meetings to discuss common concerns about their children's well-being and development. In addition, the meetings provided an opportunity for parents to share information about effective strategies for raising their children; and

• *Individual counseling.* Parents were advised how to apply information obtained through the parent groups in solving particular problems at home. Families were also referred to cooperating local agencies for more intensive interventions, as necessary for particular problems.

As part of the STORRY program, we recruited and trained family home visitors to establish communication links between parents at home and teachers at school. The basic strategy involved (1) asking teachers to identify instructional goals at school that were appropriate for parents to address and reinforce at home, and (2) having home visitors, who were able to establish rapport with family members, serve as a regular liaison between families and school. For example, if a teacher was concerned about the child's ability to follow directions at school, the home visitor could help parents work with their children in learning to follow directions at home.

STORRY's method for parent empowerment provided flexibility in varying the mix, intensity, and duration of outreach for different families. Family processes that exerted a positive influence on children were reinforced through outreach and extended by teachers at school. In addition, detrimental influences within the home environment or school were identified and addressed initially through outreach or changing the way the school dealt with families. If families required and desired more extensive support, STORRY staff linked families with more intensive treatment or support programs, as appropriate for individual families.

Student Empowerment Strategies

Table 2.4 contains a list of student empowerment strategies validated through the STORRY research program. As previously discussed, these strategies pre-

TABLE 2.4

Examples of Student Empowerment Strategies for School Restructuring

Student Empowerment Strategies	High-Risk Characteristics	Low-Risk Characteristics
Students are provided with an opportunity to develop appropriate work habits and other pre-vocational skills needed on local job sites.	Students require constant adult supervision. Students are easily distracted and often fail to complete tasks on time. Students need repeated directions and instructions. Students reject suggested habits and skills as being culturally inappropriate or are unable to integrate changes into their community life.	Students learn how to work independently. Students are taught to manage their time and complete assigned tasks. Students learn when and how to ask for follow-up assistance. Students actively adopt new habits and skills as ones that can work for them and integrate them into their lives.
Students are provided structured opportunities to explore possible career paths after high school.	Students have unrealistic expectations about their life after high school. Students lack information about where and how to apply for local jobs or support services. Students do not know what vocational skills are needed for different jobs.	Students are counseled about their likely postschool needs for job skills and financial security. Students learn about local job or support services and postschool training opportunities. Students experience the demands of regular jobs on pre-employment job sites.
Students participate in the development of transition goals and plans and in the assessment of their implementation.	Students lack self-advocacy skills. Transition plans do not respond to students' concerns. Students do not buy-in to transition plans. Students do not know how to access needed support services.	Students develop self-advocacy skills. Transition plans respond to students' concerns. Students buy-in to transition plans. Students learn how to access and control needed support services.

sume students are vulnerable to maladjustment when they lack the requisite skills for postschool success. Accordingly, students who initially required constant adult supervision to complete tasks learned to follow directions, manage their time, and work independently. Similarly, students who were unable to recognize the consequences of their social behaviors learned to anticipate how others likely would react to different social behaviors. Table 2.4 contains additional illustrations of the characteristics of students before (i.e., high-risk) and after (i.e., low-risk) student empowerment training.

Local teachers, with training and technical assistance from STORRY staff, helped develop and implement these student empowerment strategies. There were two main curricular activities:

• *Social problem-solving training.* Students were taught to solve social problems commonly found on local job sites. For example, students were taught how to accept employers' reviews and critiques of their job performance. Students also learned to handle peer pressure to leave work early or shoplift from their employer. The students received this training during regularly scheduled social problem solving classes each week; and

• *Pre-employment experience.* Students were provided pre-employment practica placements on local job sites. These placements provided youth with direct access to local employers, helped them learn required work habits and skills, and provided needed job references after high school. These practica also included career education and vocational education components at school.

These curricular activities were used successfully with different groups of high school students, including both students with disabilities and other students at risk for postschool maladjustment. Results from STORRY indicated these curricular activities help teach both groups of students the skills needed to become employed and live independently after high school.

Prior to the high school year, cooperating teachers were trained to implement the preventive education curriculum. Teachers developed Individual Transition Plans (ITPs) for each target student. The ITP listed prerequisite social and prevocational skills. The ITP also prescribed individualized sequences of coursework and practica that would help the student acquire these skills.

Staff from an alternative learning program at the local high school provided case management oversight of each student's ITP during the school year. These staff then evaluated the previous year's program and made plans for the next school year during the summer months.

Teacher Empowerment Strategies

Table 2.5 contains a list of recommended strategies that empower teachers to develop preventive education programs of transition preparation. This list reflects our observations of changes in local delivery systems that were sparked by implementation of our preventive education model. For example, local sec-

TABLE 2.5
Examples of Teacher Empowerment Strategies for School Restructuring

Teacher Empowerment Strategies	High-Risk Characteristics	Low-Risk Characteristics
Teachers participate in site-based management teams to identify local goals and objectives for transition.	Transition goals and objectives are not well coordinated across different grades. High school students have only restricted options for mainly academic programs. Secondary classrooms are poorly equipped, with mainly out-dated textbooks and limited supplies.	Specific transition goals and objectives are identified and coordinated across middle school and high school. Secondary level alternative learning programs are developed and implemented. The alternative learning program purchases new instructional materials that are directly related to transition preparation.
Teachers implement an interdisciplinary curriculum to teach prerequisite transition skills.	Existing curricula feature basic instruction in core academic subjects needed for high school graduation. Teachers work mainly in isolated classrooms with little peer interaction. Teachers lack consensus about common expectations for students' learning and behavior.	Teachers develop and implement alternative curricula to teach social problem solving, work habits, and other, transition-relevant skills. Teachers work together collegially to develop and implement transition programs. Interdisciplinary planning helps teachers identify school wide standards for student performance at school.
Teachers receive needed training and support to ensure their professional growth as transition specialists.	Continuing education courses are not relevant to a teacher's current job responsibilities. Teachers do not receive ongoing support to implement recommended instructional strategies after training ends.	Transition training is directly related to the teachers' role as transition specialists. Teams of teachers are trained together and provide each other with continuing collaboration and support after training ends.

ondary schools created alternative learning programs that supplemented basic academic training with extramural courses in social problem solving and pre-employment practica. These courses, which were developed with ongoing support from STORRY, permitted teachers to preventively address identified learning and behavior problems that would be likely contributors to difficulty in postschool maladjustment.

Experience derived from STORRY provides several additional suggestions relevant to implementation of a preventive education model at the local level:

• *Family outreach center.* We established a local, school-based center to coordinate family outreach and parent training activities. The center signaled the importance of families to the local community. The center itself was housed in several vacant classrooms in the middle school. We recruited paraprofessionals or volunteers from the community who staffed the center. Each paraprofessional or volunteer, thereby, had a small caseload of families;

• *Prescriptive student evaluations.* We provided for prescriptive evaluations of student progress over time. Youth with disabilities or at risk differ in both their transition needs and their responsiveness to prescribed training. Prescriptive evaluations helped ensure that transition training was effective and directly related to curricular sequences for each individual student; and

• *Existing school staff.* STORRY used mainly existing public school staff and resources to implement preventive education programs. This approach minimized start-up costs and helped maximize opportunities for subsequent expansion of the program. In addition, our activities complemented—rather than competed with—already established compensatory educational programs.

We are proposing that public school teachers assume a critical role in preparing youth with disabilities and youth at risk for successful postschool transitions. However, we recognize that this goal for teacher empowerment is not easily achieved.

In STORRY, key stakeholders came together in several local communities. These stakeholders included representatives from the public schools, various community-based organizations, and state agencies (e.g., the Wisconsin Department of Public Instruction). Cooperation among these stakeholders was critical in helping to provide effective transition programs for target youth and their families.

SUMMARY AND CONCLUSION

A continuing dilemma for federal and state policymakers responsible for educational programs is allocating limited resources in ways that will ensure the most effective use of the existing delivery system. Regarding youth with disabilities, the question becomes—"How can the effectiveness of instructional programs for these children, their families, and their schools be improved?" Affirmative answers to these questions are especially important today, because reduced resources may doom educational programs that cannot demonstrate effectiveness in providing services.

Research findings presented in this report have particular relevance to future initiatives to restructure our system of public education. The intent of our recommendations is to initiate a strategy for delivering transition services that preventively anticipates postschool needs—rather than only reacting restoratively after problems develop.

Preventive education prescriptively provides instruction that meets the different needs of individual students with disabilities. In addition, the use of preventive education can contribute to the effective restructuring of the educational delivery system at the local community level. We believe that such individualization and restructuring are likely to be effective where risk indices and high-risk family profiles are used in a culturally competent manner to prescribe educational and social services at a school and community-based level.

The use of a preventive education model that actively engages parents, students, and teachers will prepare students and their families for a future in which they will need to build upon natural supports and access social services. When parents, students, and teachers work together to design, implement, and monitor strengths-based plans, they do more than produce an individualized plan that will work and that families and students will apply. In addition, family and student-driven partnerships prepare students and their families for a future of independent living in which they must develop accommodations, use their own networks, and advocate for social services or assistive devices. By empowering students and their families, this approach models how they can develop their own accommodations (Osher & Hanley, 1997) or design and control invisible supports that wrap-around the individual with a disability and contribute to independent living in normalized environments (Burchard, Burchard, Sewell, & VanDenBerg, 1993; Eber, 1994).

Preventive education is a strategy for making transition services for youth with disabilities more effective and more efficient. Services can be more effective when the point of referral to particular services is moved back in time through early anticipation of the child's special needs. Services can be more efficient when parent-student-teacher partnerships are established and used to prescribe an individualized program of transition services though the secondary school years. Services can be more forceful when they are family-friendly, culturally sensitive, address the individual needs of a student and his or her family, and build upon the strengths of the student and his or her family. We believe that creating practical, culturally competent partnerships to preventively share service responsibility at home, school, and work comprises an appropriate delivery system agenda for the remainder of this decade.

REFERENCES

Affleck, J. Q., Edgar, E. E., Levine, P., & Kortering, L. (1990). Post-school status of students classified as mildly mentally retarded, learning disabled, and non-handicapped: Does it get better with time? *Education and Training in Mental Retardation, 25,* 315–324.

American Humane Association, Children's Division (1992). *An annotated bibliography of resources on cultural competence and cultural diversity in child welfare/child protection services.* Englewood, CO: Author.

Bower, B. P., Thompson, M., & Fullilove, R. E. (1990). African-American youth and AIDS high-risk behavior: The social context and barriers to prevention. *Youth and Society, 22,* 55–65.

Boyer, C. (1983). *A nation at risk: The imperative for educational reform.* Washington, DC: U.S. Commission on Excellence in Education.

Brofenbrenner, U. (1979). *The ecology of human development: Experiments by nature and design.* Cambridge: Harvard University Press.

Burchard, J. D., Burchard, S. N., Sewell, R., & VanDenBerg, J. (1993). *One Kid at a Time.* Washington, DC: CAASP Technical Assistance Center.

Chinn, P. C., & Hughes, S. (1987). Representation of minority students in special education classes. *Remedial and Special Education, 8*(4), 41–46.

Clark, H. B., & Foster-Johnson, L. (1994). Navigating rough waters: Transition of youth and young adults with emotional disturbances into adulthood. In B. A. Stroul (Ed.), *Systems of care for children and adolescents with severe emotional disturbances: Issues for the 1990s.* Washington, DC: CAASP Technical Assistance Center.

Clarke, A. M. (1980, June). Developmental discontinuities: An approach to assessing their nature. Paper presented at the Sixth Vermont Conference on the Primary Prevention of Psychopathology.

Cross, T., Bazron, B., Dennis, K., & Isaacs, M. (1989). *Towards a culturally competent system of care.* Washington, DC: CAASP Technical Assistance Center, Georgetown University Child Development Center.

Cuban, L. (1990). Reforming again, and again, and again. *Educational Researcher, 19*(1), 3–13.

Cummins, J. (1986a). Empowering minority students: A framework for intervention. *Harvard Education Review, 56,* 18–36.

Cummins, J. (1986b). Psychological assessment of minority students. In A. C. Willig & H. F. Greenberg (Eds.), *Bilingualism and learning disabilities: Policy and practice for teachers and administrators* (pp. 3–14). New York: American Library Publishing Company.

Darling, R. B. (1979). *Families against society: A study of reactions to children with birth defects.* Beverly Hills, CA: Sage.

Delpit, L. (1988). The silenced dialogue: Power and pedagogy in educating other people's children. *Harvard Educational Review, 58,* 280–298.

Dryfoos, J. G. (1990). *Adolescents at Risk.* New York: Oxford University Press.

Eber, L. (1994, Fall). The wraparound approach: toward effective school inclusion. *Claiming Children, 1,* 4–9.

Edelman, M. W. (1987). *Families in peril. An agenda for social change.* Cambridge: Harvard University Press

Edwards, P. A. (1993). Before and after desegregation: African-American parents' involvement in schools. *Educational Policy, 7*(3), 340–369.

Elmore, R. F., & McLaughlin, M. (1988). *Steady work: Policy, practice, and the reform of American education.* Santa Monica, CA: Rand Corporation.

Emrick, J. A., & Peterson, S. M. (1978). *A synthesis of findings across five recent studies of educational dissemination and change.* San Francisco: Far West Laboratory.

Federal Resource Center for Special Education. (1993). *Task force report: cultural and linguistic diversity in education.* Final draft. Lexington, KY: Author.

Focal Point. (1994). Special issue on developing culturally competent organizations. *Focal Point, 8*(2).

Franklin, M. E. (1992). Culturally sensitive instructional practices for African-American learners with disabilities. *Exceptional Children, 59*(2), 115–122.

Fullan, M., & Miles, M. (1992). Getting reform right: What works and what doesn't. *Phi Delta Kappan, 73*, 744–752.

Fullan, M. G. (1990). Staff development, innovation, and institutional development. In B. Joyce (Ed.), *Changing school culture through staff development.* (ASCD Yearbook). Alexandria, VA: ASCD.

Garber, H. L. (1988). *The Milwaukee Project: Preventing mental retardation in children at risk.* Washington, DC: American Association on Mental Retardation.

Garber, H. L., & McInerney, M. (1982). Sociobehavioral factors in mental retardation. In P. T. Cegelka & H. Prehm (Eds.), *Mental retardation: From categories to people.* Columbus, OH: Merrill.

Garber, H. L., & McInerney, M. (1989). Preventive rehabilitation: Moving the point of referral to increase program and cost effectiveness. *American Rehabilitation, 14*(4), 2–12, 24–25.

Garber, H. L., & McInerney, M. (1991). *Parental involvement in the vocational education of special needs youth: An evaluation and planning guide.* (Staff training manual). Madison: Wisconsin Department of Public Instruction.

Gersten, R. M., & Woodward, J. (1992). The quest to translate research into classroom practice: Strategies for assisting classroom teachers' work with at-risk students and students with disabilities. In D. Carnine & E. Kameenui (Eds.), *Higher cognitive functioning for all students* (pp. 201–218). Austin, TX: PRO-ED.

Ginzberg, E., & Vojta, G. J. (1981). The service sector for the U.S. economy. *Scientific American, 244*(3), 48–55.

Goodlad, J. I. (1984). *A place called school: Prospects for the future.* New York: McGraw-Hill.

Greenwood, C. R., Carta, J. J., Hart, B., Kamps, D., Terry, B., Arreaga-Mayer, C., Atwater, J., Walker, D., Risley, T., & Delquadri, J. (1992). Out of the laboratory and into the community: 26 years of applied behavioral analysis at the Juniper Gardens Children's Project. *American Psychologist, 47*, 1464–1474.

Gresham, F. M. (1981). Social skills training with handicapped children: A review. *Review of Educational Research, 51*(8), 139–176.

Harry, B. (1992). *Cultural diversity, families, and the special education system: Communication and empowerment.* New York: Teachers College Press.

Hasazi, S. R., Gordon, L. R., & Roe, C. A. (1985). Factors associated with the employment status of handicapped youth exiting high school from 1979 to 1983. *Exceptional Children, 51*, 455–469.

Hess, R. D. (1970). Social class and ethnic influences on socialization. In P. H. Mussen (Ed.), *Carmichael's manual of child psychology.* New York: Wiley.

Hilliard, A. G., III (1989). Teachers and cultural styles in a pluralistic society. *National Education Association, 7*, 65–69.

Holmes Group. (1990). *Tomorrow's schools: A report form the Holmes Group.* East Lansing, MI: Author.

Isaacs, M. R., & Benjamin, M. P. (1991). *Toward a culturally competent system of care, II.* Washington, DC: CAASP Technical Assistance Center.

Johnston, W. B., & Packer, A. B. (1987). *Workforce 2000: Work and workers for the 21st Century.* Indianapolis, IN: Hudson Institute.

Kakalik, J. S. (1979). *Issues in the cost and finance of special education.* Review of Research in Education. Washington, DC: American Educational Research Association.

Kiernan, W. E., & Brinkman, L. (1988). Disincentives and barriers to employment. In P. Wehman and M. S. Moon (Eds.), *Vocational rehabilitation and supported employment.* Baltimore: Paul H. Brookes.

Levin, H. M. (1993). Learning from accelerated schools. In J. H. Block, S. T. Everson, & T. R. Guskey (Eds.), *Selecting and integrating school improvement programs.* New York: Scholastic Books.

Louis, K. S., & Miles, M. B. (1990). *Improving the urban high school: What works and why.* New York: Teachers College Press.

Louis, K. S., & Rosenblum, S. (1981). *Linking R&D with Schools: A program and its implications for dissemination and school improvement policy.* Washington, DC: Office of Educational Research and Improvement, U.S. Department of Education.

Louis, K. S., & Smith, B. (1991). Restructuring, teacher engagement and school culture: Perspectives on school reform and the improvement of teacher's work. *School Effectiveness and School Improvement, 2*(1), 34–52.

Marjoribanks, K. (1976). Sibsize, family environment, cognitive performance, and affective characteristics. *Journal of Psychology, 94,* 195–204.

McInerney, M., Kane, M., & Pelavin, S. (1992). *Services to children with serious emotional disturbance* (U.S. Congress mandated study). Washington, DC: Office of Policy and Planning, U.S. Department of Education.

McLaughlin, M. W. (1990, December). The Rand Change Agent study revisited: Macro perspectives and micro realities. *Educational Researcher, 19,* 11–16.

Meier, T., & Brown, C. R. (1994). The color of inclusion. *Journal of Emotional and Behavioral Problems, 3*(3), 15–19.

Miles, M. (Winter 1980). School innovation form the ground up: Some dilemmas. *New York University Education Quarterly, 11*(2), 2–9.

Mithaug, D. E., Horiuchi, C. N., & Fanning, P. N. (1985). A report on the Colorado statewide follow-up survey of special education students. *Exceptional Children, 51,* 397–404.

National Longitudinal Transition Study of Special Education Students (1991). *Student statistical almanacs: Vol 3: Youth categorized as emotionally disturbed.* Menlo Park, CA: Author.

Ogbu, J. U. (1978). *Minority education and caste: The American system in a cross-cultural perspective.* New York: Academic Press

Ogbu, J. U. (1992). Understanding cultural diversity and learning. *Educational Researcher, 21*(8), 5–14, 24.

Orlandi, M. A. (1992). Defining cultural competence: An organizing framework. In *Cultural competence for evaluators: A guide for alcohol and other drug prevention practitioners working with ethnic/racial communities.* OSAP Cultural Competence Series (pp. 293–299). Rockville, MD: U.S. Department of Health and Human Services.

Osher, D., & Hanley, T. (1997). Building upon an emergent social service delivery paradigm. In L. M. Bullock & R. A. Gable (Eds.), *Making collaboration work for children, youth, families, schools, and communities.* Reston, VA: Council for Exceptional Children.

Osher, D. M., & Kane, M. (1993). *Describing and Studying Innovations in the Education of Children with Attention Deficit Disorder.* Washington, DC: U.S. Department of Education, Office of Special Education and Rehabilitative Services, Office of Special Education Programs, Division of Innovation and Development.

Osher, D. M., & Osher, T. W. (1994). Comprehensive and collaborative systems that work: A national agenda. In C. M. Nelson, R. Rutherford, & B. I. Wolford (Eds.), *Developing comprehensive systems for troubled youth.* Richmond, KY: National Coalition for Juvenile Justice Services.

Page, R. N. (1991). *Lower track class-rooms.* New York: Teachers College Press.

Parrish, T. B. (1994). Fiscal issues relating to special education inclusion. Invited paper presented at the Wingspread Conference on Barriers to Inclusive Inclusion, Racine, WI.

Pine, G. J., & Hilliard, A. G., III (1990, April). Rx for racism: Imperatives for America's schools. *Phi Delta Kappan,* 593–600.

Porter, A., Archibald, D., & Tyree, A. (1991). Reforming the curriculum: Will empowerment policies replace control? In S. Fuhrman (Ed.), *The politics of curriculum and testing*. London: Taylor and Francis.

Richardson, S. A., Koller, H., & Katz, M. (1988). Job histories in open employment of a population of young adults with mental retardation. *American Journal of Mental Retardation, 92*(6), 483–491.

Richardson, V., & Colfer, P. (1990). Being at-risk in school. In J. I. Goodlad & P. Keathing (Eds.), *Access to knowledge: An agenda for our nation's schools* (pp. 107–124). New York: College Board.

Rutter, M., & Madge, N. (1976). *The cycles of disadvantage*. London: Heinemann.

Ryan, W. (1971). *Blaming the victim*. New York: Random House.

Schalock, R. L., & Lilley, M. A. (1986). Placement from community-based mental retardation programs: How well do clients do after 8 to 10 years? *American Journal of Mental Deficiency, 90*(6), 669–676.

Seligman, M. (Ed.). (1991). *The family with a handicapped child* (2nd ed.). Boston: Allyn and Bacon.

Smey-Richman, B. (1991). *School climate and restructuring for low-achieving students*. Philadelphia: Research for Better Schools.

Smith, M. S., & O'Day, J. (1988). Research into teaching quality: Main findings and lessons for appraisal. Report prepared for the meeting of the Working Party on the Condition of Teaching, OECD, Paris, France.

Smith, M. S., & O'Day, J. (1990). Systemic school reform. *Politics of Education Association Yearbook*, 233–267.

Smylie, M. A. (1995). Teacher learning in the workplace: Implications for school reform. In T. R. Guskey & A. M. Huberman (Eds.), *Professional development in education: New paradigms and practices*. New York: Teacher's College, Columbia University.

Taylor, R. L. (1990). Black youth: The endangered generation. *Youth and Society, 22*, 4–11.

Upshur, C. C. (1991). Families and the community service maze. In M. Seligman (Ed.), *The family with a handicapped child* (2nd ed., pp. 91–118). Boston: Allyn and Bacon.

U.S. Commission on Civil Rights. (1983). Accommodating the spectrum of individual abilities. Washington, DC: Author.

U.S. Department of Education. (1992). Fourteenth annual report to Congress on the implementation of the Individuals with Disabilities Education Act. Washington, DC: U.S. Government Printing Office.

U.S. Department of Education. (1994). *National agenda for achieving better results for children and youth with serious emotional disturbance*. Washington, DC: Office of Special Education Programs, September 1, 1994.

U.S. Department of Education, Office of Educational Research and Improvement. (1993). *Educational reforms and students at-risk: A review of the current state-of-the-art*. Washington, DC: Author.

Wagner, M. (1993). *The secondary school programs of students with disabilities*. Menlo Park, CA: SRI International.

Wagner, M., Blackborby, J., Cameto, R., Hebbeler, K., & Newman, L. (1993). *The transition experiences of young people with disabilities*. Menlo Park, CA: SRI International.

Wagner, M., D'Amico, R., Marder, C., Newman, L., & Blackborby, J. (1992). *What happens next? Trends in postschool outcomes of youth with disabilities. The second comprehensive report from the national longitudinal transition study of special education students*. Menlo Park, CA: SRI International.

Wagner, M., Newman, L., D'Amico, R., Jay, E. D., Butler-Nalin, P., Marder, C., & Cox, R. (1991). *Youth with disabilities: How are they doing. The first comprehensive report from the national longitudinal transition study of special education students*. Menlo Park, CA: SRI International.

Werner, E., & Smith, R. (1977). *Kauai's children come of age*. Honolulu: University Press of Hawaii.

Will, M. (1984). *OSERS Programming for the Transition of Youth with Disabilities: Bridges from School to Working Life*. Washington, DC: Office of Special Education and Rehabilitation Services, U.S. Department of Education.

Williams, T., & Kornblum, W. (1994). *The uptown kids: Struggle and hope in the projects*. New York: Putnam.

CHAPTER 3

Lessons From the Texas–Mexico Border: Working With the Parents of Students With Mental Retardation

MICHELLE D. YOUNG
ANNA B. PEDROZA
University of Texas, Austin

PAUL KAVANAUGH
State University of Tamaulipas, Mexico

The research that the three co-authors of this chapter carried out as part of their year-long responsibilities as graduate assistants in the Effective Border School Research and Development Initiative (EBSRDI) in large part confirmed the crucial importance of parental participation in the educational achievement of students, especially students with special educational needs. This study, which was conducted in cooperation with the Texas Education Agency, the University of Texas at Austin, the University of Texas—Pan Am, and several school districts along the Texas-Mexico border, examined eight elementary, middle, and high schools, each judged to be successful, in the lower Rio Grande Valley of deep south Texas. The eight schools in this study were located in the area served by the Region One Service Center of the state of Texas and stretched from Laredo, Texas in the west to Brownsville, Texas in the east. This area is known as the lower Rio Grande Valley or "the Valley." (See Figure 3.1 for a map of the region.)

THE TEXAS-MEXICO BORDER AS AN INTERNATIONAL REGION

Although the lower Rio Grande Valley of Texas is obviously located within the geographical confines of the United States, we would like to explain why this

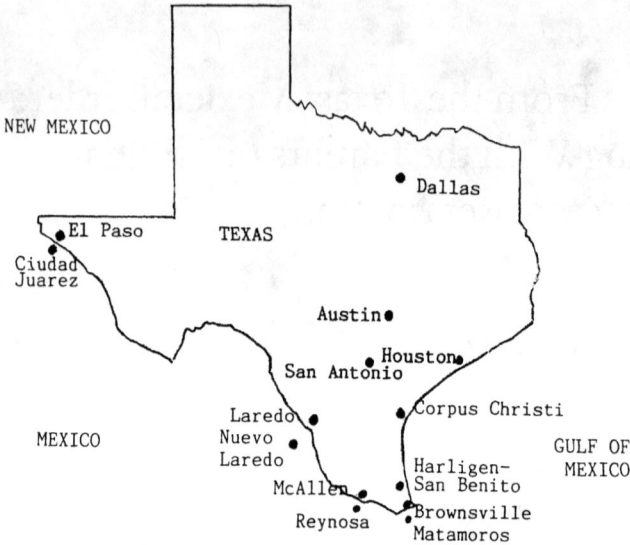

FIG. 3.1.   The Texas–Mexico border.

area can be considered an international region and, thus, justify the existence of this chapter within this book. It is not uncommon to hear from both Mexican and American visitors to the border that the border is not quite Mexico and not quite the United States, but a region unto itself—a hybrid, the result of both Mexico and the United States coming together in space and time. This ambiguity may be why the border is so confusing and disorienting to the newcomer and so fascinating to the social scientist.

Economically, the United States is by far the most influential of the two countries in the region. The average American is eight times wealthier than the average Mexican, and blatant American consumerism dominates the most visible aspects of the physical panorama of the border. Shopping mall parking lots on the American side, filled with cars bearing Mexican license plates; billboards in northern Mexico extolling the virtues of Coca-Cola, Budweiser, and the Dallas Cowboys; the ever-increasing number of U.S. manufacturing plants (called *maquiladoras*) along the northern Mexican border; these all illustrate the dominance of American capitalism along the U.S.-Mexican border.

This economic power of the United States, however, does not translate into complete social dominance of the border. Even to the most casual observer, it is not difficult to see that culturally, psychologically, and spiritually Mexico is dominant. The reasons for this identification with Mexico are historical, demographic, and geographic. It is easy for Americans to forget that the entire Southwest United States was part of Mexico hundreds of years before it became part of the

United States. It is not uncommon to encounter Americans of Mexican descent who can trace their lineage back hundreds of years to the days when what is now the U.S.-Mexico border belonged to Spain. The history of the border is not one of Puritans, Protestantism, and the Industrial Revolution. Rather, its history is replete with missionaries and explorers, Catholic mysticism, and agricultural and ranching enterprises dominated by hacienda owners and Spanish land grants.

Demographically, the U.S.-Mexican border is not Anglo, but overwhelmingly Hispanic. The U.S. side of the border contains some of the heaviest concentrations of Hispanics in the entire United States. For example, Hispanics in Brownsville and Laredo constitute over 90% of the population (U.S. Bureau of the Census, 1990). In the winter months the influx of thousands of retired Anglos from the Midwest ("Winter Texans") and university spring breakers from around the U.S. make it seem that deep South Texas has more Anglos than it really does. In fact, the border is becoming more Hispanic in spite of the fact that many Anglos are attracted to the professional employment opportunities in the burgeoning *maquiladora* industry.

> A comparison of the data from the 1980 and 1990 censuses reveals a highly significant trend throughout the U.S. borderlands: the number of Hispanics has risen much more rapidly than that of Anglos, with consequent major percentage gains by Hispanics from California to Texas. In eleven border counties the absolute number of Anglos has actually dropped. Eight of these counties are in Texas, with El Paso county experiencing the largest decline in Anglo population, from 157,842 in 1980 to 151, 313 in 1990. These population shifts reflect high birth rates among Mexican Americans, heightened immigration from Mexico, and Anglo "flight" in a number of communities. (Martinez, 1994, p. 44)

Given the fact that Mexican immigration into deep South Texas and Anglo "flight" from the region are both increasing at the same time, one can easily understand why the region is becoming more Mexican. Mexican-American teachers in one of the largest high schools in South Texas confirmed our suspicions that the area is becoming more Mexican. Two industrial arts teachers confirmed that the national character of their school was changing. One said that

> We both went to this same school when we were high school students. We rarely heard our classmates speaking Spanish in the hallways and on the school grounds. Now, Spanish is more dominant than it ever was. In the past, the Anglo population was bigger or the percentage was higher. With so many people coming from Mexico and staying here there's more of them [Mexicans] than there is of us [Mexican-Americans]. There are now more Mexican immigrants in this school than native Mexican-Americans. Now you have to look for the native born Mexican-Americans. We would guess that the population of the school now is 60% Mexican immigrant and 40% Mexican-American. Back when we were going to school here there were few people who could not speak English. Now it's very different. Students nowadays don't want to speak English.

The observations of these Mexican-American high school teachers are confirmed by census data showing the foreign-born percentage of the population at 23.5% in the Brownsville–Harlingen–San Benito area. More dramatic is the statistic showing that 96.5 % of this population speaks Spanish at home and 29.3% does not speak English well or at all (U.S. Bureau of the Census, 1980). It is likely that these statistics will steadily increase, given the significant immigration of Mexican immigrants over the past decade. Moreover, as a result of the 1986 Immigration Reform and Naturalization Act thousands of undocumented Mexican immigrants living in deep South Texas were able to legalize their immigration status and, thus, be included in later censuses.

The northern Mexican cities in the Mexican state of Tamaulipas are anything but the sleepy border towns portrayed in the movies. Whereas the three Texas cities—Brownsville, McAllen, and Laredo—have populations of 100,000, 90,000, and 120,000 respectively, the three cities in Tamaulipas—Matamoros, Reynosa, and Nuevo Laredo—are officially three times larger than their American counterparts. In addition, researchers at the Colegio de la Frontera Norte in Matamoros report that the official censuses of the Mexican government do not include the "floating populations" (temporary migrants) of the border cities. Inclusion of these populations would increase the numbers by 30–50%.

Social scientists speak about the problems of unemployment, poverty, and environmental pollution along the U.S. border with Mexico, but the veritable population explosion in this region is one of the most daunting dilemmas of all. Further, this population explosion will increase in the years to come. To illustrate, half the population of Brownsville is school age or younger and more than half the population of the northern Mexican border cities is less than 25 years of age.

Geographically, it is equally easy to see that the Hispanic Texas border cities are isolated from the more Anglo (and, thus, more American) cities of Texas. El Paso is at least an eight-hour drive to Austin or San Antonio. In fact, the city seems more closely linked to predominantly Hispanic New Mexico than it does to Texas. Laredo is a two-hour drive to San Antonio, McAllen is a four-hour drive to San Antonio, and Brownsville is a three-hour drive to Corpus Christi, Texas. Without a doubt the major Texas border cities depend more on their Mexican counterparts than they do on the state of Texas.

Our argument therefore is that, whereas the U.S.-Mexico border may be controlled by the United States from an economic perspective, and the lower Rio Grande Valley is located within the physical confines of the United States, the region is Mexican from a cultural, historical, demographic, and geographic perspective. Moreover, given the current demographic and geographic realities, the area will increasingly become more Mexican than American. Therefore, the lower Rio Grande Valley qualifies as a region whereby mental retardation must be considered from an international (and in this case, Mexican) perspective.

PARENTAL INVOLVEMENT, SPECIAL EDUCATION, AND THE MEXICAN IMMIGRANT POPULATION

Parental involvement in education reflects the logical progression of a century-old social reform movement, the roots of which date to the 1887 formation of the National Congress of Mothers. The notion of involving parents came to the fore as one of the "progressive" educational reforms of the 1920s. Since then, the underlying assumption of the parental involvement movement has been that parental involvement affects the cognitive, affective, and social development of children. Indeed, many well-known studies have concluded that a child's family is more influential on his or her education than even schooling itself (Coleman et al., 1966; Gordon, 1979).

The challenges facing children from language minority families include salient differences from those faced by non-minority families in the United States (Harry, 1992). Societal attitudes toward children who are poor or culturally, linguistically, or racially diverse make life very difficult. Parents, when sending their children to school, are concerned about the social stigma often assigned to their children because of English language skills, social status, and limited cultural capital. These children are viewed as "different" by the majority social group. This problem is compounded when the child has a disability such as mental retardation. It is well known that many minority students, whether indigenous or immigrant, do not achieve well in U.S. schools and that they are over-represented in special education programs nationwide (Kavanaugh, 1994).

It is our contention that the education and involvement of parents of Mexican immigrant students in the lower Rio Grande Valley will bring more benefits to their children with mental retardation than any other educational policy or pedagogical practice. Ours is not a proposal to simply modify the paradigm used to educate Mexican immigrant children with mental retardation. We propose to throw out the old paradigm and replace it with an entirely new one. If we really do believe that a child's parents are his or her first and most important teachers, we must design radically different policies and training programs that are congruent with that belief.

Special education programs are legally mandated to include parents in planning and decision making. The laws supporting parental involvement in special education programs represent the culmination of parent advocacy beginning in 1950 with the efforts of the National Association for Retarded Citizens (Pizzo, 1983). However, while the participation of parents is widely accepted and parents report that they are satisfied, their role is largely passive (Turnbull, 1983). In too many instances parental participation in the education of their children with mental retardation consists of parents agreeing to how their children will be educated within the formal school system. The schools, however, are not singularly responsible for this situation. Minority parents (including Mexican immigrant parents) tend to place their trust in the school and do not expect to play a substantial role in their children's education. Figler (1981) points to a traditionalistic sense of trust in school personnel and a tendency of minority families to express satisfaction with the services schools provide. Figler found that traditional respect for school authorities, however, acted in many cases as a deterrent to parental involvement. Parents preferred to let the school staff handle all education-related matters, and while those who had children in special education programs were required to attend meetings, their "participation" was often passive.

Mexican immigrant parents in the United States sometimes feel stymied in relating to the schools in the United States for two additional reasons. For the most part, parental participation in Mexican schools is neither valued nor encouraged. In most cases in the Mexican public school system there is a large divide between the schools and families. The relationship between schools and families is hierarchical; power is concentrated at the top with the director of the schools. Even in the rhetoric of Mexican public education there is no mention of the need for collegial relationships between schools and families. Consequently, the idea of parental participation in the education and management of the schools is a totally new concept for most Mexican immigrant parents.

Also, the way schools are structured in the United States is very different from the ways schools are structured in Mexico. Unlike the United States, public education in Mexico is very centralized. As a result, no matter where a Mexican lives in the country the curriculum is the same. Further, it is not difficult for Mexican students to change schools when their family must move. He or she can begin at the very point where he or she stopped at the former school. In fact, it is not uncommon for even the textbooks to be the same at the Mexican child's new school. Thus, the independence of the school systems in the United States can be extremely disorienting to Mexican parents.

During the first Binational Conference on Special Education held in Matamoros, Tamaulipas, it became very clear why parents with a Mexican cultural background in the lower Rio Grande Valley would have difficulty understanding and participating in the education of their child(ren) with mental retardation. The goal of this conference was to assist Mexican teachers in Matamoros in preparing themselves to integrate students with special educational needs into their already overcrowded classrooms. Until 1996, Mexico had a parallel system of education for students with special needs. The new policy emphasizes that students with special needs will be integrated into regular classrooms and that they will no longer be segregated. In the state of Tamaulipas, implementation of this new policy is problematic. According to the assistant director of the state department of education, Oscar Guerra, Tamaulipas has 72,000 students that require special education but only 11,000 of these students receive special services. In the coming year Mr. Guerra calculates accommodations will increase a mere 4%.

Mexican teachers in Matamoros reported that there have been significant and serious obstacles to the implementation of special education programs in Mexico. They regrettably admit that the most serious obstacle is money. In a country where unemployment, poverty, and currency devaluation and inflation are extraordinarily high, many policymakers find it very difficult to justify investing scarce pesos in the education of individuals who are unlikely to ever contribute (in a traditional sense) to the economic well-being of the country. Although there is a consensus in Mexico that all students have a right to an education regardless of whatever limitation they might have, unlike the United States, there is no law in Mexico to encourage the employment of peoples with disabilities of any kind, whether they be mental or physical.

One Mexican teacher mentioned several other obstacles to the inclusion of children with special educational needs.

In Mexico many children with special needs, whether they be physical or mental, don't attend any formal class. In many cases, it is because the parents themselves do not approve of their children going to school. Probably as many as 60% of special needs children do not go to any school. Their parents are afraid that their children will be made fun of or experience some form of rejection. Many parents do not understand the value of an education for their special needs children.

In addition, many teachers don't want special needs children in their classes. They don't think of children with disabilities as being their responsibility. Also the preparation of teachers to work with special needs children is very low. Class sizes in Mexico are already too big. (In most parts of Mexico schools are so overcrowded that students either attend morning sessions or afternoon sessions. For their part, teachers work two shifts a day, beginning at 8 o'clock in the morning and do not finish until 6 o'clock in the evening.)

There are still other problems as well, such as a lack of teaching materials for children with disabilities and the limitations of the physical school structures themselves in accommodating children with special physical or mental disabilities. Lastly, there is no transportation available to these children from their homes to the school.

Among the teachers we have a great deal of frustration with the ministry of education for making these new policies. There is a great deal of resistance to this policy on the part of teachers. They made the policy without working with parents and teachers first. They have not told us how these new policies will or should be implemented. There is a lack of consciousness among parents and teachers about all of this. People are afraid of what it means. The government is telling me to prepare myself, at my own expense, to work with special education students. You would think that with special talents it would be worth more to me but no. I will get no extra pay.

You in the United States have had thirty years experience with the design of programs for children with disabilities. You have laws to protect the rights of those individuals and you have the money to implement special programs. We have almost no history with special education, no special laws which protect the civil rights of people with disabilities, and no money for programs, training, changes in physical plants, and transportation.

Most of all teachers and parents don't fully understand or appreciate the rights of people with disabilities to a regular complete education. It would seem logical to me that we should begin at the beginning by initiating a program of consciousness raising so that people understand the value that an education has to a person with disabilities. We are trying to implement policies without changing attitudes. Consequently, the policy will fail because they do not take into account peoples' attitudes.

As this Mexican teacher in Matamoros was talking, several of her colleagues were nodding their heads in agreement. In other conversations it became apparent that this teacher was voicing the concerns of most of her colleagues.

According to a number of Mexican teachers, the major problem in the state of Tamaulipas and throughout all of Mexico is that parents and teachers do not possess a culture that recognizes and values a regular education for children with disabilities. Many parents who have children with severe or profound disabilities never even consider enrolling them in school. Moreover, the Mexican government either does not have or refuses to allocate the money to support the policies that it mandates. Thus, when children with special needs pass from Mexico into the lower Rio Grande Valley of Texas, a number of problems arise. Foremost among these problems is that the parents of the Mexican immigrant child with special needs will most likely possess little or no understanding of the special education infrastructure that exists in the United States, let alone his or her role within that infrastructure.

It is our hypothesis that a large portion of the efforts made by special education teachers on behalf of the Mexican immigrant child with mental retardation will be in vain if time is not spent teaching the parents the goals, policies, and purposes of the special education process. Further, teachers must educate parents about what they can do to support his or her child's formal schooling and why it is important that they participate.

In the following sections, we describe a number of promising practices observed during our research of effective schools in the lower Rio Grande Valley, which we believe give insight into how special education teachers can work with parents of immigrant Mexican children so as to improve the education of those children. After describing what we observed in the course of the research we conducted for the EBSRDI, we suggest strategies we believe would assist special education teachers in working with Mexican immigrant children with mental retardation and their parents.

PARENTAL INVOLVEMENT IN EFFECTIVE BORDER SCHOOLS

In serving culturally and linguistically diverse populations with mental retardation, the parent-school connection is crucial; thus, teachers must be knowledgeable of strategies such as those that we describe in the following pages. The key attributes found in the effective border schools study—parent education that is culturally sensitive, teaching advocacy, building trusting relationships, sharing resources, providing transformative learning opportunities, and sharing power— are applicable to education programs in general. That is, these strategies can be used for parents of students with and without special educational needs. Indeed, a number of the strategies were observed in both special and regular education classrooms.

Parent Education That Is Culturally Sensitive

One of the initial thrusts of the parental involvement movement was toward the education of parents in effective parenting strategies. While the target group at that time was essentially middle-class families, and participation was entirely voluntary, the emergence of anti-poverty and compensatory education programs in the 1960s refocused on educating low-income parents in effective parenting techniques (Keesling & Melaragno, 1983). This approach to parent education is based on a deficit model that posits the inherent inferiority of lower-class and culturally different parenting styles (Laosa, 1983). Further, the approach reflects the assumption that the parenting styles of Anglo, middle-class families represent the standard against which "good" parenting should be measured.

Further, the imposition of value judgments regarding what is and what is not effective parenting in a culturally diverse society is troubling. Facing issues such as these is a challenge for most educational professionals, who hold ethnocentric views of family and involvement. It is important that educational professionals learn to respect differences and to try to understand them. According to Harry (1992), it is a question of balance. That is, while we cannot put forth certain beliefs and practices as superior, we also cannot shirk our responsibility to inform parents of alternatives as well as their rights and authority.

In the special education programs in effective border schools where we observed, school staff used a number of strategies that demonstrated concern for cultural issues. Efforts were made to develop parent education programs that were culturally sensitive. Staff members reached out to the parents in an effort to find out what they wanted to learn. Parents tended to ask for classes that assisted them in working within their new environment and with their children. To illustrate, parents learned English as a second language, computer keyboarding, and parent-child communication skills. Most important, the special education teachers made an all-out commitment to communicate with the parents of his or her students. The teachers did not use the excuse that she or he did not speak Spanish as a reason for not communicating with parents.

Teaching Advocacy

Although legislative mandates have led to a dramatic increase in parental participation, the parent's role under laws such as Public Law No. 94-142 places parents in a rather passive role, that of a respondent rather than an actor. By law, parents grant permission for referral and placement and participate in planning their child's individualized education plan. For some parents and school staff members, this form of participation does not go far enough. In response, a number of parent education programs are beginning to focus on advocacy skills. Sour and Sorell (1978) created a model for establishing parent support programs that specifically focus on the needs of minority parents. Similarly, Tessier and Barton (1978) developed a program for Hispanic parents that emphasizes advocacy training.

A very important part of the advocacy training of Mexican immigrant parents is learning how they can influence their children's education. This requires that they become familiar with school rules and procedures. Further, they should understand that by voting for certain local school board candidates, they will be choosing the people who influence local school policies. This notion may be new to Mexican immigrant parents. If most of their educational experience was in Mexico, where directives came for the Ministry of Education in Mexico City, they believe that parents cannot directly influence their children's school policies.

One of the schools in the EBSRDI study demonstrated particularly well a commitment to advocating for the needs of parents and teaching parents to advocate for their own needs. In this school the parent coordinator acted more as a community organizer than anything else. She was constantly driving out into the rural community that her school served in order to organize meetings of parents in their own homes rather than at the school itself. In this very personal way she communicated directly with parents and responded to questions parents had about the school and what it was doing. One of her principal goals was also to help people in the community to get to know one another, and to be resources for one another. She realized that in a number of neighborhoods containing high immigrant populations there was no sense of community. People did not know one another and therefore there was little trust or understanding between neighbors. Through neighborhood meetings, the parent coordinator facilitated the development of a sense of community among this population and demonstrated to parents that they had a right to understand school rules and processes and that school personnel were ready to respond to any doubts or questions they had.

Building Trusting Relationships

Our experiences with the parents of children enrolled in effective border schools challenged us to consider the possibility that Mexican immigrant parents conceptualized the parent-teacher relationship differently than the literature would have us believe. At least for some Mexican immigrant parents, trust may not be an outcome of traditional respect for authority but rather a natural outcome of the type of relationships established between parents and teachers. To these parents, primarily women, the parent-teacher relationship was an extension of their worldview of community and family. They came to see teachers not solely as authorities due respect, but viewed them as people who shared with them a commitment of caring for their children's welfare. One parent's definition of parental involvement summarized this orientation: *"El envolvimiento es envolverse en todo de nuestros hijos porque el bien de los niños es el bien de todos"* (involvement is engaging in the welfare of all our children because what's good for our children benefits all of us). The success of the schools was predicated on accepting and nurturing of this orientation.

This parental framework actually makes a great deal of sense when one considers that the Mexican culture in general tends to place more emphasis on the human relationships involved in a context or activity than on the actual activities or interventions being implemented in that context. This orientation is much different than that of the Anglo culture, which tends to focus foremost on the well-being of the person not in relation with others, but in terms of the program being implemented. It is important that such differences in paradigms are understood when different cultures are working together.

It appears that the school staff in the border communities do understand this parental orientation. School staff work hard to build a sense of trust with parents. They do so by utilizing a personal touch in all their encounters with parents. Frequent personal phone calls, handwritten notes, home visits, and one-on-one conversations allow school staff members and parents to get to know one another as individuals and to develop relationships. Some parents viewed home visits as *"visitas de cortesia"* or courtesy visits. The point not to be missed is that home visits provided another way of demonstrating care and interest in the well-being of children. Home visitations are not uncommon for some children with disabilities due to the nature of their disabilities. In many cases, the home visitations are but a temporary arrangement, but the same message is conveyed: Your child's well-being is important.

Monitoring and reporting student performance to parents was also deemed important in effective border schools. Monitoring and providing feedback regarding students' skill development, whether learning to tie a shoe or articulate a difficult sound, was viewed by parents as helpful, especially if their children have severe or profound disabilities. Teachers in these schools often called parents to communicate updates on medical requirements, developmental gains, and celebrations of milestones. Additionally, the teachers at one school were required to ride the school busses of the children in their classes so they would know where their students lived as well as the conditions in which they lived. Inevitably the children were surprised and pleased that their teachers knew where they lived.

There is no doubt that making efforts such as those discussed above is initially very time-consuming, but in the long run they can save time and promote a much more positive working relationship between parents and teachers. Most people would agree that it is much easier to talk with a parent about the special needs of his or her child if the parents and the teacher have developed a trustful relationship from the beginning of their contact with one another. All too often teachers fail to see the absolute crucial importance of their relationship with the parents of the children they teach. They don't realize how much more successful they would be if they had a relationship with their students' parents as well as with the students. Within successful border schools, a high value is placed on relationships, cooperation, and the development of a common set of core values and beliefs in teachers and parents regarding the educational mission of the school. School members listen, care, understand, respect, and are honest and sensitive. The emphasis on good relationships between teachers and parents from the beginning is intended to provide a supportive environment in which all stakeholders in the schools can confidently experiment with new ideas, strategies, and roles.

Sharing Resources

The resources garnered for students and their families often went well beyond that required by law. Teachers, administrators, parent liaisons, and school counselors often looked to the community for assistance in garnering access to medical care, transportation, and donations of items such as clothing, food, and books, and they assisted parents in obtaining these resources for students with special needs. For example, at one school the counselors scheduled appointments for physical exams, the teachers would send home reminders, and the parent liaison arranged for transportation for parents and children who had none. Special efforts were also made to provide opportunities for members of social agencies and the medical community to share literature on summer camps, retreats, support groups, and other information deemed helpful by parents.

The schools communicated very clearly to the parents that the school is a resource for families, not just for children. The school counselor and school nurse saw themselves as serving the entire school community, including parents and siblings who were not immediate clients of the school. The school administrators and teachers fully realized that if a family was having difficulties with unemployment, welfare, or the Immigration and Naturalization Service, these problems would inevitably affect their children's ability to learn and to be in school. The school became involved in these types of family difficulties in order to support the education of the child.

School administrators shared other physical resources with parents as well. For example, a space in each school was allocated for parents to meet, regardless of scarcity. The school was a place for community members to come together. Offering a space for local group meetings, extracurricular activities, adult education opportunities, and afterschool child care are just a few of the ways these schools became an integral part of the community.

Further, parents and community members were invited to share their knowledge, experience, and skills with the children. For example, knowing that students of all ages need to have positive relationships with adults, parents were encouraged to volunteer in special education classrooms, on field trips, and during functional living activities to act as role models, mentors, confidants, advisors, or advocates. Having many different adults in the classroom is particularly helpful for families in which both parents work and are unable to visit the school or spend time with their children on a regular basis.

Continual, Reciprocal, and Transformative Learning Experiences

Stakeholders in the effective border school communities felt it was important that parents and special education teachers were open and willing to learn from one another. First and foremost, teachers were eager to learn about the child's home environment and his or her abilities and behaviors outside of school. Unless teachers are aware of the child's world in a holistic sense, it is likely that his or her teaching will be less well matched to each child's abilities. The best source of this information is the parent. For culturally or linguistically diverse children with disabilities, the parent-teacher relationship is of paramount importance. When their parents and teachers work together, their formal and informal learning experiences are more likely to not only complement one another but also to complement their cultural beliefs and practices. For example, special education teachers and parents openly discussed their cultural beliefs and practices and the contributions and potential contributions each could make to the education of their students with special needs. This openness facilitated the development of effective instructional programs for their children.

Similarly, members felt it important that parents be knowledgeable of the school environment, their children's abilities therein, and the skills their children are being taught. Unless skills are reinforced in both environments, it is unlikely that the skills will be long-term and transferable across environments. In one school, the principal modeled this belief by providing parents with workshops demonstrating how to reinforce questioning strategies, currently being used in the classroom, while viewing *novelas* or popular daytime dramas. In the same vein, parents were encouraged to participate in the special education classroom, especially those with younger children, as a means for learning what skills needed to be mastered and how to reinforce them at home. Thus, parents in these schools were involved in learning as well as in teaching.

In the border schools included in our study, open two-way communication was the norm. School personnel made concerted efforts to ensure that school and other pertinent information was comprehensible to parents. Additionally, care was taken to explain procedures and clarify terms in parents' native language were critical. Further, the knowledge and experience differential between teachers and parents was not used to position one above the other. Social, class, language, and educational differences between parents were ameliorated instead of emphasized, as is so often the case. Attempts to equalize relationships and build mutual respect facilitates understanding between teachers and parents. This practice helps parents understand that their child is not the only one that educators are responsible for and, thus, that teachers cannot spend all of their time with one child. Likewise educators understand that each child is very important to his or her parents and that they deserve respect, consideration, and as much assistance as can be provided.

In these schools, teachers are organized in such a way (e.g., teams, clusters, families, houses, and advisory groups) as to allow shared responsibility for a particular group of students, ensuring that each student is known well by several adults. Thus, even when students with special educational needs are mainstreamed in regular education classrooms, they are able to receive appropriate individualized instruction and modifications. Further, teachers meet regularly to discuss student progress and to share the results from portfolio assessments. Portfolio assessments, which provide a more holistic account of student progress, are used in these schools not only because they more accurately capture a student's abilities but also because they are much easier for parents to understand. Portfolios contain detailed descriptions of achievements and actual examples of student work rather than contextless numbers and percentages.

The collegial interactions described above not only ensure high quality instruction, they also affect the quality of relationships between parents and teachers (Bryk & Driscoll, 1988). In effective border schools, structures are in place that ensure teachers have an opportunity to meet together and with parents to examine their programs, solve problems, share ideas, and develop goals. Collegial relationships provide informal opportunities for personal and professional development based on individual needs and interests. Such interactions facilitate a greater sense of efficacy among school members; that is, members who work together are more likely to believe in their ability to help their students learn and to help their school become more effective in meeting the needs of all students.

Sharing Power and Authority

Power and authority lie at the heart of parent–school staff relationships. In the effective border schools we examined, principals are no longer solely responsible to a centrally controlled bureaucracy; rather, they are also responsible to the members of the school community. This change in responsibility requires that they know their community and keep informed of the needs and desires of its members. Thus, their most important role is not as manager, but as an inspirational leader and facilitator. They are "transformative" leaders (Burns, 1978). They instigate and ensure the continuation of ongoing dialogue, reflection, and change in the school. For example, the principal at one elementary school is an active listener who identifies and cultivates talents among community members, ensures that all opinions and perspectives are heard, inspires school members, and focuses them on their mission. This form of leadership is important for par-

ents, particularly those whose children are in special education, because it ensures they will be listened to and respected. Further, such a leadership style ensures parental inclusion in planning and decision-making. Not only are they are
viewed as members of the school community but they are also seen as integral to
the educational process.

In addition to their membership on Annual Review and Dismissal (ARD)
committees, parents may be called on to become a member of a decision-making committee. The teams provide an opportunity to share ideas and to develop
and implement goals and programs. This sharing is reinforced by what Comer
terms a "no-fault policy" (Anson et al., 1991). Such a policy moves away from
blame placing and toward joint problem-solving. Further, membership on such
teams allows parents to gain "voice." In the special education system, ensuring
parental voice entails helping parents become aware of their rights under the
law, to understand the basics of the system, and to develop skills for effective and
confident interaction with educational staff. In border schools, much of the information sharing is accomplished informally through discussions with teachers
and other parents. However, parents have also been offered the opportunity to
take parent training programs that focus on advocacy skill-building and distrib-
ute important information.

ADULT EDUCATION IMPLICATIONS FOR EDUCATORS
WORKING WITH MEXICAN IMMIGRANT POPULATIONS

While parents have received a great deal of attention concerning their adult education needs, recently the adult education needs of teachers regarding parental
involvement have also been addressed. Marion (1979) has outlined a model for
improved participation that emphasizes the professionals' development of respect
for minority parents and their culture as well as the implementation of a person-
alized style. Similarly, Georgetown University has recently published a manual
for professionals who work with culturally diverse parents (Roberts, 1990).

Gay (1988) stresses the need for school personnel to appreciate, respect, and
understand the differences students and their families bring to the school. Educators need to understand how family characteristics affect student behavior, relationships, and interpersonal dynamics. The life experiences of minority students,
who make up a majority of the student population in border schools, should be a
vital consideration in preparation and in-service programs. While the majority of
teachers and administrators in the communities we studied are Mexican and
Mexican-American, there are other characteristics that may separate them from
their students—for example, social class, level of enculturation or assimilation,
time in the country, and language ability. While no program can prepare educators with information about all the cultures they may encounter over the course
of their careers, teachers must have an opportunity to develop an understanding

of the impact of culture and language on self-concept, interpersonal relationships, interactions, and learning (Gay, 1988).

In his experience along the border, Paul Kavanaugh observed that it is not uncommon to see a high level of animosity as well as a high level of solidarity between people who self-identify as "Mexican-American" and those who self-identify as "Mexican." Although many Mexican-American teachers and administrators do understand and empathize with their Mexican immigrant students and their parents, this is not the case 100% of the time. (For a more in-depth investigation of the relationship between "Mexicans" and "Mexican-Americans" on the border see Martinez, 1994, pp. 67–117.) In any case, the advantage that many Mexican-American teachers in the Valley do have over Anglos, with regard to knowing parents, is that they speak Spanish. Many Anglo teachers in interviews conducted during this study said they would have a better relationship with their students and parents if they spoke Spanish.

Preparation programs should include courses in ethnography and cultural anthropology, as well as opportunities to learn how to adapt curriculum to ensure cultural relevancy. Exposure to such experiences and information will enable educators to situate learning and communication inside the culture, the aspirations, and the lives of the students. Field experiences should be viewed as an opportunity, not only to obtain supervised and guided experience, but also to become familiar with the population with whom educators will be working. Examination of the entire social context of schooling is essential for effective preparation (Liston & Zeichner, 1987), as is the opportunity to reflect on the relationship between the social context and schooling. Familiarity with social context can also be developed through the study of sociology, economics, history, and psychology courses, as well as through observation of school communities and dialogue with other educators.

Sergiovanni (1994) argues that schools too often rely on outside experts for resources and training that school personnel are capable of providing one another. The norms and practices among teachers in effective schools foster collaboration, reflectivity, and critical inquiry into teaching practices, course content, and student outcomes (Bryk & Driscoll, 1988). It is important that teachers engage in an ongoing critique of current research, rhetoric, and pedagogy, as well as their own educational goals, structures, and preferred outcomes. Teachers should seek to understand their own assumptions, values, and beliefs and then use this understanding to rethink their practice. Teachers in effective schools should share, observe and discuss each other's teaching methods and philosophies, and they must be concerned with the effects of their actions on their students and other members of their learning community.

Lastly, we suggest that colleges of education invest many more resources in preparing students to work with the parents of the students they will have in their classrooms. How can we as educators expect students to believe that the parents are the students' most important teachers when student teachers are not taught anything about working with adults? Too many student teachers think of adult education in terms of English as a Second Language, preparing adults to get their GED, and citizenship classes. There is an extraordinarily rich literature in adult education that student teachers are never exposed to during their undergraduate studies. This literature is rarely considered either important or integral in the preparation of student teachers. It is no wonder that adult education programs have such difficulty finding their place in colleges of education, where the emphasis is primarily on preparing teachers to work with students in classrooms within schools.

In this short space, we have hopefully demonstrated our principle thesis; that is, the education of parents of children with special educational needs is as important and at times more important for the welfare of the child than the education that child receives in the classroom him or herself.

REFERENCES

Anson, A., Cook, T., Habib, F., Grady, M., Haynes, N., & Comer, J. (1991). The Comer school development program: A theoretical analysis. *Urban Education, 26*(1), 56–82.

Bryk, A., & Driscoll, M. (1988). *The high school as community: Contextual influences and consequences for students and teachers.* Madison: National Center for Effective Secondary Schools, University of Wisconsin-Madison.

Burns, J. M. (1978). *Leadership.* New York: Harper and Row.

Coleman, J. S., Campbell, E. Q., Hobson, C. J., McPartland, J., Mood, A., Weinfeld, F. D., & York, R. C. (1966). *Equality of educational opportunity.* Washington, DC: U.S. Government Printing Office.

Figler, C. S. (1981). *Puerto Rican families with and without handicapped children.* Paper presented at the Council for Exceptional Children Conference on the Exceptional Bilingual Child, New Orleans. (ERIC Document Reproduction Service No. ED 204–876.)

Gay, G. (1988). Designing relevant curricula for diverse learners. *Education and Urban Society, 3,* 20.

Gordon, I. J. (1979). The effects of parent involvement in schools. In R. S. Brandt (Ed.), *Partners: Parents and schools.* Alexandria, VA: Association for Supervision and Curriculum Development.

Harry, B. (1992). *Cultural diversity, families, and the special education system.* New York: Teachers College Press.

Kavanaugh, P. (1994). Avoiding inappropriate referrals of minority language learners to special education: Implementing a prereferral process. *Issues in Special Education and Rehabilitation, 9*(1), 39–50.

Keesling, J. W., & Melaragno, R. J. (1983). Parent participation in federal education programs: Findings from the federal programs survey phase of the study of parental involvement. In R. Haskins & D. Adams (Eds.), *Parent education and public policy* (pp. 230–256). Norwood, NJ: Ablex.

Laosa, L. M. (1983). Parent education, cultural pluralism, and public policy: The uncertain connection. In R. Haskins & D. Adams (Eds.), *Parent education and public policy* (pp. 331–345). Norwood, NJ: Ablex.

Liston, D. P., & Zeichner, K. M. (1987). Critical pedagogy and teacher education. *Journal of Education, 169,* 117–137.

Marion, R. (1979). Minority parent involvement in the IEP process: A systematic model approach. *Focus on Exceptional Children, 46*(8), 616–623.

Martinez, O. (1994). *Border People.* Tucson: University of Arizona Press.

Pizzo, P. (1983). *Parent to parent.* Boston: Beacon.

Roberts, R. N. (1990). *Developing culturally competent programs for families of children with special needs* (2nd ed.). Washington, DC: Georgetown University Child Development Center.

Sergiovanni, T. (1994). *Building community in schools.* San Francisco: Jossey-Bass.

Sour, M. S., & Sorell, H. (1978). Parent involvement. In P. L. Trohanis (Ed.), *Early education in Spanish-speaking communities* (pp. 35–40). New York: Walker.

Tessier, A., & Barton, S. (1978). Parents learn to help themselves. In P. L. Trohanis (Ed.), *Early education in Spanish-speaking communities* (pp. 27–33). New York: Walker.

Turnbull, A. (1983). Parental participation in the IEP process. In J. A. Mulick & S. M. Pueschel (Eds.), *Parent-professional participation in developmental disability services: Foundations and prospects* (pp. 107–123). Cambridge, MA: Ware.

U.S. Bureau of the Census. (1980). *Census of the Population, 1980.* U.S. Government Printing Office, Washington, DC.

U.S. Bureau of the Census. (1990). *Census of the Population, 1990.* U.S. Government Printing Office, Washington, DC.

CHAPTER 4

Parents, Professionals, and the Transition Process

W. E. Hitchings
St. Ambrose University, Davenport, IA

Barbara Natelle
St. Norbert College, DePere, WI

Robert Ristow
St. Ambrose University, Davenport, IA

Graduation from secondary school, going on to employment or university, leaving home or the community and moving to our own place to live: all mark major changes in the lives of young adults. Each event signals a transition or phase in the transition process. Transition is described as "the passage or movement from one stage to another. . . . The passage from school to work . . . dependence to independence . . . from a relatively protected environment to the larger community . . ." (Patton, Hegenaver, Marinoble & Reifmen, 1984). These transitions impact not only the individual but their families as well. The impact may be more significant to families who have adolescents or young adults with disabilities, and this raises questions about the role of parents in such adolescent's transitions from secondary school to the adult world (Thorin, Yovanoff, & Irvin, 1996).

The parents in the following vignettes respond to transition in different ways. Their reactions, and how professionals can better assist parents during this critical time, are the foci of this chapter.

VIGNETTE #1: ANGELA

Angela, 18, wants to become a graphic designer because of her ability in art and interest in computers. Unlike other students in her classes, she reads lips. She communicates with her teachers and peers by using Signing Exact English (SEE).

For the last 2 years, she has played basketball (in practices and games, her mother serves as the interpreter).

Also, Angela works part time for a local deli and bakery, whose owner for many years has hired individuals with disabilities. When Angela first started working, her mother would drive her, but since Angela got her license, she drives everywhere!

Due in part to Angela's desire to continue her education at the university level, the relationship between Angela, her mother, and the school district has been at best strained. The local district has been reluctant to commit to providing interpreters proficient in the SEE system. The district personnel want to use interpreters who use an alternate sign system: American Sign Language (ASL). District personnel wanted Angela to take courses that were less challenging and more consistent with her profile based on the results of standardized testing. Furthermore, they wanted Angela to enroll in courses where interpreters were already working with other students who were deaf.

Angela's mother is a teacher of the hearing impaired in the same district, knowledgeable in language development and reading skills. In addition, she has high expectations for her daughter and believes Angela needs to have experiences that will enable her to participate in the "hearing" world. The impasse regarding the sign systems caused the mother to file for due process against the district through the state's Protection and Advocacy Agency.

When asked about transition, Angela's mother said, "When does one have time for that!"

VIGNETTE #2: CATHY AND MARY

Jean, the mother of Cathy and Mary, came to the first planning meeting for her daughters' transition to secondary school. During the meeting, Jean was most concerned about Cathy, who was identified as mildly mentally handicapped. Jean wanted her to be able to manage money better, in addition to working toward her high school diploma. Jean believed that Cathy would go on to work after graduation. On the other hand, Mary, who had a specific learning disability in reading, could probably go on for a career that required occupational training at a local community or technical college. For Mary, her mother suggested only minimal involvement from special education personnel because of Mary's ability and long-term career interests.

During the next 2 years, Jean, her husband, and their daughters participated in each girl's annual progress review meetings. For each of her daughters, Jean described their responsibilities at home and the family's expectations for each with an emphasis on increasing their daughters' independence. Jean maintained focus on applied skills for Cathy and had her participate in a summer program operated by the Joint Training and Partnership Program.

VIGNETTE #3: ANNIE

Annie, 21, presently lives at home with her parents. She is in her last year of secondary school and will graduate at the end of the school year. She has been identified as severely mentally retarded.

At 16, Annie's name was placed on a list for supervised community housing services for adults with similar disabilities. The list serves as a notice to the local county department of human services and private providers of the number of new and potential clients who may need the providers' services and government subsidy. Annie's name will be resubmitted each year until she graduates and moves on to the adult service system. Community providers, government agencies, special education personnel, and Annie and her parents have the opportunity to begin preparation early.

When Annie turned 18, she had a week-long vocational assessment at a local community service center. During her last year of school, Annie will return for a second week, in preparation for her transition at graduation. Also during that year, Annie's mother registered her for an out-of-home placement. They visited a number of group homes in order to determine the best match for Annie. After trial visits to two homes, Annie's mother made her decision.

VIGNETTE #4: DANA

Dana, 18, has 2 years until she graduates. Last summer when asked kind of work she wanted do, she replied, "A secretary for a radio station that plays rock music!" Furthermore, she wanted to get her own apartment ("but not right now") and have more friends.

The answers surprised her mother, who each year for more than 10 years went to Dana's annual meetings with school personnel to review her daughter's progress over the previous year and heard them make recommendations for Dana during the coming school year. Over time, the meetings had become a "one-sided" dialogue based on what the special education staff saw as Dana's needs and their plans or goals for her in the coming year.

This year was to be especially important for Dana and her family, as she was to be reevaluated in order to determine if she qualified for services under the disability category of mild mental disabilities. Also, it was the year that special education staff had to notify Dana and her mother about their plans to graduate Dana, 18 months before the actual termination of services.

In discussions with friends, Dana's mother indicated that she felt overwhelmed at the last year's progress meeting. The teachers and counselors had given her information about services that might be helpful to Dana and the family at some time in the future and she could contact government agencies and private services providers if she wanted to know more.

VIGNETTE #5: JOSH

By the end of fifth grade, Josh was failing mathematics and having extreme difficulties in organization skills, memory, and problem-solving. His parents felt that changes in his behavior represented a continuation of the difficulties he had been having. The school was again asked to conduct a multidisciplinary evaluation and, with support from the regular education math teacher, the evaluation was conducted in late spring.

Josh was diagnosed with a learning disability in central processing, specifically organization and problem-solving, manifested in mathematics. He did not qualify under district guidelines as a student with Attention Deficit Disorder (ADD). An Individual Educational Plan (IEP) was developed for implementation in the sixth grade. The focus was on organization skills and math concepts. Throughout sixth grade Josh continued to have difficulties in math and his behavior continued to be problematic. By the end of seventh grade, Josh's parents had been involved in several conferences with the school counselor, social worker, special education teacher and some of his regular education teachers. Josh was being seen on a weekly basis in a social development group and was on a behavioral plan for assignment completion, yet he was barely passing several of his subjects. His behavior at home had gotten more extreme. He was prone to hitting walls or slamming doors to the point of damage. His choice of friends was causing concern for his parents as well, gang-type youth rather than his original neighborhood friends from elementary school. He finished seventh grade ineligible for sports due to a low grade point average, was banned from the mall for stealing, and broke a knuckle after hitting the wall on the heels of a fight with his parents. At that time, Josh's parents chose to have him evaluated by a neuropsychologist for possible ADD.

Josh's previous diagnosis was upheld, with an additional diagnosis of impulse control disorder resulting from damage to the prefrontal cortex. The manifested behaviors appeared in the form of impulse control, organization, memory for detail, problem-solving, and decision-making. He was placed on 20 milligrams of slow-release ritalin.

His early results showed dramatic improvement. His average improved from below a 2.0 to a 3.0 in nine weeks. His teachers reported no significant behavior problems and assignments were completed and turned in on time. His behavior at home improved significantly.

Josh's transition to high school, however, was not as smooth as would be expected. During his transition IEP, which was also his three-year reevaluation, the staffing team proposed release from special education due to his progress. His parents had to argue his continued need for placement due to lack of skills in management of time, organization, and study. The staffing team acquiesced after the school psychologist agreed with his parents. Currently, Josh is in the last half of his freshman year in high school. His parents are working with his resource teacher to begin transition.

Parents react differently in their interactions with school personnel, representatives from government agencies, or private service providers, creating a range of questions and reactions:

- What kind of jobs will my daughter Cathy be able to do when she finishes high school?
- Does Dana have to leave home right after graduation? What types of living arrangements are available? When do we make them?
- What will my daughter Dana do when she is not working? How can they make friends? Do other students have the same problems?
- What about transportation? Who will help Anna learn to ride the bus? Who do I see about those things?
- They gave me information and said to contact them about getting services for Dana.
- I really think they don't want me involved! They showed me the forms and asked to me to sign.
- I have some concerns and I think Anna has some also. Who is to do all this and how do we know what Anna will need?
- What will my son Josh need to be successful in college? When will the school begin to provide him with exploration into college curriculum and career opportunities?

In Western societies, graduation from secondary school marks a significant change in the life of adolescents and their families (Marion, 1992). When someone is presented with a high school diploma, it signifies the end of childhood and adolescence. The diploma marks the end of mandated public education in the United States and Canada. At this time, parents and their sons and daughters are attempting to answer questions regarding work, living arrangements, social relationships, and the future. As parents, we do not believe the transition to young adulthood to be complete until our sons' or daughters' career plans are implemented and their initial residential choices are made (Marsh, 1992).

In the case of the authors, the transition meant continuing onto university for training as teachers. Temporarily, each left home for the university and experienced living with others of similar age. It also meant part-time employment to pay for transportation, recreation, or university-related expenses. Furthermore, it meant interacting with adults, peers, and developing new relationships.

Each of us were carrying out the expected role for adolescents and young adults in our society; that is, becoming less dependent on our parents or families and more independent in making the decisions that would shape our lives (Glidden & Zetlin, 1992; Hirst, Parker, & Cozens, 1991; Wehman, Moon, Everson,

Wood, & Barcus, 1988). Through these experiences, we were developing competencies in order to assume adult roles. We were doing what most American parents, and the systems they operate in, expect of their children—becoming self-reliant, independent, and autonomous (Jackson, 1989).

Like many other parents, our parents looked forward to the changes with great expectation, as their lives would change as well. Their roles and responsibilities would be different, as we grew up, and were preparing to leave home and create our own lives. They addressed a set of anticipations that are part of a normal, expected life cycle (Marsh, 1992). The domestic, financial, and psychological support that they had given us, could now be redirected toward younger siblings or back to their lives. Some gained the freedom to travel, return to work, further their careers, or, in some cases, change their lifestyles (Marion, 1992; Marsh, 1992; Turner, 1996).

In Western societies, the intent of the transitional period for adolescents and young adults is to increase one's options to promote satisfactory relocation and successful entry into the new setting. The transition is considered successful by individuals and their families when the young adult achieves both social and financial independence (Kleinhammer-Tramell, Rosenkoelter, & Tramell, 1994).

IMPACT OF TRANSITION ON PARENTS
OF YOUNG ADULTS WITH DISABILITIES

All families with adolescents or young adults experience challenges during this period. The transition from adolescence to the adult world can be even more traumatic for parents who have adolescents or young adults with disabilities. Families with children who are not disabled look forward to this time with anticipation, but for those whose children have disabilities, especially severe or multiple disabilities, it is a time of continued burdens and less freedoms. It is also a time of great uncertainty (Kinnison, 1987; Orlowska, 1995; Turner, 1992).

Most families with adolescents or young adults are following the cultural expectation of disengaging from the day-to-day or major responsibilities for their children. But parents whose sons or daughters are disabled can expect to have a continuing role in the lives of their offspring (Thorin, Yovanoff, & Irvin, 1996). They have been advocates, assumed a great financial responsibility, and provided social support to their children (Baker & Blacher, 1988). Many parents realize that while adolescence is a time of growing up, it is also a time of hazards. The time for preparing their son or daughter is running out and their fears grow (Lehr, 1992). As a group, parents are concerned about their sons' or daughters' welfare more than any professional (Elksnin & Elksnin, 1989).

Unlike their nondisabled peers, adolescents with disabilities are less likely to go off to college or work and parents feel a sadness at the loss of this important milestone (McCallion & Toseland, 1993). Carol Brown, a rehabilitation counselor for the state of Illinois and parent of a young adult with disabilities, said her son's graduation from high school to the adult community, as well as to a different service system, brought back feelings of grief and sadness similar to the feelings she experienced in the years following her son's birth, starting school, and when he was changing levels during his education (Brown, personal communication, 30 December 1996). She responded, in part, due to the timing of the decision, and the response of the professionals working with her son (Mendelsohn & Mendelsohn, 1988).

Graduation is more than just leaving the structured environment of school, it marks the end of a constant in many students' and their families' lives (West & Sarkees-Wircenski, 1995). For many parents, particularly those with young adults who are severely disabled, school has been an end unto itself. Just being there is more important than what is being taught (Clark & Kolstoe, 1995; Retish, Hitchings, & Hitchings, 1989). During that experience, parents gave little thought to the students' longer-term needs, including employment (Kinnison, 1987). Based on their extensive work with parents who have adolescents with mild or moderate disabilities, Jim Norris, vocational evaluator, and Stephanie Hitchings, secondary special education teacher, believe that in spite of efforts to assist parents to plan for the future, many do not want to recognize the future or view their sons and daughters as becoming adults.

ROLE OF SPECIAL EDUCATION AND REHABILITATION SYSTEM

The goals of special education and rehabilitation systems are to identify the students' future environment, where they are expected to function, and provide training for a such a setting (Everson & Moon, 1987). It is more than just skills: Lankard (1993) envisions special education personnel as advocates and role models, providing a perspective and coordinating activities. This perspective is consistent with federal mandates, which describe transition as a "coordinated set of activities for a student . . . which promotes movement from school to post-school activities" (IDEA, 20 U.S.C. 1401[A], §602[A]).

The requirement for team decision-making, including parent participation, follows a pattern established with the passage of the Education for All Handicapped Children Act, (Pub. L. No. 94-142) in 1975. In spite of the mandate, parent involvement has been minimal (Humes & Hohenshil, 1985; Lankard, 1993). In 1982, Ross found that special education paid only lip service to parent participation. Even after 15 years, the participation of parents still appears to remain at a low level (Kokjohn & Seigworth, 1994; Winton, 1990).

Four reasons may contribute to the problem. First, in the United States (and many other countries) education continues to be a professional bureaucracy that does little to develop collaboration with parents or even other agencies. The involvement of outsiders or nonprofessionals such as parents disrupts what is viewed by educators as a smoothly running system (Smith & Brownell, 1995). Second, in order to make effective use of available time, major decisions are made prior to meetings with parents (Haring, Lovett, & Saren, 1991; Kokjohn & Seigworth, 1994). Third, many professionals continue to assume they not only know more than the parents, but believe they know exactly what parents want (Everson & Moon, 1987). Fourth, some professionals in human services and education believe their systems are too complicated for parents to understand (Danek & McCrone, 1989). As a result, parents lose interest and their participation declines (Danek and McCrone, 1989). Fifth, many parents who have been in the system for years found it to be unresponsive to their son's or daughter's needs (McCallion & Toseland, 1993; Peterson, personal communication).

The problem is exacerbated by government agencies and adult service providers that relegate parents to mere permission givers (Baker & Blacher, 1988). Parent involvement is viewed as an intrusion, a refusal to allow the client to grow up. As a local provider's representative described her organization's view, "it was strictly a courtesy for them to be involved."

RESPONSE OF PARENTS

With the passage of the Education of All Handicapped Children Act in 1975, parents were to be involved in the decision-making process, including needs, goals, and setting for services. In 1990, the federal mandate included transition in the plan as a result of the re-authorization of the law, but the implementation of transition has been impaired by barriers—poorly understood roles and responsibilities of the team members, poor communication between parents and the professionals, and "turf" issues between educational and rehabilitation personnel (Didy 1987; Haring, Lovett, & Saren, 1991). The problem is compounded by limits in programming and a lack of financial resources and qualified personnel (Marion, 1992).

Recently, secondary special education teachers enrolled in a graduate course on transition were asked about the role of parents in the transition planning process, particularly the parents' degree of involvement in the decision-making. All the graduate students felt that of the parents who did come to meetings, they were just "there" and made no significant contributions. Among their observations and comments:

A father informed me [the son's teacher] that he would not come because they [educators] used $10.00 words and he didn't dress like them or have a phone and made him feel low as though they didn't want him there.

Seventeen out of 19 parents came, but they had little to say. Most just wanted to sign [the individual education/transition plan] and leave.

We tried a couple of times to reach her [the student's mother]. No response and so they met without her, then sent the forms home. I couldn't believe it!

One special educator with more than 20 years experience remarked that even though educators have been required by law to involve parents in the planning for transition, parents have not really been wanted.

The response of parents to educators and the process of transition varies from not involved to very involved, or as a mother said, "Some consider me to be a difficult parent, others have called me a pain in the butt, but I consider myself an advocate for my son. I want him to be the best he can be!" (Sue Fleck, personal communication, 22 January 1997).

Like Sue, the parents in vignettes 2, 3, and 5 have a vision for their son or daughter. Unfortunately, their vision differs with the views of the professionals. Each parent is interested in their son or daughter, but they are also knowledgable about special education and the transition process. As a result, they have become active questioners (McNair & Rusch, 1991) and facilitators of transition (Gajar, Goodman, & West, 1993).

McNair and Rusch describe a second catagory of parents, those who are not involved. In our experiences, no parent or guardian will directly admit not wanting to help their son or daughter and refuse to participate in the transition process, but their actions can reflect an apparent lack of interest. When meetings are scheduled at times convenient for them, they don't show. If transportation is made available to them, they go shopping or can't be located.

For years, Dana's mother sat in meetings and listened to educators present information on her daughter. She was then presented with a copy of the planning document and asked to sign the document. She characterized herself as "very passive" until last year, when she was overwhelmed with the whole process and the way information regarding adult service agencies and providers was "dumped" on her. McNair and Rusch (1991) describe this response as passive acceptor. Passive acceptor is very common among parents. Parents who come from non-Western cultures often respond in this manner, but the differences extend beyond cultural variation to barriers created by language and beliefs held by the professionals. There is a question of whether such parents are valued in the same manner as parents from the predominant culture (Sileo, Sileo, & Prater, 1996).

The responses of parents as they interact with professionals can, perhaps, best be explained through viewing the family from a systems model (Turnbull & Turnbull, 1997).

UNDERSTANDING FAMILIES: A SYSTEMS VIEW

Over the past several years there has been strong interest in exploring the impact of children and youth with disabilities on their families. What began as exploration into reaction patterns of mothers of children with mental retardation (Farber, 1959; Ross, 1982), has expanded to include various disabilities including epilepsy, spina bifida, autism, adolescent substance abuse, learning disabilities, and adolescent suicide (Anderson & Henry, 1994; Falik, 1995; Koopmans, 1995). While much of the earlier research focused on mother-child interactions from the mother's perceptions, recent studies have broadened their view—and rightly so—to include the complete family (Seligman & Darling, 1989). Systems theory applied to families with children and youth with disabilities along with mediational processes is a well-founded approach in the literature (Feuerstein, 1979; Minuchin, 1974).

As exploration into reactions and interactions continues, researchers must consider the vast array of confounding variables and the complexities of families relative to their method of operations (Turnbull & Turnbull, 1990). Using the systems approach provides a strong technique to delve into these complex patterns.

Systems theory is rooted in the work of Virginia Satir (1964) and Murray Bowen (1966). It addresses the complexities of family life from the angle that any change in one member of the family will impact in some way on the other members of the family (Satir & Baldwin, 1983). Systems theory exemplifies five distinct characteristics or principles: purpose, structure, rule orientation, order in operation, and perseverance. These characteristics can be applied to families through the following: all families have a purpose, each family has its own structure, its own set of rules and order in how it operates; and each family strives to perpetuate itself (Chinn, Win, & Walters, 1978, pp. 4 and 5). Coupled with the constructs of Minuchin (1974) and Feuerstein (1979), the principles of family systems provide one framework for viewing the family.

SYSTEMS AND THE TRANSITION PROCESS: A FAMILY'S VIEW

While there are many critical periods in the life of families of individuals with disabilities (Bishop et al., 1992; Turnbull & Turnbull, 1997), perhaps the transition from school to adulthood creates one of the more traumatic periods. This transition indicates the closing of one part of the family life cycle and the beginning of another. As a result, family members may need to begin to make certain adjustments within the system. It is important that professionals recognize the behaviors of family members during these times as reflective of these adjustments. As with any family whose child has grown up and is soon to leave, parents and siblings of individuals with disabilities must struggle with the impact of this change. However, unlike families of youth without disabilities, the concerns take on different proportions for the families of youth with disabilities. These concerns may be directly proportional to the type and severity of the disability

(Turnbull & Turnbull, 1997). Approaching this transition process from a systems model can be beneficial to the professional working with such a family.

In the case of Josh, the adolescent with a learning disability and an impulse control problem in vignette #5, this model helps to explain many of the adjustments his family is making toward his transition into the adult world. Josh's older brother will be graduating from high school soon. The family resources for the eldest son, who will be attending college in a few months, are expended much like those of any other family. However, the parents' resources and energies must change to accommodate the uniqueness of their younger son.

Although Josh is only a freshman, his parents are already looking at the type of skills he will need to be successful—something they weren't concerned about with their older child. They are attempting to enter into discussions with the school over such skills as decision-making, goal-setting, and self-advocacy. In order to communicate their concerns, extra time and energy is demanded on their part, thus taking away from time and energy that could be spent with other family members. Josh's parents are already talking with their son about the need for him to be more aware of his needs relative to the transition to college. This creates some disturbance in their relationship, as he does not see them sharing this type of information and energy with his older brother. In turn, his older brother sometimes does not understand why his parents are focusing their energies on the younger sibling when he is the one leaving soon for college. This dilemma causes both parents to focus more of their partnership energies on discussions about these matters, rather than usual family matters. The impact of this can be seen on the communication aspect of the family system. Often arguments crop up within the family. Both parents and children must work harder than normal to keep communication open. Professionals must recognize that the parents concerns relative to Josh may not be adequately expressed due to this disruption in the family communication system. Various techniques and models have been developed to assist the professional in collaborating with parents who are experiencing this type of system change. Some of these will be explored next.

CONSIDERATIONS

As educators, we have significant responsibilities in the transition process. One of the critical responsibilities is that we must be aware of the needs of the family relative to the future of their son or daughter. Such awareness was made evident to one of the authors at the 1985 Conference of the International Association for Special Education.

In a presentation, a father reminded his audience of special educators, social workers, rehabilitation counselors, and other human service professionals that although they had concern for and worked on behalf of individuals with disabilities similar to his son, they would never have the level of concern or work as hard as he had and would continue to do over his lifetime. This father was very committed to his son and expected to remain involved for the forseeable future. He was disappointed by the educators because they had not taken the initiative to help his son prepare for the future. Following existing procedures, the educators had scheduled transition planning to begin 60 days prior to the son's graduation. Furthermore, in his work as the director of an organization that funded local social service providers, he was aware of more than 15 programs and services available to persons with disabilities like his son. The father also knew of the difficulties a person with disabilities would encounter trying to negotiate the maze of programs in a multilayered social service system made up of agencies respresenting the county, state, and federal governments as well as private providers (see Appendix A).

While not all families possess the level of knowledge and commitment of this man, we as educators expect parents to be at least actively involved and collaborate with the professionals. There is a tendency to think less of parents when they are not involved (Aune & Johnson, 1992; Baker & Blacher, 1988; Humes & Hohenshil, 1985; Izzo, 1987).

The degree of involvement by parents is impacted by many factors. For example, in Western societies, new family patterns have been emerging over past 20 years. As a result of economic changes, there are more families with dual incomes, or parents working two or more jobs. Social factors including divorce have led to to an increase in single parents and pluralistic families (Farber & DeAllos, 1992). As noted earlier, some parents or families are trying to cope with their son's or daughter's needs as well as their own feelings of fatigue and increasing wishes for more freedom. Some parents don't have the skills to impact their son's or daughter's transition, and others don't value the purpose of transition. Furthermore, such difficulties do not consider whether the relationship between the parents or families and the educators has been positive and effective. When taken together, professionals find it difficult to get parents involved (Haring et al., 1991; Kinnison, 1987; Miles, 1987).

As one parent noted: "It's as though this [transition for her son] were my only concern. There is more to my life! I also have other children and work full time. . . ."

Therefore, it is the responsibility of educators to create an environment that is friendly and supportive, but also effective. Along with Didy (1987) and Winton (1990), we believe that professionals need to allow parents to choose a level of involvement based on the family's values. Our awareness of the family's level of commitment can come out of the student's and family's vision statements for the future. Such statements precede all other activities in the transition process (Mississippi Bend Area Education Agency, 1998). In the Special Education District of Lake County, Illinois, special educators under the direction of Tom Bartels ask parents to project 10 years ahead, or to the time when their son or daughter reaches 25 years old, and to share hopes for them in terms of employment, leisure, social opportunities, and living situations. Furthermore, the professionals want to know what parents expect for themselves by that point in their own lives.

Each organization utilizes the vision statement as a way to assess the student's and parent's view of the future. Participants have learned not to judge the initial statements in terms of realism for the student and parents, nor do they determine if the vision is within the capabilities of the transition team and resources of the community.

Following the federal mandates, both the Mississippi Bend Area Education Agency and the Special Education District of Lake County begin transition by the time a student reaches 16 years old. Educational systems in Iowa can initiate transition, if appropriate, when students are 14 years old. It may be wiser to begin a transition plan when the student enters secondary school at 12 years old. Beginning earlier may be helpful in focusing all parties' attention on the long-term needs of the individual, especially if this person is severely disabled or the services in a geographic area are limited. Furthermore, building relationships takes a long time, particularly if there has been conflict between parents and the educators or, as in some cases, parents and providers. Time permits reconciling the student's or family's vision if it is unrealistic, or developing a more constructive relationship between parents and professionals (Bishop et al., 1992; Mendelsohn & Mendelsohn, 1988; Ness, 1989; Patton et al., 1984).

During this time, parents might be introduced to a parent support group or a mentoring family who has or is successfully transitioning their son or daughter with disabilities. The purpose is not only to assist them with immediate or long term issues related to their child, but also to the parents' or family's needs.

Recognition of the behaviors and behavioral changes within the communication from school to home, and providing a listening ear as the parent shares his/her concerns is also of utmost importance (Didy, 1987; Haring, Lovett, & Sarin, 1991). Also of high importance is the professionals' insight into what skills the student in question needs to achieve self-sufficiency as an adult, and the ability to develop programming that provides for these needs in a manner that can be understood by the parents. To ascertain such information, Elksnin and Elksnin (1989) adopted a model based on the work of Heron and Harris (1987). The nine-step model begins with formulating a plan to work with the parents, then moves to establishing rapport with them before attempting to define problems and identify solutions.

Parents and students have contact with numerous professionals during their son's or daughter's secondary school experience. It is not uncommon for the professionals on a decision-making team to change each year, leaving the student and his or her parents as the only constants on the team. If developing a rapport with families is as important as gaining an understanding of their vision and needs (which can be expected to change over time), then the core membership of the team should be more consistent: at least one educator from the team should remain a constant for the student and their family. A transition guide published by the Texas Department of Education (1995) suggested a "single coordinator" to assist students and parents. Such an individual is a link to the educational system as well as to the adult service system.

The issue of a single coordinator was addressed by two of the authors, who developed a case management/primary implementer system that enabled a designated special educator to have contact with a student and his or her family during the years the student was enrolled in secondary special programs.

Whether the educator is known as a case manager, facilitator, or primary implementer, the focus is on assisting the students and their parents to bring their vision to reality through conversations during formal and informal contacts (Turnbull & Turnbull, 1997). Professionals have been taught to maintain businesslike relationships, but the conversations are designed to move away from detached, sterile approach to a more supportive, friendly relationship.

While visiting two elementary schools, one of the authors observed conferences being held in "parent centers." The centers were designed to be a comfortable environment with furnishings and decorations to create a homelike setting. Parents and teachers found such an environment preferrable to conference rooms or offices, particularly for discussing stressful topics such as discipline.

Programs that utilize group problem-solving have also proven successful (Turnbull & Turnbull, 1997). Through the use of a Group Action Plan (GAP), members of the adolescent's world, along with the adolescent, are able to move through a systematic process involving eight steps (MAPS) that provide a plan for the adolescent's future (Turnbull & Turnbull, 1977, pp. 169–170, 264–268).

A similar process, Person Centered Planning, was demonstrated for the Scott County (Iowa) Transition Planning Advisory Board (19 February 1997). As with GAP and MAPS, Person Centered Planning is predicated on the assumption that transition is shared between the individual, their family, and the professionals. Participants discovered that such efforts have positive aspects, but there are challenges (as shown in Appendix A). Yet, in spite of their effort, there is still no guarantee that parents will become more active in the transition process (Finders & Lewis, 1994).

Whatever models are used to provide parents, students, and professionals with a vehicle to make transition decisions, the authors are convinced that the following elements are needed by professionals to assure the success of the model:

1. Open-honest communication
2. Mutual respect
3. Solution searching not blame placing
4. Professional knowledge of available resources
5. Openness to ideas from all sources
6. A genuine appreciation for the problem solving process

7. A keen understanding of human nature
8. A strong understanding of the systems approach to family development
9. A strong commitment to group processes
10. A willingness to empower parents and students.

Bates (1990) developed a survey to determine the quality of transition planning in secondary special education programs (see Appendix B). While the survey does not reflect all the elements identified above, several items can be indirectly evaluated with the questionnaire. The survey could serve as a way for parents and professionals to evaluate programs, especially to determine if parents are truly part of the part of the process.

Will these ideas "play" in other cultures? That remains to be seen, because they even have a difficult time "playing" in this country. Should they work? Possibly, if we as educators and human service professionals value the individual with disabilities and role of parents in their sons' and daughters' lives.

APPENDIX A

OUTCOME-BASED PROGRAMMING AND PLANNING AREAS FOR POST-HIGH SCHOOL TRANSITIONS FOR EDUCATING EXCEPTIONAL NEEDS STUDENTS

SAMPLES OF IEP TRANSITION GOALS AND OBJECTIVES

GOAL 1: Financial/Income Security

(Topics from which to develop IEP objectives)

Earned income
Unearned income (gifts/dividends)
General Public Assistance (H&W)
Food stamps
Supplemental Security Income (SSI)
Social Security Benefits
Trust/will or similar income
Energy assistance
SSDI
SSIE
Community Integration Program (CIP)
Community Options Program (COP)
Family financial support
Medicaid, medical assistance (effect of income on benefits)

Coordination of financial resources
Tax deduction for developmentally disabled people residing at home
Other:

_____

_____

GOAL 2: Vocational Training/Job Placement/Post-Secondary Education

(Integrated Employment)

On-the-job training (OJT)
Job Training Partnership Act (JTPA)
Colleges/universities
Vocational-Technical Centers
Community-based education and training
Competitive employment
Supported work models
Volunteer work
Rehabilitation facilities
Transition employment site
Work for family business
Own business
On-the-job training programs through voc. tech. schools and/or adult agencies
Apprenticeships
Dept. of Voc. Rehab. postschool adult living
Other:

_____

_____

GOAL 3: Secure Living Arrangements

(Topics from which to develop IEP objectives)

Mental health institution
Corrections
With family
Adult foster care
Intermediate care facility
Hospital
Shelter care group home
Specialized shelter care group home (training)
Semi-independent (supervised) living
Share living (roommate)

Independent living (own house/apartment)
Other:

_____

_____

Goal 4: Adequate Personal Management

(Topics from which to develop IEP objectives)

Household management
Money management
Social skills
Hygiene skills
Personal counseling/therapy:
 Behavioral, occupational, physical, speech/language/hearing, vision, drug/
 alcohol abuse, family planning/sex education
Personal care services
Safety
Parenting skills
Dressing & grooming
Physical fitness
Food & eating
Communication skills
Organization
Self-advocacy
Crisis management
Decision-making

GOAL 5: Access to and Enjoyment of Leisure Activities

(Topics from which to develop IEP objectives)

Specialized recreation/social activities (Special Olympics, People First)
Sports or social clubs (YMCA, Scouts, Health Clubs)
Community center programs
Vocational-technical schools (craft classes, art, music)
Parks and Recreation programs
Hobby clubs
Independent activities (e.g., bowling, tennis, etc.)
Church groups
Camps, vacations
Other:

_____

_____

GOAL 6: Efficient Transportation System

(Topics from which to develop IEP objectives)

Independent (own car, bicycle, etc.)
Public transportation (bus, taxi, train)
Specialized transportation (wheelchair van)
Specialized equipment (electric wheelchair)
Street crossing/pedestrian safety
Mobility and orientation
Carpool
Parents as a transportation source
Financial resources available for transportation
Supported transportation (with peer or coworker)
Other:

_____

_____

GOAL 7: Provision of Medical Services

(Topics from which to develop IEP objectives)

Medical care: intermittent care, daily (long-term) care
Medical services: general medical services (checkups, etc.), medication supervision, dental care
Medical/accident insurance
Financial resources: group policy available, or individual policy, Medicaid, other
Mental health
Technology/equipment
Prosthetic devices
Other:

_____

_____

GOAL 8: Linkage to and Use of Advocacy/Legal Services

(Topics from which to develop IEP objectives)

Guardianship/conservatorship
Wills/trust/other
Legal Aid
OCR Office of Civil Rights
Wisconsin Coalition for Advocacy

Wisconsin Developmental Disabilities Council
Police
DVR (Division of Vocational Rehabilitation)
DCS (Division of Community Services)
PEP (Parent Education Project)
Other:

_____

_____

GOAL 9: Appropriate Personal/Family Relationships

(Topics from which to develop IEP objectives)

Counseling: genetic, family, individual, marriage, crisis
Health aide/home attendant
Support group
Respite care
Visiting arrangements to residence by parents, friends, other family members
Churches
Child care, parenting
Friends/social relationships
YMCA/YWCA
Battered women
Protective behaviors
Family planning
Community/home support networks
Divorce
Guardianship
Custody
Other:

_____

_____

GOAL 10: Community Experience

Shopping experiences
Recreation experience
Apartment management
Experience maintenance
Financial, domestic & personal skills
Banking experience
Use of public services
Use of public transportation

Street crossing/pedestrian safety
Mobility
Orientation

APPENDIX B

QUALITY INDICATORS FOR TRANSITION PLANNING

Compare the secondary special education program in your local high school to
the indicators developed by Paul Bates (1990). For a complete explanation of the
indicators, review the handout included with this document. If yes is marked, secure documentation to support the response.

QI 1: Parent Involvement with students 14 years or older

    1. Parent education plan in place   YES_____   NO_____
    2. Notification of career and vocational
       opportunities   YES_____   NO_____
    3. See Indicator
    4. Parent
       a) questionnaire of needs/goals   YES_____   NO_____
       b) identify non-school resources   YES_____   NO_____
       c) sign release for non-school entities YES_____   NO_____
    5. IEPs scheduled at a *mutually* agreed-upon time YES_____   NO_____

QI 2: Student Involvement in Transition

    1. Curriculum instruction in self-determination YES_____   NO_____
    2. Advance notice of transition needs and goals YES_____   NO_____
    3. Futures Planning Activities   YES_____   NO_____
    4. See Indicators
    5. See Indicators
    6. Participates in planning discussions   YES_____   NO_____
    7. IEPs scheduled at a *mutually* agreed upon time YES_____   NO_____

QI 3: School Personnel and Transition

    1. Inservice training
       a) Legal requirements   YES_____   NO_____
       b) Planning and service delivery models YES_____   NO_____

    2. Interdisciplinary team members
       a) Provide input on needs and goals   YES____   NO____
       b) Utilizes vision statements   YES____   NO____
       c) Invited for planning   YES____   NO____
       d) Invited to IEP   YES____   NO____

QI 4: Community Agencies and Providers

    1. Reasonable notice of transition discussions   YES____   NO____

    2. Participation at least two years before exit   YES____   NO____

    3. Reasonable notice of IEP meetings   YES____   NO____

QI 5: Transition Goals

    1. Student involvement in identfying needs and
       goals in areas of ITI   YES___   NO____
    2. Parents involved in identifying needs and goals
       of ITI areas   YES____   NO____
    3. Agencies and providers involved   YES____   NO____

QI 6: Curriculum—Career and Vocational

    1. Students needs and goals are assessed by
       a) Informal methods   YES___   NO____
       b) Community-based methods   YES___   NO____
    2. Paid work experience   YES___   NO____
    3. Staff supervision available for community
       placements   YES___   NO____
    4. Support services available for for individual
       employment goals   YES___   NO____
    5. Do students meet and maintain employment
       goals   YES___   NO____

QI 7: Curriculum (Postsecondary Education)

    1. Assess need and goals for postsecondary
       education   YES___   NO____
    2. School experiences structured to accomplish
       goals   YES____   NO____
    3. Postsecondary representatives participate in
       planning   YES____   NO____

QI 8: Curriculum (Community or Independent Living)

1. Assess needs to develop community or
   independent living goals   YES____   NO____
2. Community-based instruction   YES____   NO____
3. Support services available for for community
   or independent living goals   YES___   NO____

QI 9: SEE CATEGORY FOR INDICATORS

QI 10: Follow-up

1. See Indicator
2. Aggregate plans discussed annually and results
   monitored   YES____   NO____
3. Follow up conducted at 6 months and 1 year   YES___   NO____
4. Results shared with local transtion planning
   group   YES___   NO____

QI 11/12: School and Community Activities

1. Cooperative planning and staff development
   done with community agencies and providers   YES___   NO____
2. Community agencies and providers participate
   in individual transition planning meetings   YES___   NO____
3. Staff participate in local planning boards   YES___   NO____

REFERENCES

Anderson, A. R., & Henry, C. S. (1994). Family System Characteristics and Parental Behaviors As Predictors of Adolescent Substance Use. *Adolescence, 29*, 405–420.

Aune, E. P., & Johnson, J. M. (1992). Transition takes teamwork: a collaborative model for college bound students with LD. *Intervention in School and Clinic, 27*, 222–227.

Baker, B. L., & Blacher, J. (1988). Family involvement with community residential programs. In M. P. Janicki, M. Wyngaarden-Krauss, & M. Mailick-Seltzer (Eds.), *Community residences for persons with developmental disabilities: here to stay* (pp 173–188). Baltimore: Paul H. Brookes.

Bates, P. (1990). *Quality indicators for transition planning.*

Bishop, B., Blue-Banning, M., Holt, F., Irvin, J., & Martel, T. (1992). *Planning for life after high school* (2nd ed.). Lawrence, KS: Transition Council of Douglas and Johnson Counties in Kansas.

Bowen, M. (1966). The use of family theory in clinical practice. *Comprehensive Psychiatry, 7*, 345–374.

Brown, S. E., & Johnson, K. L. (1994). Recent federal legislation and the role of vocational rehabilitation in the transition from school to community. *Rehabilitation Education, 8*, 67–68.

Carter, E. A., & McGoldrick, M. (Eds.). (1980). *The family life cycle: A framework for family therapy.* New York: Gardner

Chinn, P. C., Win, J., & Walters, R. H. (1978). *Two-Way Talking with Parenmts of Special Children: A Process of Positive Communication.* St. Louis, MO: C. V. Mosby Company

Clark, G. M., & Kolestoe, O. P. (1995). *Career development and transition for adolescents with disabilities* (2nd ed.). Boston: Allyn and Bacon.

Danek, M. M., & McCrone, W. P. (1989). The mandate for transition; myth or reality? In T. E. Allen, B. W. Rawlings, & A. N. Schildrath (Eds.), *Deaf students and the school-to-work transition* (pp. 1–29). Baltimore: Paul H. Brookes.

Didy, D. R. (1987, October). *Transition: new challenge for special education.* Paper presented at Annual Conference of the Association for the Severely Handicapped. Chicago, IL.

Elksnin, L. K., & Elksnin, N. (1989, October). Facilitating successful vocational special education for mentally handicapped adolescents through collaborative consultation with parents. In *Life options for exceptional individuals.* Conference proceedings of the International Conference of the Division of Career Development, Atlanta, GA.

Everson, J. M., & Moon, M. S. (1987). Transition services for young adults with severe disabilities: Defining professional and parental roles and responsibilities. *The Journal of the Association for Persons with Severe Handicaps, 12,* 87–95.

Falik, L. H. (1995). Family Patterns of Reaction to a Child with a Learning Disability: A Mediational Perspective. *Journal of Learning Disabilities, 28,* 335–341.

Farber, B. (1959). Effects of a severely mentally retarded child on family integration. *Monographs of the Society for Research in Child Development. 24*(2, No. 71).

Farber, B., & DeAllos, J. (1992). Increasing knowledge on family issues: a research agenda for 2000. In L. Rowitz (Ed.), *Mental Retardation in the Year 2000* (pp. 69–84). New York: Springer-Verlag.

Feuerstein, R. (1979). *The dynamic assessment of retarded performers.* Baltimore: University Park Press.

Finders, M., & Lewis, C. (1994). Why some parents don't come to school. *Educational Leadership, 51,* 50–54.

Gajar, A., Goodman, L., & West, J. (1993). *Secondary schools and beyond: Transition of individuals with mild disabilities.* New York: Merrill.

Glidden, L. M., & Zetlin, A. C. (1992). Adolescence and community adjustment. In L. Rowitz (Ed.), *Mental Retardation in the Year 2000* (pp. 101–114). New York: Springer-Verlag.

Haring, K. A., Lovett, D., & Saren, D. (1991). Parent perceptions of their adult offspring with disabilities. *Teaching Exceptional Children, 32,* 6–10.

Heron, T. E., & Harris, K. C. (1987). *The educational consultant* (2nd ed.). Austin, TX: PRO-ED.

Hirst, M., Parker, G., & Cozens, N. (1991). Disabled young people. In M. Oliver (Ed.), *Social Work: Disabled people and disabling environments* (pp. 138–155). London: Jessica Kingsley Publishers.

Humes, C. W., & Hohenshil, T. A. (1985). Career development and career education for handicapped students: A re-examination. *The Vocational Guidance Quarterly, 34,* 31–40.

Izzo, M. V. (1987). Career development of disabled youth: The parents' role. *Journal of Career Development, 13,* 47–55.

Jackson, J.(1989). En route to adulthood: A high school transition program for adolescents with disabilities. *Occupational Therapy in Health Care, 6,* 33–51.

Kinnison, L. (1987). Do parents know best? Parents' participation: The weak link in career decision making. *Journal for Vocational Special Needs Education, 10,* 13–15.

Kleinhammer-Tramill, P. J., Rosenkoetler, S. E., & Tramill, J. F. (1994). Early intervention and secondary transition servicies: Harbingers of change in education. *Focus on Exceptional Children, 27*(2), 1–14.

Kokjohn, M. B., & Siegworth, J. M. (1994). *Parent perceptions of knowledge and involvement in the development of the individual education plan.* Unpublished master's thesis, St. Ambrose University, Davenport, IA.

Koopmans, M. (1995) A case of family dysfunction and teenage suicide attempt: applicability of a family systems paradigm. *Adolescence, 30,* 87–94.

Lankard, B. A. (1993). Parents and the school-to-work transition of special needs youth. *Clearinghouse on Adult, Career and ERIC Digest, 142,* 363–398.

Lehr, S. (1992). Integration from a parent's perspective: Yesterday was a long time ago and tomorrow isn't here yet. In K. A. Haring, D. L. Lovett, & N. G. Haring (Eds.). *Integrated lifecycle services for persons with disabilities: A theoretical and empirical perspective* (pp. 340–357). New York: Springer-Verlag.

Marion, R. L. (1992). The mentally retarded child in the family. In M. J. Fine & C. Carlson (Eds.), *The handbook of family-school intervention* (pp 134–156). Englewood Cliffs, NJ: Prentice-Hall.

Marsh, D. T. (1992). *Families and mental retardation: New directions in professional practice.* New York: Praeger.

McCallion, P., & Toseland, R. W. (1993). Empowering families of adolescents and adults with developmental disabilities. *Families in Society, 74,* 579–589.

McNair, J., & Rusch, F. R. (1991). Parent involvement in transition programs. *Mental Retardation, 29,* 93–101.

Mendelsohn, B. L., & Mendelsohn, J. Z. (1988). Families in the transition process: Important partners. In L. G. Perlman & G. F. Austin (Eds.), *The transition to work and independence for youth with disabilities* (pp. 93–106). Alexandria, VA: National Rehabilitation Association.

Miles, M. (1991). *Mental handicap services: Development trends in Pakistan, Report of a survey.* Peshawar, Pakistan: Mental Health Centre.

Minuchin, S. (1974). *Families and Family Therapy.* Cambridge: Harvard University Press.

Mississippi Bend Area Education Agency. (1998). *Transition resource guide.* Bettendorf, IA: Author.

National Transition Network (1996). Did you know you have a right to appeal any decision made by vocational rehabilitation? *Parent Brief Part 2.*

Ness, J. E. (1989). The high jump: Transition issues of learning disabled students and their parents. *Academic Therapy, 25,* (33–39).

Orlowska, D. (1995). Parental participation in issues concerning their sons and daughters with learning disabilities. *Disability and Society, 10,* 437–456.

Patton, P. J., Hengenaver, J., Marioble, R., & Reifman, L. (1984). *Transition from school to work: A guide for parents of learning disabled youth.* San Diego, CA: Department of Special Education, San Diego State University.

Retish, P., Hitchings, W., & Hitchings, S. (1989). Parents' attitudes toward the employment of the retarded: "We would rather they stayed home." In G. F. Elrod (Ed.), *Career Education for Special Needs Individuals: Learning, Earning, Contributing* (pp. 165–173). Columbia, SC: Dance Graphics.

Ross, S. A. (1982). Working with families through intentional family interviewing. In T. F. Harrington (Ed.), *Handbook of career planning for special needs students* (pp. 243–26). Rockville, MD: Aspen Publication.

Satir, V. (1964). *Conjoint family therapy.* Palo Alto, CA: Science Research Associates.

Satir, V., & Baldwin, M. (1983). *Satir step by step.* Palo Alto, CA: Science and Behavior Books.

Seligman, M., & Darling, R. B. (1989). *Ordinary Families, Special Children.* New York: Guilford Press.

Sileo, T. W., Sileo, A. P., & Prater, M. A. (1996). Parent and professional partnerships in special education: Multicultural considerations. *Intervention in School and Clinic, 31,* 145–153.

Smith, S. W., & Brownell, M. T. (1995). Individualized education program: Considering the broad context of reform. *Focus on Exceptional Children, 28*(1), 1–12.

Texas Department of Education. (1995). *Transition services from school to adult life.* Austin, TX: Author.

Thorin, E., Yovanoff, P., & Irvin, L. (1996). Dilemmas faced by families during their young adults' transitions to adulthood: A brief report. *Mental Retardation, 34,* 117–120.

Turnbull, H. R., & Turnbull, A. P. (1990). *Families, Professionals, and Exceptionality: A Special Partnership* (2nd ed). Columbus, OH: Charles E. Merrill.

Turnbull, A. P., & Turnbull, H. R. (1997). *Families, Professionals, and Exceptionality: A Special Partnership (3rd ed.).* Englewood Cliffs, NJ: Prentice-Hall.

Turner, J. S. (1996). *Encyclopedia of relationships across the lifespan.* Westport, CT: Greenwood Press.

Wehman, P., Moon, M. S., Everson, J. M., Wood, W., & Barcus, J. M. (1988). *Transition from School to Work: New Challenges for Youth with Severe Disabilities.* Baltimore: Paul H. Brookes.

West, L. L., & Sarkees-Wircenski, M. (1995). Current and future practices of at-risk programs. *Journal for Vocational Special Needs Education, 18,* 12–16.

Winton, P. J. (1990). Families of children with disabilities. In N. G. Haring, L. McCormick, & T. G. Haring (Eds.), *Exceptional children and Youth* (6th ed., pp. 502–525). New York: Macmillan.

CHAPTER 5

Disability in Australia: Policy and Practice

LORRAINE M. LING
La Trobe University, Victoria, Australia

An official Australian government report pertaining specifically to disabled people and their ability to engage in small business within the business sector of the community, was released in December 1994. The report, in describing the profile of disability in the Australian population, quotes findings by the Australian Bureau of Statistics. According to these figures, it is estimated that 18% of the population of Australia has a disability. Policy at the national and state level that pertains to people with disabilities emphasizes the philosophy of integration of people with disabilities into the community. To this end, policies of deinstitutionalization are currently being implemented, especially in the area of intellectual disability. There are mixed results emerging as this policy is implemented. There are also center-periphery tensions between the federal and state governments regarding legislation in the area of intellectual disability. Part of the concern that is expressed by professionals working in the area of intellectual disability is that the motivation for the policy of deinstitutionalization appears to be more about political and economic gain than about human welfare issues. There have been examples of institutions being closed and clients being moved to a variety of settings, sometimes in the community and sometimes in other institutions. In many instances, these closures coincide with a state election and thus, to an uninformed public, the government is deinstitutionalizing these clients and allowing them to become part of the community. Some of the experiences of such closures will be discussed in more detail later in this chapter. There is, then, in some quarters of the community, especially among professionals and paraprofessionals in areas of health, welfare, and education, a degree of cynicism about policies that purport to be about facilitating the integration of disabled people into the community.

In Australia integration of disabled people into the community may be defined as "An attempt to assimilate or integrate persons with disabilities into the nondisabled dominant culture. . . . It is about the system of values which underpin . . . everyday activities—that is how [people] see and think about themselves, of others outside their cultural circle—their art, work, leisure, politics" (Johnstone and Perry, 1993, p. 100). The concept of integration, then, involves a notion of the perceptions of the nondisabled dominant group in the community about themselves and about those who are perceived as disabled. It also involves the perceptions that the so-called disabled community members have of themselves and of the nondisabled members of the community. It is impossible to discuss any social processes such as education, health, and welfare, without recognizing the contesting and diverse values that operate within a community or social group. There are multiple meanings and perceptions operating in any social arena simultaneously and the conflicting interests, motivations, agendas, and power bases give rise to a dialectical relationship within and between all sectors and groups in a social context.

In order to understand the conflicting agendas and interests that currently operate in the disability field in the Australian context, it is necessary to address the three major subcontexts within which this issue is played out. These contexts may be labeled the political, the economic, and the social domains. Each of these domains continuously interact dialectically with one another; but it may be seen that at any one period in history, one or other of these domains may be the dominant one and the one that gives rise to the discourse of policy upon which social processes are premised.

Within the Australian context currently, the economic domain may be seen to predominate. National policy in Australia is based upon the ideology of economic rationalism and thus the processes and practices that stem from such policy will be geared towards microeconomic reform. This effectively means that systems such as health and education are regarded as tools for the process of microeconomic reform within society. The values of economic rationalism include the dominance of a market forces economy, the spirit of competition, trends towards privatization of government departments and instrumentalities, the prevalence of corporate managerialist strategies at a systemic and institutional level, the need to seek corporate sponsorship by organizations in the community, and the general thrust towards increased productivity (i.e., the imperative to produce more with less). Within this politico-economic climate of economic rationalism, previously available public resources are decreased and support systems and central administrative facilities shrink. The effects of this kind of policy are being felt and observed in many ways within the education, health, and welfare systems in Australia in the 1990s. The situation where institutions are closed in the name of deinstitutionalization, overtly motivated by welfare concerns, but covertly and more importantly motivated by economic and political factors, provides an example of economic rationalism at work. It is against this contextual backdrop that a discussion of the issue of persons with disabilities in the community in Australia will be addressed.

The discussion in this chapter will focus especially upon intellectual disability, emphasizing the state of Victoria and the policies and practices that currently exist in that state. Prior to this discussion there will be a broad outline of the policy that applies generally at a national level in the area of disability. Within this broad national context, particular concentration will be placed on disabled individuals and groups who experience special needs in addition to those resulting from their specific disability. Particular groups identified as having special needs in the Australian context include migrants from non-English-speaking backgrounds (NESB), Aboriginals and Torres Strait Islanders, rural dwellers, and women. Further discussion of the Aboriginal disability issue will follow later in this chapter.

Attention is now turned to the human services system and the approaches and policies that currently exist with regard to integration of disabled persons into the community. The opinions and perspectives of educators are not necessarily consonant with those of professionals working in the health and human services system in regard to the issue of disability. This is an important point in that, dependent upon the system and the sector of the community in which the issue of disability is approached, the strategies and philosophies on which practices are premised will vary. Whereas in education there is a view that some disabled students' needs are best served through specialist services within specialized contexts, the view of professionals who work in the area of disability in the community may be different.

POLICY AND DEINSTITUTIONALIZATION

There are currently a number of legislative documents in Australia relating to disability, and intellectual disability specifically. Relevant Commonwealth documents are the Disability Discrimination Act 1992, the Disability Services Act 1986, and the Disability Reform Package 1991.

In the Victorian state policy regarding disability, a distinction is usually clearly established between intellectual disability and other physical forms of disability. At a national level, all forms of disability tend to be combined under the same broad term. This creates a difficulty when seeking specific data about particular groups such as intellectually disabled people. Despite the homogeneous nature of national policy in the disability area, the ramifications of the policy for specific groups are different, as is highlighted in the discussion in this section. Some individuals and groups, then, despite initiatives such as the Disability Reform Package with its emphasis on increasing the participation in employment of disabled people, suffer a double disadvantage—their particular disability and their social disadvantage.

In conjunction with the federal policies, each state has its own policies.

One of the difficulties facing a country based historically on a federation of states is that government operates on a multitude of levels. . . . In addition, the tyranny of distance in a country the size of the United States but with a population of 18 million means that services have to be duplicated many times over for a small numbers of people and that the bureaucracy has to be developed further to regional administrators for both Commonwealth and state programs. (Conway, 1992, p. 66)

Thus, although states must adhere to the Commonwealth legislation, they may also have their own more specific legislation that is followed in conjunction with federal law. To this end the Commonwealth/State Disability Agreement 1991 was established. One of the major policies to emerge in the current period is the Disability Discrimination Act (DDA) of 1992.

The DDA 1992 contains three objectives:

a) to eliminate as far as possible, discrimination against persons on the basis of disability

b) to ensure, as far as practicable, that persons with disabilities have the same rights to equality before the law as the rest of the community

c) to promote recognition and acceptance within the community of the principal that persons with disabilities have the same fundamental rights as the rest of the community. (Commonwealth of Australia, 1992, p. 1)

This act is in line with overall principles of the Racial Discrimination Act (1975) and the Sex Discrimination Act (1984).

The DDA goes on to list specific areas in which disability discrimination is prohibited. These are: employment; education; accommodation; goods, services, and facilities; clubs; and sport. Such terms as "discrimination", "harassment," and "victimization" are defined at length and related back to the areas of discrimination prohibition. Specific official persons—for example, the Commissioner—are given responsibilities and guidelines to ensure the administration of the Act.

As is the case with the DDA, a more recent policy, the Disability Services Act (DSA) 1986, focuses on the assumption that people with disabilities have the same rights as the rest of society. "The Disability Services Act was formulated to enable organisations to assist people with disabilities achieve their aspirations and respond to consumer needs, as well as to overcome the restrictions of the previous legislation on innovation in service development and delivery" (Commonwealth of Australia, 1995, p. 14). The objectives of the DSA are based on the fundamental principles of "normalization" and "least restrictive alternative." It supports deinstitutionalization, integration, and the right for all to live in the community and have access to community services, generic services, and specialized services. The objectives of this act are:

a) to replace provisions of the Handicapped Persons Assistance Act 1974

b) to assist persons with disabilities to receive services necessary to enable them to work towards full participation as members of the community

c) to promote services available to persons with disabilities

d) to ensure that the outcomes achieved by persons with disabilities by the provision of services for them are taken into account in the granting of financial assistance for the provision of such services

e) to encourage innovation in the provision of services for persons with disabilities

f) to assist in achieving positive outcomes, such as increased independence, employment opportunities and integration in the community, for persons with disabilities who are of working age by the provision of comprehensive rehabilitation services. (Commonwealth of Australia, 1986, p. 1)

Again, the DSA is specific in designating responsibility through positions of authority in an attempt to promote the success of the objectives.

In 1991, a policy that was specifically designed to address the issue of employment for disabled people was introduced. This policy was the Disability Reform Package (DRP) 1991. The DRP "sought to introduce a more active system of income support for people with disabilities while encouraging participation in a range of mainstream community activities, with an emphasis on employment" (Commonwealth of Australia, 1995, p. 17). The general aim of the DRP is to assist people with disabilities to contribute to the workforce, whether this be full-time, part-time, or supported. Vocational training and income support for those who require it was also considered.

The primary objectives of the DRP for people with disabilities are as follows:

1. to reduce the level of dependence on income support;

2. to increase their participation in employment, education, training and rehabilitation; and

3. to achieve long term reduction in Government outlays on income support payment. (Commonwealth of Australia, Evaluation of the Disability Reform Package, 1995, p.17)

The Commonwealth/State Disability Agreement (CSDA) was introduced in 1991 in an attempt to coordinate federal and state legislation regarding disability within Australia. This had never been attempted before in a national manner. The broad aims of the CSDA were to

set out the framework for better resource use and minimize duplication in the sphere of disability services. Under the Agreement, the Commonwealth Government administers employment services for people with disabilities while State Governments are responsible for accommodation and other support services. The Agreement also requires that all States and Territories pass Disability legislation consistent with the Commonwealth's DSA. (Commonwealth of Australia, Evaluation of The Disability Reform Package, 1995, p. 15)

The CSDA also required that all states initiate their own legislation based on the principles and philosophies of the DSA. Funding and legislative responsibilities are stated and delegated. For example, "responsibility for accommodation, respite care and recreation are to be administered by the states, while employment and TAFE training are to be administered by the commonwealth" (Conway, 1992, p. 68).

The wording in these various legislative documents at state and national level is not only idealistic but also ambiguous and vague. Phrases such as "as far as possible" and "as far as practicable" ensure that achievement of goals is unable to be measured, thus disqualifying sentences using these phrases as objectives by definition. Conway (1992) addresses this issue of language when discussing the document that contains amendments to the Disability Services Act: "Amendments to the Disability Services Act soften the terminology used, by changing the objectives in the Act from enable to assist and from achieve to assist in achieving" (Conway, 1992, p. 67). Terms such as these are so vague and open that any government agency or other body can state that they are conforming to the current legislation. In the light of these various government policies, one may ask if it is realistic to think that we can change the opinions of the wider society to enable acceptance and integration of disabled people. Stern, commenting upon the impact of government policy and legislation, states, "Unfortunately the Disability Services Act has done little to change community attitudes and this is crucial, if the lot of people with intellectual disabilities is to be improved" (1993, p. 19).

The ultimate question to explore may be how people with disabilities are benefiting from this act directly. Deinstitutionalization can be seen to have occurred as a consequence of the DSA. However, the movement to deinstitutionalization started in the early 1980s before the introduction of the DSA. Deinstitutionalization theoretically leads to integration, normalization and improved quality of life. Again, this is a generalized ideology and is not necessarily the case for each individual with a disability. Community acceptance is not achieved merely by people with disabilities residing in the general community. Education and support programs need to accompany such moves both at a state and local level. A greater understanding of the rights, needs, and abilities of people with disabilities by the general public is required before assimilation can be made possible. "If these rights and freedoms don't exist in practice, then legislating them to happen changes nothing. We have begun to change community attitudes and perhaps it is better to do this by action not decree as has occurred in some of our state racial vilification laws" (Conway, 1992, p. 73). The federal legislation is designed to establish services, define already existing services, and assist people with disabilities to access these services. Many services have been established to aid the integration and improve quality of life of people with intellectual disabilities since the introduction of the act. Access to these services is often difficult. Generally, entry requires undergoing a specific assessment, being assigned a case worker, joining a waiting list, and possessing defined prerequisites. This is all time-consuming and often contributes towards dissuading people with disabilities, or their carers, from even attempting to access these services.

Australian laws and regulations such as the Disability Services Act, the Disability Discrimination Act and other potential legislation reflect the importance placed on ensuring that persons with a disability receive appropriate services. The problems of translating legislated services and rights into adequate practices can, however, be a source of frustration for all players in the field—persons with a disability, carers, advocates, service providers and governments. (Conway, 1992, p. 65)

The Acts themselves are only relevant and effective if they, in fact, help people with disabilities in various life areas directly. In order to achieve this, a commitment of funding and services is necessary. "The lack of proper financial planning to accompany the introduction of new policies would seem to be a serious flaw in the whole process. In some cases transition funding has served the purpose well, while in others it has failed, in that overall, services have been depleted, while the number of people requiring these services continues to grow" (Stern, 1993, p. 18). It is questionable how much importance a government places on a social justice issue such as disability when there is so much political pressure revolving around economic issues and unemployment. The stated policies regarding people with disabilities are pushed even further back on the agenda and may thus be perceived as disingenuous attempts on the part of governments to win votes but not to make a commitment to carrying through the stated policies in any practical and genuine sense. An analysis of government policy in the area of disability provides a view of the rhetoric but not of the practice. What follows here relates to research and observations in the field of intellectual disability in Australia and specifically in the state of Victoria.

DEINSTITUTIONALIZATION

Since the first half of the 1980s there has been a strong movement toward deinstitutionalization in Australia. Before this time people with intellectual disabilities were housed in large institutions, or "hospitals" as they were more commonly called. There was no legislation focused directly on people with intellectual disabilities, as their "care" fell under the Department of Health. Australia was slow to follow the process of deinstitutionalization of clients that was occurring in other parts of the world. This could be attributed to many facts, not the least of which may be the influence of the Liberal government, which was in power until 1983. Intellectual disability was not a high-profile issue and did not attract public interest. Indeed, the public in general preferred not to have to think about people with disabilities, and this was achievable by having them "locked" away en masse far from the community eye.

People with intellectual disabilities are still a low-profile group of citizens, not considered by people in general (unless disabled people are moving into their community or there is a high-profile event surrounding disabled people). Such an event, propelling people with intellectual disabilities into the Australian—and indeed world—spotlight, was a devastating fire that occurred at a large institution in Melbourne early in 1996. There were nine fatalities (all clients) and the public was outraged. Living conditions were questioned with regard to the particular residential service, which houses over 600 clients. Much political mileage was made of this event both from the government in support and defence of their policies and also by lobby groups that were against recent government cutbacks to funds and staff. Within six months, however, all was forgotten and the conditions of people with intellectual disabilities once again faded into the background.

Deinstitutionalization, however, is an inevitable process due to many factors, including its economic benefits for the government. It can be argued that client personal preference is not necessarily one of these factors: "This process of de-institutionalization is generally undertaken with little or no client choice; an action which relies for its empirical justification on studies which have demonstrated an object improvement in life quality following such relocations" (Cummins, 1993, p. 64).

In Melbourne, extensive research was undertaken into the quantitative improvements to clients' lives after they had been relocated from a large hospital setting to a number of Community Residential Units (CRUs). "The closure of St Nicholas Hospital was part of the Victorian Government policy of deinstitutionalization in the state and as of June 1989 a total of 170 CRUs had been created in Victoria housing about 850 people with intellectual disabilities" (Cummins, Polzin, & Theobald, 1990, p. 305). Baseline data were gathered six months prior to deinstitutionalization and just before the clients moved to the community setting. Follow-up data were gathered 6 months, 12 months, and 4 years after the closure of St. Nicholas. The results of this study indicated that in general, deinstitutionalization had a positive effect on the clients involved. The life area that showed the highest level of improvement was that of living skills, such as adaptive behavior. "Over the four year period these people had gained the equivalent of 2.3 developmental years over what they would have experienced by remaining at St Nicholas. This translates into a 46% advantage in skill development over this period. . . . Other results demonstrated a normalisation in daily routines and activities" (Cummins, 1993, p. 65).

Living in CRUs allowed the clients to experience varied routines that were not possible in the hospital setting. On weekends in CRUs they generally slept in late. Breakfast times were varied and they went to bed later. There was a higher participation in active leisure activities such as gardening. Short-term family visits increased, but long-term family contact remained constant—at a low frequency. Clients experienced many more holiday opportunities, especially to venues interstate.

Similar research carried out in New South Wales found that "the relocation of people with a developmental disability in New South Wales has been demonstrated to lead to increases in overall adaptive behaviour over a one year period, when compared with changes over the same period in people who were not transferred from hospital wards to the community" (Molony & Taplin, 1990, p. 156). This study found that clients who had been deinstitutionalized demonstrated an increased level of age-appropriate functioning compared with those who remained in the institution. The study also revealed that the clients' self-help and socialization skills improved and that there was no long term increase in maladaptive behavior.

> There seems no doubt that the CRU's are continuing to develop in ways that develop a more normative environment for the residents. The increased personal freedom that this provides, together with the enhanced opportunities for personal development, and more frequently social contact with family and friends, are all indicative of a higher quality of life as defined by these variables than was available within St Nicholas Hospital. (Cummins et al., 1990, p. 320)

However, the question can be raised: How does one really measure quality of life? "We must stop judging success simply on the basis of objective criteria and start asking the recipients of the service how they feel, how their lives have been improved, what they would like to happen and so on" (Cummins, 1993, p. 67). Quantitative research has led to findings of an increase in life skills and adaptive behavior, but how do we know if the clients themselves feel happier than they did while living in an institution?

> While both the St Nicholas Project in Victoria and the Richmond Program in New South Wales clearly recognise the importance of the gains that have been identified so far, the objectives of deinstitutionalization go further than this. What is required in addition is evidence that persons with developmental disabilities actualise these various adaptive skills and behaviours so as to exercise more control over their own affairs and fulfil their own aspirations and needs. (Molony & Taplin, 1990, p. 150)

To ask people with intellectual disabilities where they would most like to live and what would make them most happy would be the obvious answer, and to this end the Comprehensive Quality of Life Scale (Cummins, 1992) could be employed. This test, however, requires an understanding of abstract concepts such as "importance" and "desirability," thus reducing its worth when considering the more profoundly intellectually disabled population. It is tempting to be idealistic and to state that "our duty should be to provide people with an informed choice; to provide them with the opportunity to experience different living arrangements if they choose to do so and for them to make the final choice" (Cummins, 1993, p. 70). This line of thinking is commendable when referring to people who can obviously make an informed choice. But what of those that can't? It is unrealistic to assume that all people with intellectual disabilities are either able to make an informed choice or are able to adequately communicate it. This being the case, it may be that the most effective method of determining what is best for individuals who can not speak for themselves is research and experience, both of which indicate that quality of life is improved when a client moves from a dormitory-style institutional setting to a house in the community shared with three or four other residents.

The ease with which a client assimilates into community life will be affected by the method by which they are transferred from institution to CRU. For a majority of clients, institutional life is all they have known. For them, it is a safe way of life with regular routines and procedures. The move to a house can be a frightening proposition. A client should not be forced to move to a CRU without adequate training and preparation. When an entire institution is closed en masse it is unlikely that all clients will have the opportunity to experience adequate preparation or even to be given the time to come to terms with their forthcoming change in lifestyle.

An Example of Deinstitutionalization

The closure of the last remaining large institution in Melbourne seems inevitable. Rather than waiting until the eleventh hour, however, when relocation of clients is a necessity instead of an option, clients are slowly moving to the community and being given the opportunity to come to grips with this reality. This method of step-by-step deinstitutionalization allows the clients to have the luxury of choice and time.

A unit on the grounds of the institution was converted into a setting more similar to that of a typical residential house, with the greatest difference being that of client numbers—14 as opposed to 5 in a CRU. The clients living in this unit or "House Hostel" are given training in independent living skills and adaptive behavior skills. Due to the location of the unit, the clients are not isolated from all they have known or from the friends they have made within the institution. They are given time to come to grips with being assigned chores, having a varied routine, and having to make choices for themselves on a regular basis. Clients are also encouraged to visit already existing CRUs and to participate in community activities while also utilizing community services.

When a client is deemed to be ready to move to a CRU, based on the client's expressed wishes and the observations of staff, they are selected along with four other residents from the unit. Selection is based on personal relationships and compatibilities. The clients move to a CRU, which is a rental property selected by staff and management. The property is in the vicinity of both the institution and other CRUs established in the same manner, thus not isolating the clients from already established friendships and familiar settings. The clients are given an initial trial period of 3 months. If after this time they are unhappy, exhibiting maladjustive behaviors, or disrupting the lives of co-residents, they are given the opportunity to move back to the institutional setting they are used to and another client is offered the placement in the CRU. If, however, a client expresses a wish to remain in the community setting but is nonetheless displaying challenging behaviors, every effort will be made to accommodate them, including providing them with behavioral strategies, counseling, and developmental programming.

This deinstitutionalization program has been in operation for over 2 years. From professional observation it can be said that clients have more ability in the areas of living skills, interpersonal relationships, community access, communication, and self-confidence than was previously exhibited in the institutional setting. More importantly, these clients express a desire to remain in the community and do not wish to return to the daily routines of the institution.

In order to gain a more complete picture of the integration of disabled people into the community, a discussion that focuses upon the education system and its responses to the issue will follow.

EDUCATION

In addition to initiatives regarding employment of people with disabilities, there have been major policy initiatives in the field of education with regard to mainstreaming or integration into normal school settings of people with a disability. In 1988 in Victoria, the policy that directed the process of integration of students with disabilities in the government school system was based upon five principles.

1. Every child has a right to be educated in a regular school
2. Non-categorization
3. Resources and services should, to the greatest extent possible, be school-based
4. Collaborative decision-making processes
5. All children can learn and be taught. (Ministry of Education, 1988, p. 7)

The government policy in 1988 placed emphasis on the process of integration of students with disabilities. It was stated that there should not only be an effort to increase the participation of persons with disabilities in the mainstream education system, but also that those students seen to be at risk were not to be segregated.

As the integration process developed in Victorian schools, the previously designated "Special schools" were reduced in number. Special schools were seen as contradictory to the concept of mainstreaming, assimilation, and increased participation in the community, and thus were not in line with the government policy regarding integration. Following the implementation of the policy, there are still centers operating in the community for students whose disabilities are of such a profound nature as to render it inappropriate to attempt to mainstream them. In general, however, wherever appropriate, students are not segregated, and thus are not withdrawn from mainstream classrooms for special classes or programs.

Since 1988 in Victoria, there has been a change of state government from a Labor to a Liberal conservative government. (In Australia, the Liberals are considered to be the conservative party as distinct from Labor). The incoming Liberal government articulated its own policy in the area of integration, and while there were some minor changes to the processes, the spirit of the 1988 policy remained largely unchanged. With the induction of the Liberal government in late 1992, there was a major upsurge in the process of microeconomic reform in Victoria and the education and health systems were severely affected by this. Critics of the government and its strategies in the area of disabilities perceived that the efforts to close special schools and institutions where persons with disabilities were accommodated was motivated more by an economic than a social agenda. While in the popular press and in the public arena the government espoused a social justice agenda with regard to the reduction of public resources and decreasing of specialist support services for disabled persons, it was felt by critics that the major drive was towards cutting costs by withdrawing support in the disability field at all levels.

> Some agencies, in the pursuit of the 'normalization' ideal have gone to the other extreme and have abrogated their responsibility for providing very necessary services. People who are dependent upon a range of medical/therapy supports now have to seek access to generic 'normal' services, whether the generic services have the expertise that people with disabilities require or not. For people with disabilities there remains a constant uphill battle for resources and support. (Johnstone & Perry, 1993, p. 105)

Criticism was commonly voiced that the government had devised and mandated a policy for disabled persons in the community without providing the necessary resources to support it. This resulted in a situation where classroom teachers and school personnel, operating from a social justice agenda, felt considerable stress and frustration in their efforts to best serve the needs of integration students in their schools. In general, educators are strong in their support for the principles of integration, but are highly critical of the resources and support that are provided in this respect. Thus, it has been seen as another example of the trend in Australian education systems to push the crisis down the line from governments and bureaucratic level to the local level, and is part of the continuous tension that exists between the center and the periphery of systems in society.

Further pursuing the need to adequately support moves to integrate persons with disabilities in the community, and stating the situation in the state of South Australia, Johnstone and Perry (1993) claim

> There are a lot of independent persons with an intellectual disability, who, in the name of normalization are more isolated from human contact then they were in institutions. . . . The actions of well-meaning people are perpetuating the abandonment, isolation, lack of care and lack of personal relationships which were supposedly characteristic of living in institutions. Normalisation has meant that there are no longer any institutions which provide permanent accommodation for

children with disabilities in South Australia. . . . Given the social, political dominance of the mainstream culture, it is inevitable that it will continue to have the effect of people with disabilities coming to see themselves as inherently inadequate, with or without mainstreaming programmes. (p. 105)

In this statement, the authors are asserting that there is still no challenge to the dominant elite system of values, which further entrenches perceptions that mainstream society holds regarding people with disabilities in the community. Johnstone and Perry (1993) asserted that the ideology of integration has not changed existing negative social attitudes to disability. Another critic of the integration attempts within the education system (Ramsay, 1992) states that "Mainstreaming neglects and marginalises the needs of such students by constructing and reinforcing their invisibility and inaudibility. . . . We have learnt and are now well aware that treating people who are different as if they are the same actually perpetuates inequality" (in Johnstone & Perry, 1993, p. 110). The issue of integration of people with diasabilities into mainstram education remains contested and under-resourced. As microeconomic reform strategies become more widely practiced—and as the education system contends with reductions in funds and staff, school closures, and demands for increased productivity and greater accountability for outcomes—the debate about the feasibility of successful integration of people with disabilities continues.

In concluding this discussion of the Australian perspective and policy pertaining to disability and the normalization of people with disabilities, some of the groups with special needs that require even deeper consideration when examining disability will be addressed.

DISABLED PEOPLE WITH SPECIAL NEEDS

With regard to employment of disabled people with special needs such as have been identified in this section, a number of issues emerge, despite the DRP programs that have been initiated at national level.

The data for 1993 and 1994 suggest that approximately 2% of DRP clients were disadvantaged migrants. For all CES clients, the number of disadvantaged migrants approximated 6% of unemployed clients. . . . Qualitative research findings suggested that recently arrived non-English-speaking migrants with English language difficulties may not be accessing the DRP because of the bureaucratic nature of the reforms. . . . Data on DRP Aboriginal and Torres Strait Islander clients are also low when compared to DEET [Department of Employment Education and Training] data for all clients. Aboriginal and Torres Strait Islanders were the other main group identified in the qualitative research as having difficulty accessing the DRP. Reasons were stated to be, once again, the bureaucratic nature of the reforms and the lack of information available to clients. (Commowealth of Australia, 1995, p. 68)

It is also stated in the DRP Evaluation Report (1995) that it is likely that, for cultural reasons, some of the special needs groups such as the Aboriginals and the non-English-speaking population may be hesitant to report disabilities; thus, data pertaining to these groups is to be treated with caution. In the case of Aboriginals and Torres Strait Islanders, an additional disadvantage is that they are excluded from participation in the Community Development Employment Programs. This stems from the fact that Aboriginals are, in general, supported by a Disability Support Pension and funding for people receiving this pension to participate in the Community Development Programs is currently not available. Groups with severe intellectual and psychiatric disabilities are also seen to miss out in many DRP programs due to the high level of funding necessary to achieve successful outcomes for these groups.

> Around half of the peak disability and welfare groups which responded to the questionnaire [administered as part of the evaluation of the DRP] stated that people with severe disabilities had not benefited at all from the DRP. These groups also felt that clients with lower support needs, who were likely to achieve positive outcomes received a disproportionate share of the resources . . . people with high support needs did not receive adequate assistance . . . people with high support needs, sensory and/or multiple disabilities were being screened out of the process. (DRP Evaluation Report, 1995, p. 185)

For programs to assist Aboriginal and Torres Strait Islander disabled clients to be successful, it is regarded by welfare agency staff that these programs need to be implemented within the local Aboriginal community and that they need to be conducted and accessed in a less bureaucratic manner.

In terms of gender and disability, 37% of women (as distinct from 63% of men) gain assistance through employment support services in general and DRP places in particular. The labor force participation rates in 1993 for females with a disability was 39.9%, as compared with 52.6% for disabled males (DRP Evaluation Report, 1995, p. 64). Another disadvantaged disabled group identified in the DRP Evaluation Report (1995) were those with intellectual disability. It was revealed through data collected at a national level that the "proportion of people with an intellectual disability assisted by Disability Services Program funded services has declined, with access improving for people with psychiatric and physical disabilities" (p. 71).

CONCLUSION

In Australia the issue of deinstitutionalization and of integration of people with intellectual disabilities into mainstream social settings is complex and contested. There are, as with any area of public policy, many special interest groups and lobby groups operating within the arena of policy construction for the provision of these services. The political motivation for what on the surface may appear to be social justice agendas is more likely to stem from an economically and politically driven base. This disjunction between what governments purport to be attempting to achieve in the rhetoric of policy and what they covertly contrive to achieve in practical terms creates ongoing difficulties for those who work in the area of intellectual disability and for those who are themselves intellectually disabled. Families and carers of intellectually disabled people are also often caught in a no-win situation between a policy that states one agenda and acts out another.

Despite the political nature of the area of intellectual disability, there have been some major advances in terms of moving these people into the community. This has been largely due to the commitment and lobbying of those people who are genuinely concerned for the care and welfare of intellectually disabled people and who are prepared to enter the arena of contest and struggle to change policies and change attitudes. In the case of changing attitudes, while there has been some positive breakthrough in community perception, in general there are still prejudices and myths abounding that require much concentrated effort to dispel. In some cases the public media exacerbates the negative attitudes of the public and, in some sense, even constructs negative attitudes. Misinformation, whether deliberate or accidental, is not uncommon in reporting issues regarding intellectual disability; this serves to further entrench biases and fears about these people and their entry into the mainstream of the community. The key to changing attitudes may lie in the need to communicate through well-established networks throughout the community so that correct information reaches the public rather than distorted or incorrect information.

In an era of economic rationalism such as is in evidence currently, the health systems and the education systems appear to be the ones where the greatest cuts to funding occur. Within this climate of constraint, then, the challenge to work creatively and innovatively within and through these constraints is clear. New approaches to new situations are needed, and it is to this task that the attention of professionals working in the area of intellectual disability must now turn.

APPENDIX A

A CASE STUDY OF COMMUNITY LIVING AND INTEGRATION

The training centers throughout Victoria are closing, in line with the current political agenda of deinstitutionalization. Those training centers are large, institution-style establishments that accommodate people with intellectual disabilities. The last remaining training center in Victoria is the largest in the state, and is now moving towards closure, following the path of the other institutions in the state of Victoria.

This case study is an outline of the deinstitutionalization of five men with intellectual disabilities. For the sake of this case study, they will be called George, Derek, Alex, Ned, and Bob.

In 1993 a unit in the training center was earmarked for closure. This involved the relocation of 22 clients who resided in this unit. Eighteen of these clients were placed in other units within the training center, which resulted in a lower staff-client ratio and higher numbers of beds per room. Four of the clients, however, were selected to live in a house that was owned by and adjacent to the training center. This house was staffed on a needs-based roster system. This meant that when the clients were at home, the house was staffed by one staff member. When the clients were at work or on placements during the day, the house was unstaffed. In this sense, the house was less costly than that of a regular unit.

George, Alex, Ned, and Bob moved into this house in late 1993. A base staff of four people was selected to work in the house, one acting as house supervisor and liaison with the unit manager at the training center. The clients paid a total of 80% of their disability pension to the training center for rent and payment of bills. The training center was responsible for the house upkeep and improvements. As the house was situated immediately to one side of the training center, a gate opened through the fence, providing direct access. The clients, therefore, did not have to make any environmental adjustments as far as the local community was concerned. Similarly, the neighborhood was used to dealing with people with disabilities, so there was no adjustment to be made by the surrounding members of the community.

All four of the clients settled in well to their new location. They had to learn new daily living skills in order to assist in maintaining their new home. In the units of the training center, some staff members worked purely on a domestic basis, cooking and cleaning. In the new arrangement, these tasks became the responsibility of the clients and staff working in the house. The clients were placed on formal developmental programs in order to learn these skills. All the clients participated willingly and were eager to assist the staff. All four of the clients had some form of day placement, either paid employment at a sheltered workshop located within the training center grounds or a placement at a local Adult Training Support Service. This assisted the clients to maintain their previous vocation.

A year later it was decided by staff and management that the four clients and an additional client from a transitional unit would move to a house out in the community, which they would privately rent. It was perceived that this option would be more financially viable for the clients and that it would also provide them with a more socially typical and independent lifestyle. A house was duly found in a suburb near the training center. Staff did not want to move far from the training center, as the clients' placements were all within the local area and transport costs would become a problem. It was also considered to be a benefit to the clients if they could recognize similar features in their new environment and still be able to easily visit their friends in the training center.

George, Ned, Alex, Bob, and Derek relocated to a privately owned house in 1995. The regular staff also relocated with them, and the same management regime with which they had become familiar still applied. Clients divided the monthly rental costs between them and the rent was paid directly through their financial administrators. Bills were also divided among the clients. All clients continued in their full-time placements. The neighborhood to which the clients relocated is considered to be one of the more affluent in Melbourne. The community was not familiar with people with disabilities and the staff thus used a variety of strategies and techniques to enhance integration of these clients into the mainstream community.

A housewarming party was organized soon after the clients moved into the house. All families of the clients and other interested parties were invited. The party itself was a success, but it is significant to note that despite invitations, none of the immediate neighbors chose to attend. As a means to acclimatize the clients to the local area, staff accompanied clients to the local shops where they would be doing their shopping. The clients were introduced to the workers in the shops, who displayed an extremely positive attitude to the clients. Clients were trained to access these shops independently, thus increasing their ability to integrate in the community. The five clients also attended local activities such as fêtes, Neighbourhood Watch meetings, and sporting events. They also utilized local facilities such as the swimming pool, doctors, clinics, as well as dental and other specialist services. All of these activities helped to raise the public awareness and understanding of the community residential living program that was being introduced within their own community.

Despite these efforts to integrate the community house within the community, the staff received a complaint from the local council. Apparently, one of the immediate neighbors had complained about the clients. The neighbor was not named by the council, and the staff could not approach him or her and discuss the issues. The council was asked by the staff to issue an invitation to the concerned parties to come and join the clients and staff for afternoon tea the following week so that they could meet the clients and, hopefully, dispel any fears that may be based upon irrational concepts. The staff heard no more about the issue and the invitation was never accepted.

Over the next 3 years the clients lived in this same rented property. They learned numerous life skills and their independence increased enormously. Staff noted a general improvement in behavior and attitudes of the clients. Day to day issues relating to client compatibility arose, and personality clashes inevitably occurred. However, these were not out of the ordinary in terms of interpersonal relationships and remained manageable.

After 3 years at the rental property, and with no further community negativity noted after the initial complaint, the landlord who owned the rented property decided to sell the property. Purchasing the property was not a viable financial option for the clients and thus another move was necessitated. Again, a privately rented property within the same local area was sought. A large house in the same area as two other rented community houses that had developed as a result of the success of the first house was secured. This provided increased social opportunities for the clients, although they were faced with a fresh environment to conquer. Again a housewarming party was organized and neighbors were invited. On this occasion, one neighbor attended but the other neighbors neither declined the invitation nor attended the party.

Within one day of the clients moving into the house, the real estate agent rang to inform staff that there had been a complaint made to the owner of the house regarding the clients' move to the house and to the neighborhood. The complaint was not related to any specific incident, but was rather a reaction to the presence of intellectually disabled people in the street. The real estate agent advised the complainant that it was not based upon any logical argument, and therefore, it was dismissed.

It is now a number of months since the clients moved to their new location. There have been no further complaints and clients are settling in effectively. They have quickly adapted to their new surroundings and are enjoying the independence of community life. Overall, the deinstitutionalization of these five men can be seen as a very positive and successful experience. All have gained an increased self-confidence and a higher self-esteem. The community as whole also appears to be accepting the presence of disabled people in their neighborhood. As a result of the success of this process of integration into the community, two more houses have been established and more are planned in the near future.

REFERENCES

Commonwealth of Australia. (1986). Disability Services Act. Australian Capital Territory: Australian Government Printing Service.

Commonwealth of Australia. (1992). Disability Reform Package, focus of ability. Australian Capital Territory: Australian Government Printing Service.

Commonwealth of Australia. (1995, March). Evaluation of the Disability Reform Package. Main report, Disability Task Force. Australian Capital Territory: Australian Government Printing Service.

Conway, R. N. F. (1992). Disability and legislation: Between changing policy and changing practices. Australia and New Zealand Journal of Developmental Disabilities, 18(2), 65–73.

Cummins, R. A. (1992). The community living support service: An operational overview. Australian Disability Review, 3, 51–59.

Cummins, R. A. (1993). On being returned to the community: Imposed ideology versus quality of life. Australian Disability Review, 2, 64–72.

Cummins, R. A., Polzin, U., & Theobald, T. (1990). Deinstitutionalization of St Nicholas Hospital. IV: A four year follow-up of residential life-style. Australia and New Zealand Journal of Developmental Disabilities, 16(4), 305–321.

Department of School Education, Victoria. (1993). Educational opportunities for students with disabilities and impairments. Victoria: DSE.

Johnstone, P., & Perry, J. (1993). The social justice of "mainstreaming" students with disabilities:

Two critical views. In A. Reid & B. Johnson (Eds.), *Critical issues in Australian Education in the 1990s* (pp. 100–111). Adelaide: Painters Prints.

Ministry of Education, Victoria. (1988). *Integration support group procedures for regular schools.* Melbourne: VGPS.

Moloney, H., & Taplin, J. E. (1990). The deinstitutionalization of people with a developmental disability under the Richmond Program: 1. Changes in adaptive behaviour. *Australia and New Zealand Journal of Developmental Disabilities, 16*(2), 149–159.

Ramsay, E. (1992, April). All students are special: An equity in education perspective [Newsletter]. Australian Association of Special Education, South Australian Chapter.

Stern, W. (1993). A further plea for rationality: Author's response to reviewers comments. *Australian Disability Review, 1–93,* 14–21.

Personal and Social Inclusion

Leisure and Persons With Developmental Disabilities: Empowering Self-Determination Through Inclusion

RICHARD D. MACNEIL
University of Iowa

STEPHEN C. ANDERSON
University of Florida

In the early 1970s, one of the authors of this chapter, Richard MacNeil, was working in the vocational rehabilitation department of a large Massachusetts institution, designed for the care of individuals with developmental disabilities. At this time, the philosophies of deinstitutionalization and mainstreaming were beginning to be emphasized. As a result, the institution staff's efforts were directed toward preparing clients to adjust to a life outside our facility. As part of their preparation, our clients received rigorous training that emphasized vocational competence and independent living skills, and focused upon activities of daily living (i.e., grooming, cooking, shopping, etc.).

While many of our clients successfully completed the transition to an independent life in the community, many others did not. Upon analysis, it was discovered that one of the most important factors associated with the failure to adapt to community living was the inability of our clients to use their free time in a personally satisfying manner. It was found that many of them suffered from loneliness, boredom, and anxiety brought on by too much unstructured free time and a lack of knowledge about what to do with it. In retrospect, it appears that we had successfully prepared many of our clients to meet the vocational and domestic demands of community living, but we had failed to prepare them for leisure.

Our failure to recognize the importance of leisure is not uncommon. While most of us willingly claim that participation in leisure and recreation activities is an important aspect of "normal," everyday life in our society, in practice leisure is frequently trivialized. Traditionally, leisure services have had relatively low priority in programs for person with disabilities, and only recently have specific recreation and leisure skill educational techniques (Voeltz, Wuerch, & Wilcox, 1982) and leisure curricula (Dattilo & Murphy, 1991; Wehman & Schleien, 1981) been developed. The neglect of relevant leisure programming and services for persons with developmental disabilities is particularly unfortunate, because appropriate participation in recreation activities is an important factor in successful community adjustment (Bedini, Bullock, & Driscoll, 1993; Hill & Bruininks, 1981) and the development of collateral skills that enhance quality of life (Dattilo, 1993; Dattilo & Rusch, 1985; Gollay, 1981).

The focus of this chapter will be upon leisure opportunities and resources and how they are utilized by persons with developmental disabilities. We will present our viewpoint that personally satisfying leisure is a critical component of mental health and life satisfaction. Moreover, we will argue that leisure contributes to personal empowerment through self-determination, a quality essential to community adjustment.

The chapter will be divided into three main sections. The first section will be used to present our explanation of leisure and its contribution to our sense of well-being. The next section will discuss a variety of factors associated with the historically documented exclusion of persons with developmental disabilities from community-based leisure opportunities. In the chapter's final segment, we will consider general suggestions meant to facilitate the development of inclusive leisure services.

LEISURE AND WELL-BEING

The concept of leisure is perhaps best understood by considering the origin of the word itself. It derives from the Latin *licere,* which means *to be permitted.* Implicit in this meaning is the notion of personal freedom; the license to do what one wants, when one wants. In this context, *leisure* refers to both freedom *from* (work, chores, and so on) and freedom *to* (do as one chooses).

The Greek word for leisure, *schole,* is the origin of the word for school or scholar in many modern languages. As used by Plato, *schole* referred to the ultimate purpose of education, to liberate one from the toil of work. Once free from unnecessary labor, humans could participate in distinctly human forms of activity such as contemplative thought, creation, or appreciation of the arts. To the Greeks, involvement in these experiences represented leisure.

The Greek conceptualization of leisure has been largely forgotten since the Industrial Revolution. The Platonic notion of leisure has been replaced by concepts that define leisure in terms of time or diversionary activity. In the first context, the term *leisure time* has become synonymous with unobligated time: the "free" time left over after the "necessary" tasks of life (i.e., working, eating, and sleeping) have been completed. In this context, the identifying quality of leisure is the period of time in which one engages in it. Thus mowing one's lawn, washing one's clothes, and similar tasks are commonly considered forms of leisure if one participates in them during one's otherwise unobligated hours.

In the second context, leisure is identified in terms of the activity in which one engages rather than in terms of the time of engagement. Most people would have no trouble responding to the request, "Name your favorite leisure activities." This perspective assumes that leisure refers to freely chosen, nonutilitarian activities that provide enjoyment and satisfaction to the participant. The underlying assumption is that the enjoyment we associate with leisure is inherent in the activity itself.

However, we encounter a dilemma when we attempt to explain the preponderance of empirical findings (Mancini & Orthner, 1980; Ragheb & Griffith, 1982, Riddick, 1985; Russell, 1987) that link leisure satisfaction with a high level of life satisfaction. If leisure is merely unobligated time, why is it that all retirees do not have a high level of satisfaction? Or for that matter, why is it that unemployed or underemployed individuals who cannot find satisfactory employment usually have low levels of life satisfaction?

If leisure is defined as nonessential activity, how might we explain the fact that a particular activity may be identified by a participant as leisure at one time, but as work, a chore, or drudgery at another time? For instance, satisfaction in a game of tennis may be thought of as leisure when one is playing up to his or her perceived skill level or in the company of friends, but it does not seem like leisure if one is playing poorly or is playing with others whose company one does not enjoy. The activity has not changed, but the perception of leisure has. So again we ask: What might account for the finding that leisure is a primary contributor to perceived life satisfaction?

In an effort to resolve this quandary, the authors propose an alternative way of looking at leisure. Rather than conceiving of leisure in terms of time or activity, we may more appropriately view it in relation to an individual's emotional and cognitive response to an activity or experience. Thus, we may conceive of leisure as an emotional condition within an individual that flows from a feeling of well-being and self-satisfaction. This condition is characterized by feelings of mastery, achievement, success, personal worth, and pleasure.

What is the source of the feelings described above? Iso-Ahola (1980) and Neulinger (1981) have suggested that the most distinguishing features of leisure involvement are the perception of freedom/personal choice on the one hand and involvement motivated by intrinsic rather than extrinsic factors on the other. In other words, the underlying characteristic of a leisure experience is the perception of personal control. Leisure is what one does because one wants to do it. As an intrinsically motivated behavior, it is done simply for its own sake. The feelings of well-being and self-satisfaction that are produced are the result of an awareness of potential pleasure stemming from associated feelings of competence and control over one's life, which are manifested in intrinsically motivated behavior.

We may now have the answer to our question, Why might leisure be a vital contributor to life satisfaction? Studies have consistently produced findings that indicate that personal perceptions of control may be influenced by the provision of choice (Langer & Rodin, 1976; Mannell, Zuzanek, & Larson, 1988; Rodin & Langer, 1977; Shary & Iso-Ahola, 1989). More significantly, three studies, one conducted by Peppers (1976) another by Ray (1979), and a third by MacTavish and Searle (1991), have shown that perceived control over activity choices can have a positive influence on life satisfaction.

Iso-Ahola and Weissinger have summarized the evidence as follows:

> Empirical research leaves little doubt about the fact that intrinsically motivated leisure is positively and significantly related to psychological or mental health. Those who are in control of their leisure lives and experiences and feel engaged in and committed to leisure activities and experiences are psychologically healthier than those who are not in control over their leisure lives and feel detached and uncommitted. (1984, p. 41)

LEISURE AND PERSONS
WITH DEVELOPMENTAL DISABILITIES

Participation in leisure and recreation activities is an important aspect of life for all members of society. Most individuals welcome time away from work, school, or other responsibilities and carefully plan ways to use their free time in a personally satisfying manner. Kraus (1990) maintains that the potential benefits derived from leisure involvement include the reduction of stress, emotional satisfaction, physical health, enjoyable social contacts, and feelings of achievement. Leisure seems to be a primary contributor to both personal and community well-being.

Persons with developmental disabilities are no different in their need for leisure and recreation. Unfortunately, this population has historically been excluded from community-based leisure programs and services.

The consequences of exclusion have been widely discussed in recent decades. Efforts to integrate persons with disabilities into community leisure services are generally regarded as an outgrowth of the normalization principle and the resulting movement toward community placement. Normalization, a concept defined by Nirje (1969), involves making the societal patterns and conditions of everyday life available to persons with disabilities. Wolfensberger (1972) expanded upon the concept to include "the utilization of means which are as culturally normative as possible in order to establish or maintain personal behaviors or characteristics which are as culturally normative as possible" (p. 28).

Normalization is governed by the belief that persons with disabilities should be accepted as equal members of society and should be permitted to participate in the norms and patterns of the community. One of the patterns of mainstream community life recognized by Wolfensberger is recreation. Elaborating on this idea, he wrote: "In a normalizing program scheme, their is a need not only for meaningful work, but also for recreation, each to be conducted at appropriate places and appropriate times" (Wolfensberger, 1972, p. 86). In addition to being consistent with the principles of normalization, involvement in community recreation and leisure programs may be a vitally important contributor to the development of skills needed for independent functioning by individuals with developmental disabilities. Research has shown that improvements in language, cognition, and physical fitness can be realized by this population during participation in leisure-related experiences (Schleien & Wehman, 1986). Green and Schleien (1991) have convincingly argued that the development of friendships between individuals with developmental disabilities and their nondisabled peers may be fostered by skills developed during recreational activities. Moreover, factors such as self-concept (Van Andel & Austin, 1984), social skill development (Novak & Heal, 1980), and successful transition from school to adult life (Bedini, Bullock, & Driscoll, 1993) can be enhanced through participation in recreational activities and leisure education programs.

It is also interesting to review the findings of international projects concerned with efforts to define "quality of life" as it applies to persons with disabilities (Goode, 1994). Several of these efforts, including two studies conducted in Canada (Brown, Brown, & Bayer, 1994; Woodill, Renwick, Brown, & Raphael, 1994) and one in the United States (Connally, 1994) specifically identify leisure opportunities as an essential component associated with quality of life for people with disabilities. Furthermore, independent investigations conducted in nations such as Finland, Denmark, Australia, and Germany consistently identified the conditions of perceived choice and the right to self-determination as the theoretical underpinning of the definition of quality of life (Goode, 1994). These conditions are consistent with the conceptualization of leisure advanced previously in this chapter and add support to the hypothesized relationship between leisure opportunity and its significance in the lives of individuals with developmental disabilities.

INCLUSIVE LEISURE SERVICES: THE NEXT STEP

Advocating for the principle of normalization, Wolfensberger wrote the following comments in 1972:

> Today, we conduct special camps for the handicapped, reserve bowling alleys for occasions when the handicapped bowl by themselves, and reserve swimming pools on a similar basis. Other examples of segregation in recreation can readily

be cited. Often, such segregation is practiced not intentionally or from lack of alternatives, but from a neglect to pursue a strategy of integration consciously and
systematically. (p. 53)

Comments made in the previous section of this chapter identified possible benefits of providing leisure and recreation opportunities for people with disabilities. However, if the philosophy of normalization is to be realized, it is clear that
recreation activities provided for these individuals must not be segregated from
society as a whole. Normalization demands, to the fullest extent possible, full
participation in mainstream community life. Full participation means that people with disabilities have the same chances as their nondisabled peers to use community leisure resources, to participate in the same community recreation activities, and to live, learn, and enjoy life in contact with other people.

The unfortunate reality is, however, that the majority of persons with disabilities participate in segregated recreation services if they participate at all. Studies
conducted in the United States (Rynders & Schleien, 1991), in Hungary (Gollesz,
1994), and in the United Kingdom (Moss, 1994) lend support to this claim. In Australia, Suttie and Ashman (1989) found that less than 30% of people with a mild
or moderate level of disability participate in general community recreational activities on a regular basis. Likewise, investigators in Western Canada claimed that
leisure and recreation activities that promote social and community involvement
are not encouraged by agencies or homes concerned with the care of individuals
with disabilities (Brown, Brown, & Bayer, 1994).

The time has come to adapt a new way of thinking, one founded on the prem-
ise that the community belongs to everyone, and everyone—regardless of level
and type of ability—belongs to the community. Inclusive community leisure
services can be powerful vehicles for promoting this ideal (Schleien, 1993). The
term "inclusive" leisure services is used to capture the full acceptance and integration of individuals with developmental disabilities into the recreation mainstream. Inclusion infers that "diversity is valuable—not just a reality to be toler-
ated, accepted, or accommodated, but a reality to be valued" (York, 1994, p. 11).

Inclusive leisure services are beneficial to all community members. The benefits of inclusion for people with disabilities would include: (1) the cultivation of
friendships; (2) the development of a sense of affiliation; (3) the acquisition of social skills; (4) the provision of positive role models; and (5) the development of
life-long skills. For the nondisabled, inclusive recreation would help the development of positive attitudes, encourage understanding and acceptance of people
with differences, and promote personal growth (Dattilo, 1994).

OVERCOMING BARRIERS TO INCLUSIVE RECREATION

Given the desirability of inclusive leisure services, one may ask why they remain
rare. In this section we will outline some of the major barriers that prevent or in-

hibit the provision of inclusive leisure services. For organizational purposes we have divided these obstacles into two categories: external barriers and intrinsic barriers. External barriers are composed of the many forces in the environment that impose limitations on people with developmental disabilities. Intrinsic barriers are those obstacles that result from an individual's own limitations. We will briefly describe each barrier, discuss how it may inhibit recreation inclusion for persons with developmental disabilities, and present a few ideas that may help to overcome the barrier.

Extrinsic Barriers: Societal Attitudes

Fishbein and Ajzen (1975) describe an attitude as a learned predisposition to respond in a consistently favorable or unfavorable manner with respect to a given object. Attitudes influence behaviors; the more negative our attitude toward an object, the more likely we are to display behaviors that reflect our disdain for the object. Thinking or feeling negatively about a particular disability or a person with a disability generates an attitudinal barrier. Unfortunately, persons with developmental disabilities may often be less valued by nondisabled persons because of their disabilities. Nondisabled persons may accentuate these differences in the manner in which they interact, or choose not to interact, with persons with disabilities. Included among the variety of unpleasant behaviors are paternalistic attitudes, apathy, avoidance, or negative behaviors such as mocking or name-calling (Schleien & Ray, 1988).

When asked to describe the most difficult barrier to overcome, people with disabilities consistently state negative attitudes. Of all the barriers faced by individuals with disabilities, attitudinal barriers are probably the most far-reaching. Not only are negative attitudes in part responsible for the prejudices and discrimination that limit equal participation of persons with disabilities, they also can have much broader consequences. For instance, Heyne, Schleien, and McAvoy (1993) found that "fearful and negative attitudes about people with disabilities" was one of the most frequently reported obstacles to friendship development between persons with and without disabilities. It stands to reason that if negative attitudes could be eliminated most, if not all, other barriers would follow.

Experts (Dattilo, 1994; Schleien & Ray, 1988; Smith, Austin, & Kennedy, 1996) agree that negative attitudes held by the public toward individuals with developmental disabilities have contributed to lack of access to inclusive leisure services. Fortunately, specific strategies to help people without disabilities develop more positive attitudes about people with disabilities have been identified. One of the more effective means of changing attitudes toward people with disabilities was reported by Hamilton and Anderson (1991). They found that people without disabilities often positively alter their attitudes about people with disabilities as a result of joint participation in leisure activities. According to Hamilton and Anderson, since leisure activities often offer a greater opportunity for close personal contact than either education or employment, participation in inclusive leisure services can provide an effective channel for changing the attitudes of the general public toward people with disabilities. By encouraging joint participation of people with and without disabilities and thereby facilitating inclusive leisure services, professionals can make a substantial contribution to the acceptance of persons with special needs.

Based upon a review of relevant research, Dattilo (1994) proposed a number of other useful strategies for promoting more positive attitudes toward individuals with developmental disabilities. Among the actions Dattilo suggests are (a) the use of structured interactions; (b) extensive personal contact; (c) joint participation; (d) facilitating equal status contact; (e) fostering cooperative interdependence; and (f) encouraging age-appropriate behaviors. Additionally, employing the principles of Wolfensberger's (1983) "social role valorization" theory would seem applicable to the formation of more positive attitudes.

External Barriers: Reasonable Accommodations

"Reasonable accommodations" is a broad term that we will use to describe a series of external barriers that separately and in combination impair efforts to ensure inclusive leisure services. Although many such barriers exist, we will confine our comments to three; architectural, transportation, and communication.

Architectural barriers are man-made structures that present obstacles for people with disabilities. Individuals with disabilities cannot successfully participate in leisure programs if they are unable to enter or make their way around recreation facilities. The California Quality of Life Project recently recognized the lack of accessibility to public recreation facilities and programs as a continuing obstacle preventing people with disabilities from integrating socially in the community (Connally, 1994).

Problems associated with architectural barriers may be addressed in several ways. Legislative action may be used to mandate compliance with accepted standards of accessibility. (This solution, is of course, much more effective if supported by financial incentives and deterrents.) Architectural accessibility surveys of both indoor and outdoor recreation environments to help identify potential barriers to leisure participation should be conducted. If used, such surveys should be conducted in consultation with potential consumers with disabilities. In addition, in situations where facilities cannot be made totally accessible, program modifications/adaptations designed to facilitate access and participation should be considered.[1]

Transportation barriers refer to obstacles that inhibit individuals from getting to and from sites and programs. The lack of usable and affordable methods of

---

[1] For readers interested in specific examples of program modifications and adaptations, the authors recommend chapter 12 in Dattilo's text, *Inclusive Leisure Services* (1994).

transportation is one of the most prevalent concerns that persons with disabilities have, and is recognized as a barrier to enjoy a satisfying social life (Schleien & Ray, 1988). The problems associated with transportation include physical accessibility, conveniences of schedules, lack of awareness or understanding of transport systems, and cost. Whatever the nature of the barrier, the ultimate result of transportation problems is that some individuals who have disabilities cannot benefit from available community sources, including leisure services.

Several solutions are possible. Governments could adopt sensible polices on transportation of persons with disabilities. Canada is a leader in this regard, as it adopted a national policy in 1983 that guarantees individuals with disabilities "reasonable, reliable, and equitable transportation services and facilities" (COPOH, 1987). Persons with developmental disabilities—or their advocates or organizations representing their interests—could conduct community-wide surveys to determine the availability, costs, and scheduling or transportation agencies within a local area. Efforts could be made to secure low-cost or donated transportation from community service agencies, churches, or corporations. Privately owned taxi companies could offer rate reductions and convenient services for users of community leisure services. Most importantly, individuals with developmental disabilities could be taught to independently use available transportation systems within the community (Schleien & Ray, 1988).

Communication barriers, according to Smith et al. (1996), result from reciprocal interaction between individuals with disabilities and their social environment. Of course, communication is a two-way street. For individuals whose speech and language abilities are affected by certain developmental disabilities, communication may be limited. Their problems may be compounded when leisure service personnel lack the necessary skills (e.g., sign language or interpreting communication boards) to "talk" to them. Ultimately, communication problems may limit access to leisure opportunities that are available within the community and may prevent participation in social interchanges required in many leisure contexts.

Schleien and Ray (1988) offer a variety of strategies to help resolve communication barriers. Among their suggestions are the following:

1. Networking with allied health professions such as Speech Pathology or Communication Disorder Specialists to make in-service presentations on communication disorders and alternative communication systems.
2. The use of volunteer advocates who understand the participant's communication system to serve as liaisons or intermediaries between recreation staff and the participant.
3. Enrollment of recreation staff in sign language classes at local educational institutions.
4. Arranged meetings between potential clients (or their advocates) and leisure services personnel to explain the participant's communication needs for the recreation activity in which he or she is planning to participate.

With respect to communication barriers, the authors feel compelled to mention the work of Professor John Dattilo from the University of Georgia. Recognizing the social contexts in which leisure is often experienced, Dattilo has studied the use of augmentative and alternative communication competencies among individuals with mental retardation. In a series of studies (Dattilo & Camarata, 1991; Dattilo & O'Keefe, 1992), he has demonstrated that communication skills for many individuals with developmental disabilities can be improved by means of a relatively simple intervention strategy. If communication forms a barrier for leisure opportunities for some individuals, Dattilo's strategy merits further investigation.

Intrinsic Barriers

Although intrinsic barriers often derive from external factors, they are internal to the individual and can handicap persons with developmental disabilities when they attempt to participate in leisure services. One example of an intrinsic barrier is lack of knowledge or deficient skills. Many persons with developmental disabilities are not able to realize their maximum leisure functioning because they lack necessary information about community recreation resources or the support systems available to make recreation opportunities accessible. Indeed, both Bedini, Bullock, and Driscoll (1993) and Connally (1994) identified a lack of awareness of recreational opportunities among individuals with developmental disabilities as well as among their guardians. When knowledge of recreation resources or support services are insufficient, the ability to make informed choices about leisure opportunities will obviously suffer.

Closely related to lack of knowledge as a barrier to leisure participation are deficiencies in skills necessary for recreation involvement. Enjoyment of a recreation activity is often possible only if the participant perceives the challenges of an activity to be in balance with his or her skills (Csikszentmihalyi, 1975). If the challenges are thought to be too great, anxiety may limit the chance for enjoyment. If the challenge is too easy, boredom often results. Sometimes the nature of their impairment limits individuals from developing appropriate skills; however, often persons with developmental disabilities do not get the opportunity to develop skills necessary to succeed in leisure. As a result, they correctly perceive that many recreation activities are too challenging for their present skill level and sense of helplessness develops. With this perception comes fewer attempts to participate. As attempts decrease, opportunities to experience enjoyment also decline. The result is usually nonparticipation (Dattilo, 1994; Smith et al., 1996).

An appropriate response to deal with lack of knowledge or deficient skills would be the implementation of a leisure education program. The term *leisure education* was first used by Chinn and Joswiak (1981) to describe the application of comprehensive models focusing on the educational process to enhance an individual's leisure lifestyle. While a variety of leisure education models exist, they all share the common goal of "exposing all people to the possibilities that leisure may hold for them to live creatively and give expression to the wide assortment of their capabilities" (Bucher, Shivers, & Bucher, 1984, p. 290).

Leisure education programs typically employ a variety of components that directly address barriers associated with lack of knowledge or deficient skills. Among the components often included in leisure education programs are (1) leisure appreciation; (2) awareness of self in leisure; (3) self-determination; (4) leisure decision making; (5) knowledge and utilization of leisure resources; and (6) social interaction (Dattilo & Murphy, 1991).

Although empirical support for the effectiveness of leisure education in broadening participation of persons with developmental disabilities remains limited, promising results were reported in at least two studies: Anderson and Allen (1985) and Lanagan and Dattilo (1989). Facilitating a leisure education program for individuals with developmental disabilities could be a primary responsibility of community recreation agencies or local school systems.

A second intrinsic barrier to leisure experienced by many persons with special needs related to social ineffectiveness. This may be particularly true for individuals with mental retardation. Parental overprotection and segregation from people without disabilities are two reasons that account for deficiencies in interpersonal skills. As a consequence, persons with developmental disabilities often lack the ability to meet the social demands required for positive engagement in many community leisure settings.

Learning how to engage in recreational activities with peers without disabilities can greatly expand the opportunities available to persons with mental retardation (Schleien et al., 1995). Therefore, teachers, parents, and caregivers should be encouraged to provide social skills training in age-appropriate leisure situations at school, at home, and in community settings. Programs should be designed to encourage socialization among participants. It has been shown that recreation activities that are based on cooperation between participants with and without disabilities, are usually more effective than activities of a competitive or individualistic nature when social interaction is the goal (Schleien et al., 1997). Therefore, professionals should plan activities that are grounded in cooperation rather than competition or solitary involvement. An example of this would be for persons with and without developmental disabilities to work together on building a birdhouse or complete a puzzle rather than to engage in a game of table tennis or painting a picture.

A final barrier to be considered is dependency. In the process of physical and psychological development, individuals in most societies are expected to move from a state of dependency to one of independence. Whether limited by disability, by overzealous care providers, or by restrictive social service systems, people with developmental disabilities often never gain the ability to function independently in the community. As a result, they often become deficient in their abilities to make decisions and choices and, thus, depend upon others to have their leisure needs met.

Physical dependency is obviously problematic for some people, but because it is readily visible it may be easier to deal with than psychological dependency. Psychological dependency is associated with a perceived inability to control events and situations in one's life. Seligman's (1975) pioneering work with "learned helplessness" has demonstrated that exposure to uncontrollable events may lead to feelings of futility and despair. Thus, learning of helplessness reduces the incentive to respond, which decreases motivation. Learned helplessness undermines a person's motivation to respond, reduces the ability to learn that responding works, and results in psychological dependency.

As we mentioned, one consequence of helplessness is dependency upon others to meet one's leisure needs. Fortunately, leisure experiences may also be part of the solution to dependency. A theoretical model suggesting this perspective was first proposed by Iso-Ahola, MacNeil, and Szymanski in 1980. Known as the "attributional analysis" approach, this model demonstrated how the careful selection of recreational activities may be used to combat perceptions of helplessness. According to this model leisure professionals can combat helplessness by:

(a) Exposing clients to leisure experiences in which uncontrollability cannot be inferred (i.e., arts and crafts, cooperative games)
(b) Emphasizing the role of discriminated helplessness
(c) Providing a supportive social environment. (Iso-Ahola et al., 1980)

EMPOWERING SELF-DETERMINATION
THROUGH LEISURE INCLUSION

Throughout this chapter, we have argued that the opportunity to experience leisure is a primary contributor to the quality of life. We discussed a variety of possible benefits, from physical fitness to mental health, that may be accrued as a result of participation in leisure experiences. We also spoke of leisure's role in assisting persons with developmental disabilities in successful community adjustment. At this point, however, we will discuss what we believe to be leisure's most important contribution to the lives of persons with developmental disabilities: empowering self-determination.

Empowerment is a term commonly used to refer to the transfer of power and control over values, decisions, choices, and directions of human services from external entities to the consumers of services (West & Parent, 1992). The intent of empowering consumers is to provide them with the freedom (and responsibility) to make decisions with respect to the conduct of lives. This freedom may also be referred to as *self-determination*. As described by Ward (1988), self-determination refers to attitudes and abilities that lead individuals to define goals for themselves, and their ability to take the initiative to achieve their goals. Self-determination is associated with personal dignity on the one hand, and increased motivation to participate and succeed on the other. When self-determination is achieved, increases in learning and perceptions of competence occur (Dattilo, 1994). People who perceive themselves as capable and self-determining are able to effectively deal with the challenges of day-to-day life (Iso-Aholo & Weissinger, 1984; Shary & Iso-Ahola, 1989).

Some theorists (deCharms, 1968; Deci & Ryan, 1985) have concluded that self-determination is associated with intrinsic motivation. Motivation that is intrinsic energizes behavior and results in feelings of perceived control. Because a sense of perceived control is linked to enjoyment and satisfaction, performances that are intrinsically motivated do not require external rewards. Thus, intrinsically motivated behaviors are enjoyable to the individual because they induce feelings of autonomy and control, which in turn lead to the perception of self-determination.

What does this have to do with leisure? The reader may recall an earlier section of this chapter in which we had an extensive discussion of the meaning of leisure. At that time we concluded that in spite of an expanding body of evidence that identifies leisure as a critical component in life satisfaction, leisure is frequently trivialized. We explained this trivialization as a product of society's insistence on defining leisure in terms of time or activity rather than as an emotional and cognitive response to an activity or experience.

While this distinction may seem insignificant, it is essential to our discussion of self-determination. As we said at the time, the distinguishing quality of the leisure experience, the dimension that sets leisure apart for all other experiences in life, is its association with perceptions of personal control. Stated succinctly, to experience leisure is to experience self-determination. Consequently, efforts to promote inclusive leisure services may legitimately be justified as an issue of equality and civic responsibility, but more significantly, it is a means to empower individuals with development disabilities to gain control over their lives to the greatest extent possible.

CONCLUSION

In 1992 the American Association of Mental Retardation approved a new definition for mental retardation. Although the changes in wording between this definition and its 1983 predecessor are subtle, its impact may have a profound effect on the way society views individuals with developmental disabilities. The new definition stresses the interaction between an individual who is classified as mentally retarded and his or her environment; that is, that mental retardation now refers to a level of functioning that requires from society significantly above-average training procedures. As a result, the tendency to concentrate on a person's IQ as representative of mental retardation is removed, and the focus shifts to the degree of support society should provide so the individual may achieve personal growth and development. The underlying intent of this change is to acknowledge the worth of these people as human beings and to lessen the discomfort that more pejorative terms might cause them and their families.

This isolated change is representative of a much broader shift in the views of professionals in the field of developmental disabilities. In previous decades the focus of concern of most professionals in the field was directed toward classification and the specification of the needs and characteristics of people with developmental disabilities. This modified definition symbolizes the start of a new era in which the focus will shift to quality of life issues for individuals with disabilities.

Efforts to define quality of life for people with developmental disabilities are well under way. Spearheaded by the efforts of David Goode, an extensive international collection of papers on the subject were published in the book *Quality of Life for Persons with Disabilities: International Perspectives and Issues* (Goode, 1994). Writers from ten different countries provided contributions to Goode's text.

While the expressed views on quality of life were diverse, one common theme emerged: the ability to exert influence over one's own life. There was general agreement among the writers that just like their nondisabled peers, most persons with disabilities have expectations and dreams, and like others they want to control decisions concerning their lives as much as possible.

The international support for the importance of individual choice as a vital component of quality of life may be garnered in the following representative statements.

• Living a "good life" in Denmark means "that one is able to determine the course of one's own life and has the opportunity to create an existence based on one's own dreams, visions, wishes and needs" (Holm, Host, & Perlt, 1994, p. 10).

• The Disability Services Act, an important piece of civil rights legislation passed in Australia in 1986, emphasizes the principle of choice and participation in personal decision-making as a right for the disabled (Parmenter, Cummins, Shaddock, & Stancliffe, 1994, p. 81).

• Efforts to define quality of life of persons with developmental disabilities in Ontario, Canada were based on the assumption that "quality of life must incorporate the notion of maximizing the personal control each person has over his/her own life" (Woodill, Renwick, Brown, & Raphael, 1994, p. 60).

It is clear that having the right and opportunity to make choices is expressed or implied in most conceptualizations of quality of life for all individuals. Similarly, it is also clear that persons with developmental disabilities are frequently limited in their capacity to control events in their lives due to restrictions in personal resources or the resources provided to them by their environment. It follows that given the desirability of personal choice and the inherent limitations associated with disability, that opportunities for persons with developmental disabilities to experience control and self-determination should be optimized.

What route to optimization? The authors of this chapter would suggest leisure opportunities! As we have argued throughout this work, a strong theoretical relationship exists between leisure and perceived feelings of personal control and competence. From a pragmatic perspective, involvement in leisure experiences offers many social, emotional, physical, and intellectual benefits to participants. The provision of leisure opportunities is consistent with the principles of normalization, can help fill free time with personally satisfying experiences, and fosters a sense of empowerment and self-determination.

Given this scenario, it is disappointing to review the international perspectives on quality of life documents in the Goode (1994) text and find such little attention paid to leisure. As mentioned earlier in this work, only the quality of life documents produced by Canadian and American authors specifically targeted leisure opportunities as essential components for enhancing life quality among persons with developmental disabilities. While nine quality of life assessment instruments for persons with disabilities were identified in a recent review, only two of these instruments included leisure and recreation components (Schalock, 1994). When leisure is addressed in quality of life documents, it is variously described as "segregated" (Gollesz, 1994), "supervised" (Paramenter et al., 1994), "passive" (Matikka, 1994), and "spectator-oriented" (Brown, Brown, & Bayer, 1994). Although emphasis is rightfully placed upon academic and vocational training in many nations, there is apparently no attention paid to education for leisure. This void exists despite convincing evidence that leisure education has been shown to help eliminate many of the intrinsic barriers that prevent persons with developmental disabilities from engaging in leisure opportunities within their communities.

A person becomes an individual partly through the choices he or she is allowed to make. For those identified as developmentally disabled, personal choices are often very limited. While opportunities for personal choice in some areas of life (such as work and education) may be extremely difficult to equalize for everyone, providing equal opportunities for leisure involvement should not be difficult.

In the final analysis, few would disagree that all people, regardless of level of ability, deserve the opportunity to develop their full potential. As the focus of professional concern for persons with developmental disabilities shifts to an emphasis on quality of life, the responsibility for promoting conditions necessary for a quality life increasingly shifts to the community. It is in this context that we propose that inclusive leisure opportunities should be considered a basic civil right for all human beings. In the end, achievement of this dream can only enrich all of our lives.

REFERENCES

Anderson, S., & Allen, L. (1985). Effects of a leisure education program on activity involvement and social interaction of mentally retarded persons. *Adapted Physical Activity Quarterly*, 2(2), 107–116.

Bedini, L., Bullock, C., & Driscoll, L. (1993). The effects of leisure education on the successful transition of students with mental retardation from school to adult life. *Therapeutic Recreation Journal*, 27(2), 70–83.

Brown, R., Brown, P., & Bayer, M. (1994). A quality of life model: New challenges arising form a six year study. In D. Goode (Ed.), *Quality of life for persons with disabilities: International perspectives and issues.* Cambridge, MA: Brookline Books.

Bucher, C., Shivers, J., & Bucher, R. (1984). Leisure education and counseling. *Recreation for today's society* (2nd ed., pp. 290–303). Englewood Cliffs, NJ: Prentice-Hall.

Chinn, K., & Joswiak, K. (1981). Leisure education and leisure counseling. *Therapeutic Recreation Journal*, 15(4), 4–7.

Connally, P. (1994). The California quality of life project: A project summary. In D. Goode (Ed.), *Quality of life for persons with disabilities: International perspectives and issues.* Cambridge, MA: Brookline Books.

COPOH. (1987). Transportation and disabled citizens: Policies on eligibility and reciprocity. *Journal of Leisurability*, 14(1), 4–12.

Csikszentmihalyi, M. (1975). *Beyond boredom and anxiety.* San Francisco: Jossey-Bass.

Dattilo, J., & Rusch, F. (1985). Effects of choice on leisure participation for persons with severe handicaps. *Journal of the Association for Persons with Severe Handicaps*, 10, 194–199.

Dattilo, J., & Murphy, W. (1991). *Leisure education program planning: A systematic approach.* State College, PA: Venture Publishing.

Dattilo, J., & Camarata, S. (1991). Facilitating conversation through self-initiated augmentative communication training. *Journal of Applied Behavioral Analysis*, 24, 369–378.

Dattilo, J., & O'Keefe, B. (1992). Setting the stage for leisure: Encouraging adults with mental retardation who use augmentative and alternative communication systems to share conversations. *Therapeutic Recreation Journal*, 26(1), 27–37.

Dattilo, J. (1993). Facilitating reciprocal communication for individuals with severe communication disorders: Implications for leisure participation. *Palaestra*, 10(1), 39–48.

Dattilo, J. (1994). *Inclusive leisure services: Responding to the rights of people with disabilities.* State College, PA: Venture Publishing.

deCharms, R. (1968). *Enhancing motivation: Change in the classroom.* New York: Irvington.

Deci, E., & Ryan, W. (1985). *Intrinsic motivation and self-determination in human behavior.* New York: Plenum Press.

Fishbein, M., & Ajzen, I. (1975). *Belief, attitude, intention and behavior: An introduction to theory and research.* Reading, MA: Addison-Wesley.

Gollay, E. (1981). Some conceptual and methodological issues in studying community adjustment of deinstitutionalized mentally retarded people. In R. Bruininks, C. Meyers, B. Sigford, & R. Larkin (Eds.), *Deinstitutionalization and community adjustment of mentally retarded people.* Washington, DC: American Association of Mental Deficiency.

Gollesz, V. (1994). Quality of life of people with disabilities in Hungary after leaving school. In D. Goode (Ed.), *Quality of life for persons with disabilities: International perspectives and issues.* Cambridge, MA: Brookline Books.

Goode, D. (Ed.). (1994). *Quality of life for persons with disabilities: International perspectives and issues.* Cambridge, MA: Brookline Books.

Green, F., & Schleien, S. (1991). Understanding friendship and recreation: A theoretical sampling. *Therapeutic Recreation Journal*, 25(4), 29–40.

Hamilton, E., & Anderson, S. (1991). Effects of leisure activities on attitudes toward people with disabilities. *Therapeutic Recreation Journal, 17*(3), 50–57.

Heyne, L., Schleien, S., & McAvoy, L. (Eds.). (1993). *Making Friends: Using recreation activities to promote friendship between children with and without disabilities.* Minneapolis: Institute on Community Integration (UAP).

Hill, B., & Bruininks, R. (1981). *Family, leisure and social activities of mentally retarded people in residential facilities.* Minneapolis: Developmental Disabilities Project on Residential Services and Community Adjustment, University of Minnesota.

Holm, P., Holst, J., & Perlt, B. (1994). Co-write your own life: Quality of life as discussed in the Danish context. In D. Goode (Ed.), *Quality of life for persons with disabilities: international perspectives and issues.* Cambridge, MA: Brookline Books.

Iso-Ahola, S. E. (1980). *The social psychology of leisure and recreation.* Dubuque, IA: William C. Brown.

Iso-Ahola, S., MacNeil, R., & Syzmanski, D. (1980). Social psychological foundations of therapeutic recreation: An attributional analysis. In S. Iso-Ahola (Ed.), *Social psychological perspectives on leisure and recreation.* Springfield, IL: Charles C. Thomas.

Iso-Ahola, S., & Weissinger, E. (1984, June). Leisure and well-being: Is there a connection? *Parks and Recreation, 18,* 40–44.

Kraus, R. (1990). *Recreation and leisure in modern society.* New York: HarperCollins.

Lanagan, D., & Dattilo, J. (1989). The effects of a leisure education program on individuals with severe disabilities. *Therapeutic Recreation Journal, 23*(4), 8–17.

Langer, E., & Rodin, L. (1976). Effects of choice and enhanced personal responsibility for the aged: A field experiment in an institutional setting." *Journal of Personality and Social Psychology, 342,* 191–198.

MacTavish, J., & Searle, M. (1991). Older individuals with mental retardation and the effect a physical activity intervention on selected social psychological variables. *Therapeutic Recreation Journal, 25*(2), 55–71.

Mancini, J., & Orthner, D. (1980). Situational Influences on leisure satisfaction and morale in old age. *Journal of the American Geriatrics Society, 281,* 466–471.

Mannell, R., Zuzanek, J., & Larson, R. (1988). Leisure states and 'flow' experiences: Testing perceived freedom and intrinsic motivation hypotheses. *Journal of Leisure Research, 20,* 289–304.

Matikka, L. (1994). The quality of life of adults with developmental disabilities in Finland. In D. Goode (Ed.), *Quality of life for persons with disabilities: International perspectives and issues.* Cambridge, MA: Brookline Books.

Moss, S. (1994). Quality of life and aging. In D. Goode (Ed.), *Quality of life for persons with disabilities: International perspectives and issues.* Cambridge, MA: Brookline Books.

Neulinger, J. (1981). *To leisure: An introduction.* Boston: Allyn and Bacon.

Nirje, B. (1969). The normalization principle and its human management implications. In R. Kugel & W. Wolfensberger (Eds.), *Changing patterns of residential services for the mentally retarded.* Washington, DC: President's Committee on Mental Retardation.

Novak, A., & Heal, L. (Eds.). (1980). *Integration of developmentally disabled individuals into the community.* Baltimore: Paul H. Brookes.

Paramenter, T., Cummins, R., Shaddock, A., & Stancliffe, R. (1994). The view from Australia: Australian legislation, service delivery, and quality of life. In D. Goode (Ed.), *Quality of life for persons with disabilities: International perspectives and issues.* Cambridge, MA: Brookline Books.

Peppers, L. G. (1976). Patterns of leisure and adjustment to retirement. *The Gerontologist, 16*, 441–446.

Ragheb, M., & Griffith, C. (1982). The contribution of leisure participation and leisure satisfaction to life satisfaction of older persons. *Journal of Leisure Research, 14*(4), 295–306.

Ray, R. O. (1979). Life satisfaction and activity involvement: Implications for leisure service. *Journal of Leisure Research, 11*, 112–119.

Riddick, C. (1985). Leisure satisfaction determinants of older males and females. *Leisure Sciences, 7*(1), 17–27.

Rodin, L., & Langer, E. (1977). Long term effects of a control relevant intervention with institutionalized aged. *Journal of Personality and Social Psychology, 35*(12), 897–902.

Russell, R. (1987). The importance of recreation satisfaction and activity participation to the life-satisfaction of age-segregated retirees. *Journal of Leisure Research 19*(4), 273–283.

Rynders, J., & Schleien, S. (1991). *Together successfully: Creating recreational and educational programs that integrate people with and without disabilities.* Arlington, TX: Association for Retarded Citizens of the United States.

Schalock, R. (1994). The concept of quality of life and its current applications in the field of mental retardation/developmental disabilities. In D. Goode (Ed.), *Quality of life for persons with disabilities: International perspectives and issues.* Cambridge, MA: Brookline Books.

Schleien, S., & Wehman, P. (1986). Severely handicapped children: Social skills development through leisure skills programming. In G. Cartledge & J. Milburn (Eds.), *Teaching social skills to children: Innovative approaches* (2nd ed., pp. 219–245). Elmsford, NY: Pergamon.

Schleien, S., Ray, M. (1988). *Community recreation and persons with disabilities: Strategies for integration.* Baltimore: Paul H. Brookes.

Schleien, S. (1993). Access and inclusion in community leisure services. *Parks and Recreation, 28*(4), 66–72.

Schleien, S., Meyer, L., Heyne, L., & Brandt, B. (1995). *Lifelong leisure skills and lifestyles for persons with developmental disabilities.* Baltimore: Paul H. Brookes.

Schleien, S., Ray, M., & Green, F. (1997). *Community recreation and people with disabilities: Strategies for inclusion* (2nd ed.). Baltimore: Paul H. Brookes.

Seligman, M. (1975). *Helplessness: On depression, development and death.* San Francisco: W. H. Freeman.

Shary, J., & Iso-Ahola, S. (1989). Effects of a control-relevant intervention on nursing home resident's perceived competence and self-esteem. *Therapeutic Recreation Journal, 23*(1), 7–16.

Smith, R., Austin, D., & Kennedy, D. (1996). *Inclusive and special recreation: Opportunity for persons with disabilities.* Dubuque, IA: Brown and Benchmark.

Suttie, J. N., & Ashman, A. F. (1989). *An acceptable standard of living and quality of life: Fact or fiction for aging persons with intellectual disability.* Paper presented to the 25th Annual Conference of the Australian Society for the Study of Intellectual Disability.

Van Andel, G., & Austin, D. (1984). Physical fitness and mentally handicapped: A review of literature. *Adapted Physical Activities Quarterly, 3*, 207–220.

Voeltz, L., Wuerch, B., & Wilcox, B. (1982). Leisure and recreation: Preparation for independence, integration and self-fulfillment. In B. Wilcox & G. Bellamy (Eds.), *Design for high school programs for severely handicapped students* (pp. 175–209). Baltimore: Paul H. Brookes.

Ward, M. (1980). The many facets of self-determination. *National Information Center for the Children and Youth with Disabilities: Transition Summary, 5*, 2–3.

Wehman, P., & Schleien, S. (1982). *Leisure programs for handicapped persons: Adaptations, techniques and curriculum.* Austin, TX: PRO-ED.

West, M., & Parent, W. (1992). Consumer choice and empowerment in supported employment services: Issues and strategies. *Journal of the Association for Persons with Severe Handicaps, 17*(1), 47–52.

Wolfensberger, W. (1983). Social role valorization: A proposed new term for the principle of normalization. *Mental Retardation, 21*(6), 235–239.

Woodill, G., Renwick, R., Brown, J., & Raphael, D. (1994). Being, belonging, becoming: An approach to the quality of life of persons with developmental disabilities. In D. Goode (Ed.), *Quality of life for persons with disabilities: International perspectives and issues.* Cambridge: Brookline Books.

York, J. (1994). A shared agenda for educational change. *Newsletter: The Association for Persons with Severe Handicaps, 20*(2), 10–11.

CHAPTER 7

Teaching the Mentally Retarded Parenting Skills: International Perspectives

MICHAEL F. SHAUGHNESSY
Eastern New Mexico University

THERESA GLOVER
College of St. Scholastica, Duluth, Minnesota

MARCI GREENE
Florida Gulf Coast University

RAY Y. L. CHOY
City University of Hong Kong

With the advent of deinstitutionalization and "mainstreaming," more and more mentally retarded individuals are being served in the community rather than in large psychiatric facilities or developmental centers. Services to these individuals have expanded and become more relevant to their needs.

One area of need has been the social and interpersonal realm. Mentally retarded individuals have needs for social stimulation, as well as sexual and emotional needs, which must be addressed. Many individuals want as normal a lifestyle as possible; that may include, in certain instances, marriage and a family. With marriage comes the possibility of offspring. It is incumbent upon our society to provide the skills needed for these mentally retarded individuals to adequately parent their children. The children may or may not be mentally retarded, and one of the married couple may not be mentally retarded. One of the couple may have adaptive behavior deficits but not cognitive deficits, or vice versa. Thus, program planning must include a high degree of individualization.

There is little in the literature regarding the efficacy of programs regarding the teaching of parenting skills to mentally retarded parents. There is also little regarding long term follow-up and evaluation of the efficacy of said programs. Further, there is little regarding what specific skills should be taught to parents regarding the rearing of their children. Indeed, even average and normal parents have different concerns as their children grow from infants to children to young adults. Bornstein (1995) has recently edited a multivolume text on parenting that delineated various aspects of parenting different types of children at different stages in the life cycle (e.g., infants, gifted children, adolescents, those with aggressive behavior, children with Down syndrome, twins, etc.).

In this chapter, we will attempt to review the existing literature, discuss international perspectives and philosophies, and delineate future research agendas. It should be recognized that it is difficult to procure primary sources on this subject, even with the Internet and modern technology.

Feldman, Case, Towns, and Betel (1985) conducted an early exploratory study in Toronto, wherein they examined the development of 12 two-year-old children who had been reared by mentally retarded mothers. They did find evidence of language delays, but also found that in cases where a mother had previously lost custody of a child, there was also slow development. This study only examined these children at two years of age and did not include any long-term follow-up.

Budd and Greenspan (1985) explored the parameters of successful and unsuccessful interventions with mothers seen to be mentally retarded. They concluded that parent training programs had to be lengthier, more intricate, and more directive than those for nonhandicapped parents. Limited generalization was also a concern relative to other parenting domains.

Fantuzzo, Wray, Hall, Goins, and Azar (1986) investigated the training of mentally retarded mothers who had been identified as "maltreaters." Using the work of Foxx and his colleagues (Foxx & McMorrow, 1985; Foxx, McMorrow, & Mennemeier, 1984; Foxx, McMorrow, & Schloss, 1983; Foxx, McMorrow, Storey, & Rogers, 1984), Fantuzzo et al. worked with three mothers to enhance performance, self-monitoring, and response-specific feedback. The efficacy of treatment was supported by generalization data.

Seagull and Scheurer (1986), based on their review of the literature and their data, concluded that "given the complexity of the problems, and the lack of readily available solutions . . . the needs of the children to be nurtured and protected, must, at least be better served" (p. 500). Their research showed that of 64 children (seen from 1 to 7 years earlier), only 11 remained with their low functioning parents. Six had been relinquished for adoption, nine were placed in foster care, two had died, and two had been awarded to a nonretarded parent. For 34, courts had terminated parental rights.

Heighway, Kidd-Webster, and Snodgrass (1988) described the Positive Parenting Project and delineated many of the problems of working with mentally retarded parents. Often, these parents are unable to access the human services system and have difficulty learning parenting skills or even coping with life itself. In addition, they have not made routine such basics as immunizations and physical exams, and have trouble differentiating developmental difficulties from discipline problems. Anecdotal evidence was presented to indicate the improvement of parenting skills as well as the need for intensive ongoing follow-up.

Pomerantz, Pomerantz, and Colca (1990) discussed a Specialized Family Program for deinstitutionalized disabled individuals. Recognizing the 1977 Proceedings of the White House Conference on the Handicapped, which indicated the right of persons with disabilities to marry, procreate, and rear children (Proceedings, 1977), the authors attempted to provide appropriate support services for several families. One case study served to exemplify the need for permanent support structures for certain families. The case study did not end on a positive note: the child in the family had multiple medical problems and died in intensive care. This dramatically indicated the magnitude of need that some families may represent, and the negative outcomes if extensive supportive services are not forthcoming.

Dickerson, Eastman, and Saffer (1984) produced a child care training manual for adults with mental retardation. Illustrated with 68 pictures, this manual is written at a very simple level and is employed in Canada as an aid to working with mentally retarded parents. This manual can be used for education and training purposes in group homes, residential treatment centers, and institutions.

Muccigrosso (1991) examined pregnant teenagers enrolled in special education classes for the retarded. She advocates sex education for the mentally handicapped as the pregnancy rates are disproportionately high. Preparation for future vocational/social life is also indicated.

Bakken, Miltenberger, and Schauss (1993) investigated the training of parents with mental retardation and delineated the difference between knowledge and skills. In their study, they found it imperative to assess criterion specific skills in the home. Concern was raised as to generalizability and long-term effects of training. Training in the home with follow-up appears to be the most needed aspect of training.

Feldman (1994) has reviewed outcome studies relative to parenting education for parents with intellectual disabilities. He examined parenting education programs in 20 studies, wherein 190 parents with intellectual disabilities served as subjects. The primary focus was behavioral. The initial training, follow-up, and some social validity results were noted to be encouraging. However, generalization and child outcomes data were felt to be weak. Feldman concluded his review of 20 program reviews by advocating five areas that require additional research: (1) how to increase confidence in the effectiveness of parent training; (2) how various individual, family, child, and environmental variables affect initial parenting problems and responsiveness to intervention; (3) what innovative programs need to be developed and evaluated; (4) a comparison of cost effectiveness and long-term impact to the child; (5) the need to develop and evaluate preventative and remedial interventions that focus on teaching parents supervision, positive-based child behavior management, stress/anger management, noncorporal discipline, and cognitive stimulation.

Tymchuk (1992) reviewed the literature on the issue of parenting by parents with mental retardation. Certain specific variables were examined: parental knowledge and skills, health care and safety, decision-making, interaction, and child outcomes relative to cognitive delays and emotional delays.

There are however, some research studies that indicate concern. Seagull and Scheurer (1986) followed 64 neglected or abused children, seen approximately 1 to 7 years prior, and found that six children had been given up for adoption; in 34 cases, parental rights had been terminated and an additional nine were placed in foster care. The authors conclude that the parents' cognitive limitations seemed to prevent these mentally retarded parents from employing services to assist them in caring for their children.

Currently, involuntary sterilization of persons with disabilities is banned by courts, upholding that parenting is a basic right of all adult citizens (Hayman, 1990).

Mathews (1992), Espe-Sherwindt (1991), Espe-Sherwindt and Kerlin (1990), and Tymchuk, Andron, and Rahbar (1988) have all indicated that people with mental retardation are capable of parenting. There are, of course, concerns with an operational definition of adequate parenting, and even of mental retardation. There are some individuals with deficits in cognitive skills but not adaptive behavioral skills. Others have adaptive behavioral and social deficits, but may not lack intellectual or cognitive skills. Many have been misdiagnosed in the past.

PARENTING AND SEXUALITY EDUCATION
FOR THE MENTALLY RETARDED

Parents are most children's primary teachers, and as such are responsible for much of their children's education. The goal of most parents is for the positive growth and development of their children as they understand it. Most often this includes the critical aspect of appropriate sexuality education. When parents are proactively involved in sexuality education over the course of their child's education, this goal is met more effectively. Mentally retarded individuals, however, may lack certain nuances of understanding and the ability to communicate in this intimately personal realm.

How should parents, especially mentally retarded ones, talk to their children about sexuality? Most normal parents often have urgent questions and valid concerns about this. These include how to discuss sex without giving their children permission to have sex, whether talking about sex give young children "ideas," and exactly when should a parent talk about sex with their children. Adolescents often have questions about sex, including what exactly is the right age to have sex. One could, as an example, respond with a counter-question: When exactly is the "right age" to be emotionally intimate?

If parents are intent upon the positive growth and development of their children, they can do the following:

1. Parents should think of sexuality as a human characteristic to be nurtured like any other human characteristic; sexuality is a part of, not separate from, being human.

2. Parents should begin when children are young. Parents teach children everything else about being a person and do so throughout their development. Parents offer information and opportunities to learn, whether intentionally or through teachable moments. Parents answer questions and respond to children's reactions to what they observe in the world around them, even questions regarding sexuality. Mentally retarded parents can do this as well, but they may need additional training, education, and feedback.

3. Parents typically do not instruct their children in a vacuum: they offer their children moral and ethical guidance. Parents instruct children how to protect themselves and how to be safe. Any education about sexuality would also involve this kind of support and education.

4. Parents can and should rely upon any resource that is available to them to help support teaching their children. Resources should be made available to the mentally retarded at a reading level appropriate for their needs.

5. Parents should realize their children will learn about sex, and possibly experiment, regardless of the lack of parental support. Humans do not need "permission" to do what comes naturally. The mentally retarded are no exception. However, for children to be safe and become responsible, guidance must be provided. Parents are in an ideal situation to offer this guidance, but many mentally retarded individuals may need assistance and skills in this area (Glover, 1987).

An important issue when dealing with the sexuality of those afflicted with mental retardation is that of safety and protection. There is nothing unusual in the teaching of sexuality to those with mental retardation: the principles of sound sex education for all children also apply. Knowledge and experience, however, may be limited in those with mental retardation. To the degree that instruction can be offered, it should be. A key component of sexuality education for the mentally retarded is the education of those charged with their care (when applicable).

As with any parent or teacher, knowledge and understanding of that which must be imparted is critical to helpful instruction. It should be seen as an ongoing process and curricula should be made available. Books, tapes, and high-interest, low-vocabulary materials are needed. Ongoing training is needed rather than quick, time-limited programs (Glover, 1986).

INTERNATIONAL PERSPECTIVES

Llewellyn (1990) recently reviewed the literature regarding adults with intellectual disability serving as parents, both after deinstitutionalization and after having been identified as needing assistance. In Australia, Llewellyn notes a great disparity in terms of the definition of "adequate parenting" and a great heterogeneity in terms of parenting experiences, supportive familial networks, and socioeconomic backgrounds.

Llewellyn and Brigden (1995) have explored the factors affecting service provision to parents with intellectual disabilities. Client characteristics were examined, and limited resources and interagency involvement were seen as crucial factors leading to provision of mainstream support services.

In Canada, one program that bears mentioning is the Parent Education Program (PEP) of Surrey Place Centre in Toronto. PEP is a nonprofit, community-based facility, the purpose of which is to help parents with cognitive challenges to become more effective and to conduct research toward developing criteria for training programs and evaluating their effectiveness. In this program, referral can come from parents, advocates, child welfare workers, public health nurses, and family physicians. After a referral is received, a PEP therapist visits the home several times so that an idea of what a typical day is like can be surmised. Observations are made of feedings, bathing, dressing, playing, and so forth, to determine how well these activities are being performed. Referrals are also made for older children, where the problem usually centers around behavior. The next step is for the parent and workers to identify parenting skills that will be targeted for instruction. Checklists are used to facilitate this process. The checklists are based on a task analysis approach. Each step is scored correct or incorrect. Topics might include bottle feeding, crib safety, and toilet training.

A typical training session schemata is as follows:

Step 1: PEP therapist demonstrates the task step by step.

Step 2: Parent practices the task and the PEP therapist gives feedback. Sometimes a manual is given to the parent with pictures depicting each step in a task as well as a written description of what to do.

Step 3: Repeat this process until parent knows how to perform the task well.

Step 4: Observe the parent performing the task once a month over the next 12 months.

Step 5: Parent receives reward for improving performance; gift certificates are used.

The PEP program also has an ongoing assessment program for the child, to catch any developmental problems early on. The PEP therapist visits at least once a week. Visits can last from 1 to 2 hours. Once a month parents and children are also invited to a parent group meeting at Surrey Place Centre. At these meetings, the therapist, in addition to dealing with parenting issues, provides assistance on issues such as housing, leisure activities, and social skills.

In Jordan, researchers and concerned professionals are beginning to realize the need for planning and needs assessment. Qaryouti (1984) conducted research to assess the country's needs in terms of social services and educational needs. Two questionnaires, informal interviews, and a review of materials from the Ministry of Social Development constituted this investigation.

In East Germany, Herrfurth and Herrfurth (1986) examined heterosexual partnerships of severely mentally retarded patients. Since East Germany no longer exists at this time, the practices cited in this article may be obsolete.

In the former Soviet Union, Danielov and Utin (1986) studied the parents of 402 oligophrenic subjects. This study revealed a high degree of marital homogeneity in terms of intellectual development. Gender, cultural, and familial factors were also seen as important.

Ann Craft and Michael Craft (1979) conducted a study in Wales that examined marriages wherein the couples were handicapped from birth by mental, physical, or personality disorders. This study found certain patterns of concern relative to each of these marriages.

In Australia, Booth and Booth (1995) examined case studies from 20 families wherein one or both of the parents had a learning disability or difficulty. In many cases, children were taken from parents, and there was a constant fear of surveillance; inadequate supports were also noted. Smith, Bland, and Grey (1993) further examined the situation of handicapped parents having nonhandicapped dependents. A book by Hall (1986) addressed ten topical areas relative to mentally retarded individuals and their rights in Australia. The three most salient to this discussion are marriage, the right to have children, and the right to adopt.

In New Zealand, Chapman and Pitceathly (1985) investigated the issues regarding sexuality and mentally handicapped individuals. Marriage was one concern and their report indicated the many mentally retarded individuals are capable of initiating a marriage and raising children. Pitceathly and Chapman (1985) further reported on programs dealing with psychosexual growth, sexual difficulties, and marital and parental concerns. This report also reviewed the importance of counselors in assisting the mentally retarded with several issues.

In Pakistan, group homes and community living arrangements are common, but there are still institutions for the mentally retarded. Little formal information is available from this country. In Israel, Chigier (1992) has written on sexuality and mental retardation and offered a perspective on marriage, parenting, and sex education in that country. In Finland, there are international conferences regarding various syndromes (Pyysalo, 1996) where treatment and parenting issues are addressed. Finland is currently in a state of transition away from institutions. Physicians are taking a more active role in prenatal screening, and are assisting parents by giving information and helping with support groups. Institutions still exist, but transition to group living arrangements are in progress.

In Korea, there is no proper system established, but there are parent education programs regularly scheduled in three steps, with each step lasting approximately 16 weeks. These programs include sex education. Apparently there is much more familial and parental involvement in the rearing of children at the current time in Korea than in western countries. Rhee Jong-Hee is the director of the Seoul Welfare Center for the Mentally Retarded; she reports that there is continuous family involvement in such situations in terms of responsibility. In Korea, the extended family accepts responsibility for children as a matter of pride, honor and duty. She directs the therapy and education department and oversees the parent education program in 13 major cities in Korea. Families are more apt to accept responsibility for their children and seek consultation.

In Hong Kong, Leung (1995) has written about the need for "other social welfare services" that are more unconventional. These include self-help groups (Wong, 1989), informal social networks, and the reality of 1997 as a revolutionary year for Hong Kong. Further, social welfare concerns are being confronted with a deficit-ridden government system and increasing migration and legal concerns.

Yau and Chang (1993) have addressed the need to assess the ability to consent to marriage in those with mental retardation. In general, if a mentally retarded person is going to marry and they are known to an agency, that specific agency would prepare that individual for marriage. Parenthood is another issue. Yau and Chang also indicate that the U.N. Declaration on the Rights of Mentally Retarded Persons (1971) states that the "mentally retarded person has, to the maximum degree of feasibility, the same rights as other human beings." In Hong Kong, the government has reaffirmed in the Green Paper on Rehabilitation (1992) that "disabled persons should enjoy the same basic rights as other members of the community." With regard to marriage, there is no law in Hong Kong preventing a mentally retarded person from contracting a valid marriage (Marriage Ordinance, 1984). It is essential, nevertheless, to satisfy the Registrar of Marriages that both parties in the marriage are capable of understanding the meaning and responsibilities of marriage (Hoggett, 1990). The clinical psychologists at the Social Welfare Department are sometimes asked to assess this ability. In Hong Kong, anyone can marry if they have reached the legal age of consent for marriage and understand the nature and effect of marriage. Nevertheless, if anyone with developmental disabilities would like to get married, they have to abide by the legislation governing all marriages. Yau and Chang (1993) have defined the most basic meaning and responsibilities of marriage to include the following:

1. That one will enter into a sexual relationship with the spouse.
2. That one will live together with the spouse with at least some degree of permanency.
3. That it will be a monogamous relationship, and

4. That the relationship is legally binding; that is, it can only be terminated by the Court.

A clinical psychologist must ascertain the individual's ability to understand these concepts. There is no objective test or instrument available for these purposes. Yau and Chang have developed a set of open-ended questions to ascertain how mentally retarded individuals understand the above concepts. The questions are:

1. Why do people want to get married?
2. What constitutes a marriage?
3. If you were to get married what would be your plans afterward?
4. What is the difference between marriage and cohabitation?
5. Can you marry another person while already married?

In light of the fact that there is no objective measure, the skilled clinician can rely on the mentally retarded individual's comprehension and understanding of these as at least a baseline or preliminary measure of their ability to understand their responsibilities.

Other people such as parents or professionals can provide advice for people with developmental disabilities to help them exercise their rights in getting married and having children sensibly. The parents of children with developmental disabilities (especially the parents of a female child) in Hong Kong are very cautious about letting their children marry, although the parents legally may have nothing to do with their children's decision if the latter have reached the legal age of consent for marriage. Yet parents' support and concern are always of vital importance in children's marriage. If those with developmental disabilities are known to other professionals such as psychologists, social workers, or occupational therapists, they would most likely get some help from these professionals in preparation for marriage. This may include housekeeping, contraception, family planning, and parenting.

In discussing family life and community involvement, the White Paper indicates that

> Family life education impresses upon the public the importance of family life and how it can be sustained. The principal target groups are adolescents, young adults about to marry, parents-to-be and parents. . . . People with a disability and their families may take advantage of family life education in the same way as anyone else. (Hong Kong Government, 1995, p. 83)

Obviously, problems often arise for married people with developmental disabilities if they want to have children. Having children often puts financial and emotional strain and stress upon the couple. Again, professionals and social service organizations may provide extra help for the couple if required.

If a child of a parent with developmental disabilities is neglected or abused, like any other suspected child abuse cases the Social Welfare Department may become involved in deciding what should be done to help the child and the family concerned. Though the paramount concern is for the welfare of the child, every effort will be made to keep the family together. Professional help and community support services will be tapped to strengthen the parental capacity and ensure the quality of care of the child. The child may be temporarily taken away from the parents or, in extreme cases, committed to the care of the Director of Social Welfare as a ward.

In India, non-governmental organizations are basically responsible for looking after mentally retarded children and citizens. Often the various state governments in India award grants to such institutions. Community-based rehabilitation is the program that is currently in vogue in many parts of India.

It is very rare in India that mentally retarded individuals are allowed to marry. In some cases, if the family bonds are very strong, individuals are allowed to marry, but the families shoulder much of the burden of rearing the children and helping the parents cope. In India, mothers assume a great deal of the burden of rearing children, often with the aid of the community-based rehabilitation staff. Such organizations are termed "Sewa-in-Action," "CADABAM," and Spastoes Society of India, and these organizations assist the families and extended families in coping with these situations. Specific programs to teach parenting skills are not formally recognized or distributed.

Procuring specific information from European and Asian countries is problematic. In addition, a questioner is often given the "official position" when the reality may be somewhat different. Procuring specific information for the teaching of parenting skills is difficult. Further, the little information available is accessible only to certain professionals. There are advances in networking and communication, however, via the Internet. There is an Americans with Disability Act Information Center that provides a link to other international disability sites on the World Wide Web. The address for this is http://www.idir.net/%7Eadabbs. This site is maintained by the Kansas Commission on Disability Concerns. It is anticipated that this source of information will expand substantially over the next few years.

SUMMARY AND CONCLUSION

This chapter has attempted to review some of the existing literature regarding the teaching of parenting skills to mentally retarded parents. There is a lack of systematic research in this area, and nations vary greatly in their definition of mental retardation and how best to address these issues.

As we approach the year 2000, it may be necessary to take a more systemic view of this problem and standardize procedures internationally. The ultimate concern is for the welfare of all children, in all nations, of all parents.

ACKNOWLEDGMENTS

Thanks to the following individuals for their assistance: Raj Nivas, Kaarina Jager, Dr. S. Bhaskara, Dr. Kimmo Lehtonen, Kang Mee-hee, Veronique Parker, Jeremy Martin, Brackston Taylor, Brad Imrie, and Arthur Cropley.

REFERENCES

Bakken, J., Miltenberger, R. G., & Schauss, S. (1993). Teaching parents with mental retardation: Knowledge versus skills. *American Journal on Mental Retardation, 97*(4), 405–417.

Booth, T., & Booth, W. (1995). Unto us a child is born: The trials and rewards of parenthood for people with learning difficulties. *Australia and New Zealand Journal of Developmental Disabilities 20*(1), 25–39.

Bornstein, M. H. (1995). *Handbook of parenting. Vol. 1: Children and parenting.* Mahwah, NJ: Lawrence Erlbaum Associates.

Budd, K. S., & Greenspan, S. (1985). Parameters of successful and unsuccessful interventions with parents who are mentally retarded. *Mental Retardation, 23*(6), 269–273.

Chapman, J. W., & Pitceathly, A. S. (1985a). Sexuality and mentally handicapped people: Issues of sex education, marriage, parenthood and care staff attitudes. *Australia and New Zealand Journal of Developmental Disabilities, 11*(4), 227–235.

Chigier, E. (1992). Sexuality and mental retardation. *Semin Neurol (SEJ), 12*(2), 129–134.

Craft, A. & Craft, M. (1979). *Handicapped married couples: A Welsh study of couples handicapped from birth by mental, physical or personality disorder.* London: Routledge and Kegan Paul.

Danielov, M. B., & Utin, A. V. (1986). Problems in the assortedness of marriages in mental retardation. *ZH Nevropatol Psikhiatr, 86*(3), 389–393.

Dickerson, M. U., Eastman, M. J., & Saffer, A. M. (1984). *Child care training for adults with mental retardation: Volume I, infants.* Downsview, Ontario: National Institute on mental retardation.

Espe-Sherwindt, M., & Kerlin, S. L. (1990). Early intervention with parents with mental retardation: Do we empower or impair? *Infants and Young Children, 2*, 21–28.

Espe-Sherwindt, M. (1991). The IFSP and parents with special needs/mental retardation. *Topics in Early Childhood Special Education, 11*(3), 107–120.

Fantuzzo, J. W., Wray, L., Hall, R., Goins, C., & Azar, S. (1986). Parent and social-skills training for mentally retarded mothers identified as child maltreaters. *American Journal of Mental Deficiency, 2*, 135–140.

Feldman, M. A., Case, L., Towns, F., & Betel, J. (1985). Parent education project I: Development and nurturance of children of mentally retarded parents. *American Journal of Mental Deficiency, 90*(3), 253–258.

Feldman, M. A. (1994). Parenting education for parents with intellectual disabilities: A review of outcome studies. *Research in developmental disabilities, 15*(4), 299–332.

Foxx, R. M., & McMorrow, M. J. (1985). Teaching social skills to mentally retarded adults: Follow-up results from three studies. *The Behavior Therapist, 8*, 77–88.

Foxx, R. M., McMorrow, M. J., & Mennemeier, M. (1984). Teaching social/vocational skills to retarded adults with a modified table game: An analysis of generalization. *Journal of Applied Behavior Analysis, 17*, 343–352.

Foxx, R. M., McMorrow, M. J., & Schloss, C. (1983). Stacking the deck: Teaching social skills to retarded adults with a modified table game. *Journal of Applied Behavior Analysis, 16,* 157–170.

Foxx, R. M., McMorrow, M. J., Storey, K., & Rogers, B. (1984). Teaching social/sexual skills to mentally retarded adults. *American Journal of Mental Deficiency, 89,* 9–15.

Glover, T. (1986). Effects on children's social development through positive parent-child interactions. Paper presented at the annual meeting of the Speaking for Children Conference University of Nebraska. Lincoln, Nebraska.

Glover, T. (1987). A model for positive parent–child communication toward fostering appropriate decision making skills in children. Paper presented at the annual meeting of the Building Family Strengths Symposium University of Nebraska. Lincoln, Nebraska.

Hall, J. (Ed.). (1986). Legal rights and intellectual disabilities: A short guide. Redfern, Australia: Redfern Legal Centre Publishing.

Hayman, R. L. (1990). Presumptions of justice: Law, politics and the mentally retarded parent. *Harvard Law Review. 103,* 1201–1271.

Heighway, S. M., Kidd-Webster, S., & Snodgrass, P. (1988). Supporting parents with mental retardation. *Children Today,* 24–27.

Herrfurth, R., & Herrfurth, D. (1986). Heterosexual partnerships of severely mentally retarded patients. *Z Gesamte Hyg, 32*(7), 432–433.

Hoggett, B. (1980). *Mental health law.* Sweet & Maxwell.

Hong Kong Government. (1994). Marriage Ordinance. Chapter 181. Hong Kong: Government Printer.

Hong Kong Government. (1995). *White paper on rehabilitation. Equal opportunities and full participation: A better tomorrow for all.* Hong Kong: Government Printer.

Leung, J. C. B. (1995). Social welfare. In S. Y. L. Cheung & H. Sze (Eds.), *The other Hong Kong reports.* Hong Kong: Chinese University Press.

Llewellyn, G. (1990). People with intellectual disability as parents: Perspectives from the professional literature. *Australia and New Zealand Journal of Developmental Disabilities, 16*(4), 369–380.

Llewellyn, G., & Bridgen, D. (1995). Factors affecting service provision to parents with intellectual disability: An exploratory study. *Australia and New Zealand Journal of Developmental Disabilities, 20*(2), 97–112.

Mathews, J. (1992). *A mother's touch.* New York: Henry Holt.

Muccigrosso, L. (1991). Double jeopardy: Pregnant and parenting youth in special education. Exceptional children at risk. CEC Mini Library, Council for Exceptional Children Reston, VA.

Pitceathly, A. S., & Chapman, J. W. (1985). Sexuality, marriage and parenthood of mentally retarded people. *International Journal for the Advancement of Counseling, 8*(3), 173–181.

Pomerantz, P., Pomerantz, D. J., & Colca, L. A. (1990). A case study: Service delivery and parents with disabilities. *Child Welfare, 69*(1), 65–73.

Proceedings From the White House Conference on the Handicapped. (1977). Washington, DC.

Pyysalo, R. (1996). NCL-sairaus vie kuolemaan. *Suomen Kuvalehti, 27,* 32–35.

Qaryouti, Y. F. (1984). Special education in Jordan: A present status and needs assessment study. *Dissertation Abstracts International, 45*(07A), 2067 (Michigan State University).

Seagull, E. A. W., & Scheurer, S. L. (1986). Neglected and Abused children of mentally retarded parents. *Child Abuse and Neglect: The International Journal, 10*(4), 493–500.

Smith, N. J., Bland, R., & Grey, C. (1993). Handicapped parents with non-handicapped dependents. *International Journal of Rehabilitation Research, 16,* 157–159.

Tymchuk, A. J. (1992). Predicting adequacy of parenting by people with mental retardation. *Child Abuse and Neglect: The International Journal, 16*(2), 165–172.

Tymchuk, A. J., Andron, L., & Rahbar, B. (1988). Effective decision making/problem solving training with mothers who have Mental Retardation. *American Journal on Mental Retardation, 92,* 510–516.

Wong, S. M. (1989). *Parent's group—A way of helping families with mentally handicapped children.* Hong Kong: Hong Kong Caritas Centre.

Yau, P., & Chang, S. (1993). *How to assess the ability to consent to marriage in a person with mental retardation.* Hong Kong: Clinical Psychology Unit Social Welfare Dept.

CHAPTER 8

Challenges and Complexities of Introducing Western Models of Service Delivery for People With Disabilities in Eastern and Central Europe

AVI RAMOT
Joint Distribution Committee, Israel

PESACH GITELMAN
American Jewish Joint Distribution Committee
International Development Program

All societies, from the least developed to the most advanced, must provide a range of essential services for their citizens in order to enable the society to continue functioning. The methods and approaches selected for providing these services and the priorities assigned to each obviously vary in different societies, according to a wide range of considerations and societal values.

Among the population groups for which societies need to consider making services available, are "people with special needs." Current terminology uses this phrase to relate to a broad range of individuals—including those with mental retardation, physical disabilities, and mental illness. This phrase tends to redirect the responsibility to the needs-providing mechanisms and not necessarily to the weaknesses or difficulties of the individuals involved. It further implies that this population is not necessarily defined by negative capacities or qualities but rather appears along a continuum of "needy" people—that is, the entire society, which is in need of one kind of support or another. At the same time it is evident that by combining various population groups, there is a great danger in generalizing the elements of policy and service provision and the individual or small group needs may be overlooked.

In a review of historical developments, it is clear that societies have differed greatly in their approach to service provision and to the nature and extent of services offered. Certain societies deal with issues in this area by developing a broad range of special services for the special needs population. From the positive perspective, this orientation is explained as a effort to assure that these citizens will be offered the services that meet their individual needs in the best, most comprehensive manner possible. However, this approach may lead to the isolation of members of this group from the broader society and its service provision network. It has been claimed (though often dismissed by many observers as apologetics), that members of this group actually prefer to remain isolated with others like themselves rather than being integrated into broader society. Observers critical of this approach have stated that this orientation will prevent society from having to see and therefore deal with the problems generated by this especially "needy" population.

At the other extreme, certain societies have consciously decided to enable their special needs citizens to take part in the broad range of "regular" services available to all citizens, recognizing the rights of individuals with special needs to participate fully in society.

Both the separation and inclusion approaches noted above have in common the stated goal of providing of adequate services, if not better. At the same time, many societies, both in the past and to this day, make available only the bare minimum of services, either separate or combined, to people with special needs. The bases for determining the minimal nature and extent of services offered may be claims of limited resources or decisions to support different priorities.

Historically, comparable levels of service development may develop for completely different reasons. For example, special services may exist not for the benefit of the people with special needs but in an effort to isolate them and keep them away from the "normal" society. Similarly, societies may have maintained their special needs citizens in "regular" services not with a aim of integrating them into society but in an attempt to limit societal expenses for people whose contribution to society is viewed as minimal at best.

In a similar fashion, societies that are simpler and less sophisticated may offer more possibilities for those people with even limited productive capacity to fill useful roles in the society. In the more complex, achievement-oriented, fast-paced modern environment, the special needs population may find itself with almost nonexistent marketable skills.

This chapter seeks to present experiences of introducing Western models of services for people with special needs into two Central European countries, the Czech Republic (Czechoslovakia until January 1993) and Romania. The experiences involve both theoretical and practical components and, despite the uniqueness of each, they have much in common. The planning and implementation phases in both countries involved an understanding and sensitivity to the elements involved in the determination of the nature and extent of existing services as outlined previously.

Following the major upheavals of the late 1980s, the countries of Eastern and Central Europe opened their societies (to a greater or lesser extent) to visitors from Western countries. Until that time all but the most astute students and observers of these societies had been unable to understand and appreciate the developments taking place. The "opening to the West" initially and most dramatically involved the recognition of political and economic developments and their impact on the formerly closed societies. More slowly, but perhaps no less profoundly, the areas of education and welfare services have opened up, revealing the developments that have taken place. Western input has had a dramatic impact toward the profound changes that have taken place. Similarly, this "opening" has enabled citizens to become receptive to the input of ideas from outside sources. Those who would seek to take advantage (in a positive sense) of this change in approach and the openness that has taken place must be sensitive to the implications of the new situations that have developed. These individuals and the organizations they may represent must be aware that the possibility of providing useful assistance must be based on a clear understanding of the dynamics of the situations that exist, and an appreciation of the developments that have taken place.

In this chapter, the Romanian experience will be presented first, followed by the experience in the Czech Republic and a summary and conclusion.

ROMANIA

Until the revolution of December 1989, the only option offered in Romania for people with special needs was institutional care. This approach was common in communist societies, and Romania did not deviate from the Eastern European norm. The term for these facilities in Romanian is *camin-spital* or "home-hospital." Generally, these facilities housed between 80 and 140 children and adults with a variety of disabilities, including mental retardation, mental illness, and behavior and personality disturbances. The institutional approach well matched the generally low scientific and technological level of the country (not just in comparison to Western countries but also in comparison to other communist countries like Hungary and Czechoslovakia). For example, disposable medical equipment only reached Romania in 1994. At the same time it should be noted that unlike the former Soviet Union, the institutions weren't used for punishment but only for professional treatment alternatives for individuals who were significantly deviant from the norm.

Community treatment services for people with special needs did not exist. The institution was seen as the ultimate solution for a broad range of disturbances, including orphans who were identified only as having a "social problem." This issue reached the headlines due to an ABC network television program anchored by Barbara Walters. This program, while misrepresenting the social

orientation of the Romanian people, shed light on the professional solutions
that characterized the Eastern European regimes, with particular emphasis on
Romania.

With the downfall of the communist regime in December 1989, there began an
influx of representatives from Western voluntary organizations. By 1991, dozens
of voluntary organizations, including those from the U.S., Denmark, Holland,
Germany, and France were already operating in the country. Each organization
brought its own social ideology, professional approaches, and methods of operation. All felt a deep sense of commitment to help the Romanian people, just
released from the chains of the communist regime, get a new start. Each organization also brought its own substantial funds with which they sought to set up
social welfare services, mainly community-based, which didn't exist in the past.
The new Romanian regime welcomed all the organizations and even the busi-
nessmen who came from all over. The government didn't have any screening and
control mechanism to deal with the influx, nor were there any criteria to study
and measure the various programs and projects.

It is necessary to understand these developments from a broader perspective.
The previous communist regime collapsed suddenly, in one day. The democratic
elections that took place shortly thereafter were an initial indicator of the type of
regime that would be installed in the future, but they weren't an indication of a
carefully planned new system of government. Thus, it happened that the communist regime was replaced by an unidentified void that had elements of democratic tendencies, enthusiasm for change, a lack of structure, and workers who
couldn't "read the map" and either continued to operate as in the past or became
paralyzed waiting for the new regime to coalesce.

One of the interesting characteristics of this period was that a Western visitor,
if a professional or businessman, could quite easily meet almost any Romanian
minister with only brief prior notice, but couldn't meet the supervisor of industrial plants in a geographic area or the supervisor of facilities for special needs
populations in a particular region. The ease of access dramatically influenced the
reaction of people at different levels of government to the ideas that came from
Western sources. These new ideas brought about the collapse of the communist
concept that "all is well" and brought a new definition to the needs of people
with special problems. This redefinition of needs is a deep process: it generally
upsets the self-confidence of a professional who was, for many years, responsible
for maintaining the illusion of stability. In Romania at the beginning of the 1990s
this process was not only deep and serious but also very painful, and it brought
about great confusion at various levels. The new leaders accepted the change
with enthusiasm. They welcomed any organization or entrepreneur who came
with a new program, especially if there was money to implement the idea. In addition, many "field people," especially the younger ones (some of whom were already exposed to these new ideas), were very interested in learning about new
professional approaches from the West. At the bureaucratic and professional lev-

els, those individuals who were in between the political and field levels were the most resistant to new approaches. At this level, the workers generally retained their positions from the previous regime. They were surrounded by the enthusiasm of those at the political level and the workers from the field, who anticipated sweeping changes. Because the statements of the politicians weren't converted to operative programs, the middle level remained without self-confidence or any clear direction, almost in "deep freeze." This situation resulted in all workers responding aggressively to changes wafting in the air.

A positive spirit came from the direction of university social science students, who were exposed to professional literature and lecturers from the West and who publicly attacked the bureaucratic level for its rigid approaches and the political level for "talking and not doing."

One of the voluntary organizations that decided to operate in Romania was Project Concern International (PCI). This organization had a history of thirty years of humanitarian activities in various countries including Guatemala, Bolivia, Indonesia, and Mexico. In 1991 the organization came to Romania, initially focusing on improving medical care for newborn infants. In 1992 a decision was taken to work with people with disabilities who were then living in *camin-spitals* but who could live in the community. The decision was to develop a project combining residential and vocational services. To develop the initial concept PCI involved experts from the U.S., Europe, and Israel, with funding from their own sources and from the U.S. Department of State. Several basic principles were adopted:

1. The target population is those living in institutions diagnosed as having "oligophreny." This diagnosis, most closely related to mental retardation, has not been used in the West for about fifty years but remains central in the Romanian system.

2. A model project, appropriate to the Romanian culture but involving Western values and treatment approaches, would be prepared.

3. The project would be implemented by local personnel with guidance from American staff and experts from the U.S., Europe, and Israel. The experts would meet the Romanian minister responsible for services for people with disabilities and other senior personnel, and tour institutions meeting supervisors, directors, and local psychiatrists.

4. The project would be implemented with the cooperation from the senior political level (ministers and directors-general), middle-management level (supervisors and regional directors), and "field" personnel (psychiatrists and directors of institutions).

5. From the outset, it would be made clear to all the participants that the central goal is to develop a new model that would be slowly spread throughout Romania.

The site chosen for the project was a private house in the village of Malda-reshti, near the town of Horezu in the Vilcea district, three hours west of Bucha-rest. A generous donation from Monaco was used to refurbish the house. The re-modeling process engendered many ideological discussions involving issues of the level of repairs: Should the level be higher than that of the neighbors? Should running water be installed? What kind of entrance ramp should be put in? Should central heating be put in or, like in the surrounding houses, should a fire-place be installed in each room? In the end, it was decided to accept the common Romanian level with some improvements to make life more comfortable.

At the same time, a professional staff was recruited, mainly young and enthu-siastic teachers, but also including social workers and others from the field of ed-ucation. The staff underwent several months of training, based on a model pre-pared by two Israeli experts who also participated in teaching several of the units.

In the middle of 1993 the project staff, in cooperation with workers from the institutions, began interviewing candidates. There was a sense that the institu-tion staff members were cooperating based on their hope that something good was to take place without really understanding the process.

At the same time steps were being taken to guarantee even partial govern-ment funding for the project. This expectation was hard for the government representatives to appreciate and even harder to accomplish. Budget transfers, flexible budgets, and alternative funding weren't concepts being used in 1993 in Romania. As a result, PCI made preparations to identify alternative funding sources and donations for the project.

At the beginning of 1994 the first six residents entered the project. Four of them were able to find work in the village or nearby town, and two were em-ployed (for minimum wage by the a contractor) to help remodel a building on the grounds that was to serve as a sheltered workshop for the project. In 1995 the residence was fully occupied by 14 residents, of whom six worked in the village and the rest in the workshop.

CZECH REPUBLIC

From even a preliminary review of the situation it must become clear to all that it is not simply an issue of the "progressive" Western societies graciously offering fruits from their wisdom and experience to the "backward" Eastern societies. As the following statement indicates, the situation is much more complicated than that:

> The problem of disabled persons in the past forty years [in Czechoslovakia] was not in their social security which was/in relation to our mean population/of even a higher standard than in most western countries. Disabled people in this country also had far smaller problems with job finding than the disabled in the West.
>
> The problem, however, lay in the fact that they were literally segregated from

the healthy population and concealed from the public. We have had probably the most extensive system of special schools in the world in which children with even smallest disability were placed / missing fingers, slight hearing impairment, etc. / . They were ghettoes in which the disabled were literally concealed. The majority of [the] healthy population practically did not meet their disabled fellow citizens at all. Seriously disabled people, as well as old people, were concentrated in large capacity and mostly isolated social welfare institutions even in the cases in which the creation of elementary prerequisites would have enabled them to live in their own environment. Particularly difficult was the situation of the mentally handicapped, mentally ill and their families. The problems of disabled people were practically not published at all. Due to segregation there was no interest in the elimination of architectural, orientation, communication and psychological barriers which would enable the disabled persons to live in a normal society. (Government of the Czech Republic, 1993)

This clearly states that the issue of nature and distribution of services for people with disabilities in the Czech Republic (and in the former Czechoslovakia) was not simply an issue of availability of sufficient resources but one of service delivery policy priorities that were ultimately based on values. The society decided to develop, at not inconsiderable expense, a range of segregated services, "probably the most extensive system of special schools in the world . . . ghettos in which the disabled were literally concealed" (Government of the Czech Republic, 1993). This approach indicated the priority in this society was to exclude people with disabilities from being part of it. Their presence was determined by decision-makers to be counter-indicated to the functioning of society. At the same time, it would seem that a decision was made that educational services for the children with physical disabilities needed to be offered and maintained at an "acceptable" (in other words, minimal) level, while those for children and others with mental disabilities could be of much lower quality.

In the aftermath of the Velvet Revolution of 1989, these decisions were opened to scrutiny, and the newly appointed policymakers (many of whom were actively in opposition to the previous regime) as well as many citizens, particularly those with direct connections to the system, weren't pleased with what they saw. It should be noted that despite their previous active roles in opposition, the new decision-makers weren't necessarily the best qualified to introduce and manage the reforms for which they so actively fought. In fact, many of the leaders who entered office after the revolution (in Czechoslovakia and other Eastern and Central European countries) did not succeed in introducing the changes they sought and many did not remain in their positions for a long time.

When the opportunity to benefit from outside assistance became possible (through a project supported by the United States Agency for International Development and implemented by the American Jewish Joint Distribution Committee Inc.) the local partners approached this "generous offer" with appropriate hesitation. The local experts correctly understood that while outside support could be vital in enabling them to advance an agenda for change, at the same time the control of and responsibility for ongoing developments needed to be in the hands of local authorities. The minister of health, who subsequently became an ardent supporter, described the large number of visitors and entrepreneurs who came to his office as "humanitarian tourists" who sought to "add another country to their list." Only after being convinced that this project would not impose outside models, standards, and approaches did he agree to support and assist the activities.

As a direct result of the hesitations noted above, the project's managers guided the activity with a conscious effort to involve the local partners in defining priorities and specifying goals. In addition, the project adopted certain guidelines that were basic to the range of activities and programs developed. Among these guidelines were:

1. Utilize a nonjudgmental approach: alternative (not necessarily better) approaches were being presented;

2. Promote questioning, issue-based attitudes: for review and discussion and adoption if deemed appropriate, and change and adaptation to local conditions, priorities, and values;

3. Encourage the development of a range of services. Rather than concentrating on one specific service, an effort should be made to service a specific program in a broad context and thus deal with a range of service needs;

4. Promote the creation of alternatives. Individual choice, at all levels and positions, should be encouraged,

5. Develop needs assessment techniques, in order to help develop services that meet individual needs—not merely matching individuals to services already developed;

6. Stimulate both the "bubble-up" and "trickle-down" approaches, with a focus both on direct services and policy developments;

7. Promote professional networks in various parts of the country, and encourage ongoing professional and personal contacts among colleagues. The opportunity for assuring continuity of the project goals could best be served by developing a cadre of trained committed professionals. The need for peer support was evident to all who sought in the past to make changes in aspects of their work and met with lack of support and understanding.

8. Emphasize the implementation of multi- and interdisciplinary approaches. The focus here is both on the need for interventions from a variety of modalities and professions and on the support from colleagues indicated in the previous item;

9. Avoid focus on single geographic area despite its possible centrality and significance. The condition of "Pragocentrism," a reality of many previous en-

deavors where programs were designed to serve only the capital city, was to be avoided to the extent possible;

10. Encourage public airing of related issues—bringing the topic to broad public attention. Attention was devoted to developing media contacts—newspaper, radio, and even TV—to open the subject to public scrutiny. The previous approach of isolating the special needs population both physically and emotionally was seen, by local partners, as a basic element enabling the services to develop as they had in the past.

The project as conceived had two basic components: a training aspect and a direct service model. The training aspect was developed in coordination with the prestigious Charles University in Prague. It involved the creation of a core curriculum of areas that were identified by the project team and outside experts as basic to the Western approach to services for people with special needs. The four key elements that were ultimately selected, after a comprehensive process, to complete the core aspects, were family support services, integration, adult services, and legal elements in services. Experts from the United States and Israel were invited to present the latest in Western ideas in each of the areas for the students review and assessment. In addition, in each of the topic areas presented, the experts were guided to focus on the value-based components, which provided an underpinning to the actual services that developed. This approach was essential, because the ultimate goal was for the local participants to relate not only to the services that developed but also to the rationale and underlying elements that enabled or encouraged the various services to develop as they had (Svestkova, Nemcik, Hutar, & Odehnal, 1994; Ministry of Labor and Social Affairs, 1995). In addition to the core curriculum a wide range of topic areas were suggested by the local participants and tailor-made training programs were prepared for specific audiences. This participatory component was identified as significant by the local participants, as it clearly demonstrated that, knowledgeable though the visiting experts may be, their contribution could only be worthwhile if it related to local needs and interests. As such, the visiting experts were not simply teachers presenting information but role models and concerned colleagues who accepted a broad responsibility for helping making the lives of people with disabilities better. During the course of the project 161 students graduated from the core program and 3,107 participated in short-term training programs (American Jewish Joint Distribution Committee, 1995).

The second component, the direct service model, was designed to test out in practice some of the basic elements that were being presented in the training component. From the outset, the project defined its mandate to include practical, hands-on elements that could be tested and adapted as needed to the local situation. The specific aspect selected in this regard was a "community living arrangement" (CLA) for individuals with mental retardation. The CLA represented a community-based residential alternative to institutional placement for adults with mental retardation or other disabilities who could no longer live with their families. Prior to the project the only out-of-home alternative available for this population was a large, impersonal institutional facility, often far from family. The CLA, implemented by a newly created, local, parent-run voluntary organization, demonstrated that alternatives were possible and, with appropriate support, viable and even desirable for many. The newly reorganized Ministry of Health, which was dealing with the issue of maintaining professional mental health services in very large, antiquated mental hospitals (some resembling villages with up to 2,000 patients), was interested in possibly adopting this model as an alternative to inpatient services. The existence of the CLA model in Prague, managed by a local organization and staffed by local personnel, offered the opportunity for skeptics and supporters alike to observe, monitor, criticize, and help to adapt the service to existing local circumstances. The value of this exposure, both from professional and educational perspectives, cannot be underestimated. For the first time this new model of service was being presented not as a foreign trend but as a viable, local alternative designed to meet the needs of people with special needs in the Czech Republic. In fact, a wide range of professionals and family members have visited the CLAs (by the end of the project period 5 were operating and more were planned), in order to learn about its operation and determine whether it might be applied to other places. No amount of foreign "wisdom" and experience could have accomplished this change.

Subsequent to the operation of the CLAs and as the result of continuing interventions of the local voluntary association, the Ministry of Labor and Social Affairs agreed to provide monthly maintenance for the operation of the CLAs. Although the funding level was insufficient, the decision to provide funding was seen as a formal acknowledgment by the social welfare authorities that this service model was a valid alternative worthy of receiving government support.

SUMMARY AND CONCLUSIONS

The material presented in this chapter sought to identify the key common elements involved in two separate projects in Romania and the Czech Republic, shortly after each country underwent major changes following the downfall of the communist regimes. Each project attempted to assist in the process of enhancing the lives of people with disabilities in these countries. Each project sought to be sensitive the cultural traditions and values of the country, to relate to currently existing service patterns, and to develop cooperative relationships with key local partners. The projects relied on substantial (particularly by local standards) outside resources to enhance opportunities for service development. At the same time each project team was particularly concerned that these funds be used sensitively, with careful reference to local patterns and procedures. Each project planned its activities by taking into account the short-term nature of its own involvement and the commitment that the programs implemented would be continued by local authorities following the completion of the project period.

In attempting to draw conclusions in regard to the achievements of the projects, several issues should be noted. First of all, each of the funding sources appointed independent evaluators to review project accomplishments. In each case the overall assessments were generally very positive and supportive of the work that had been done. Specific suggestions were made regarding changes and adaptations that could be made to assure maximum achievements. In addition, other measures may be introduced including whether the programs begun by the projects have been maintained despite the ending of the project period. Information regarding this has been gathered from a variety of sources. For example, in a speech given by Senator Edward M. Kennedy to the United Nations International Symposium on Intellectual Disability (cited in the AAMR News and Notes), he states the following: "In the Czech Republic, there is growing use of community residences for people with mental retardation . . ." (Kennedy, 1996). This independently confirms the continued implementation of a basic component of the project. This continuation clearly reflects that local authorities have sufficiently accepted key elements of the projects and adopted them as a component of the routine services being offered to citizens with disabilities.

Without meaning to sound overly optimistic, the authors believe that the combination of factors, including timing, resources, appropriate professional and personal contacts and partnerships, and the basic common human needs and concerns that characterize all societies have made it possible to transfer and adapt experiences and approaches from one society and culture to another.

REFERENCES

American Jewish Joint Distribution Committee. (1995). Final quarter report—Training institute/ community living arrangements. Project Prague, Czech Republic Cooperative Agreement No. Eur-0032-A-00-1023-00 (October–December).

Government of the Czech Republic. (1993). National plan of measures to reduce the negative impact of disability. Document approved by Resolution No. 493, Czech government sources.

Kennedy, Edward M. (1996). From disability to capability. *AAMR News and Notes* 9(4), 5–6.

Ministry of Labor and Social Affairs, Prague. (1995). State employment policy—Organization and tasks of employment services in the Czech Republic. Czech government sources.

Svestkova, O., Nemcik, J., Hutar, J., & Odehnal, M. (1994). The problems of comprehensive rehabilitation and the origin of rehabilitation centers in the Czech Republic. *Legislation for Disabled Persons and their Integration to [sic] the Community. Proceedings of IV National Seminar with
External Participation* (pp. 37–40).

CHAPTER 9

Disability Arts: Developing Survival Strategies

JENNY CORBETT

Institute of Education, University of London

There has been an increasing development of organizations run by disabled people for disabled people in the United States and in the United Kingdom. This has grown out of a general dissatisfaction with the many powerful and influential organizations run by nondisabled people who act on behalf of the disabled. It has been just one effect of the dynamics of empowerment and the demands for rights, choices, and opportunities by people with disabilities.

This chapter is concerned with the self-help area of disability arts. Over recent years a disability culture has emerged in the U.S. and in the UK, which is reflected in music, poetry, dance, art, and drama. It is owned by disabled people as their means of self-expression and pride in identity. There are tensions between those who feel that disability culture ghettoizes disability arts and those who want it to remain separate and free from external censure.

The key issues explored under the broad heading of disability arts are:

- How people with learning disabilities and additional mental illness are supported by disability arts;
- the extent to which disability arts is a form of empowerment;
- the ways in which people learn skills for survival;
- the limitations of this form of empowerment.

DUAL OPPRESSIONS

Over recent years, a heightened sensitivity has developed among staff who work with people with learning disabilities, which alerts them to see their clients as adults who are more than usually vulnerable to social risks. Where they had so often been regarded as simply adult-size children in the past, there has been much research that reveals the extent of their adult status, requiring that they learn to speak out against exploitation. This has been particularly powerfully documented in the delicate and uncomfortable area of sexual abuse (Corbett, Cottis, & Morris, 1996).

There has been a gradual recognition of the impact of dual oppression on people who are already the targets of social discrimination. This applies, for example, to people with learning disabilities who are also Black (Baxter, Poonia, Ward, & Nadirshaw, 1990) and to women with learning disabilities who may be seeking refuge because of sexual abuse (Brown, 1996). A more recent area that has been addressed in relation to preventative medical care and awareness training about HIV and AIDS is that of the dual experience of having learning difficulties and being gay (Davidson-Paine & Corbett, 1995; Cambridge, 1996).

Among people with learning disabilities, there are some who also experience mental illness. Recent research on the combined effects of having both a learning disability and schizophrenia have indicated that they tend to present difficulty in diagnosis, which can delay the onset of appropriate support (James, Mukherjee, & Smith, 1996). However, group therapy was found to be of particular value here. The combination of limited language skills, mental confusion, and anxiety makes self-expression extremely difficult, and the need to help people to know their own minds becomes a major priority.

THE INFLUENCE OF EMPOWERMENT AS A CONCEPT

Professionals who support empowerment as a learning concept often recognize that this difficult process must involve addressing imbalances in the area of power relationships and moving towards a re-evaluation of the nature of human worth. The simplistic notion of the powerful transferring knowledge and skills to the powerless is now acknowledged as a facile and arrogant assumption. What is empowering for one person may be potentially destructive for another, and each of us has to find our own path to self-empowerment.

Mosley (1994) has been influential in the United Kingdom in developing workshop activities that help staff and clients, professionals and service-users, to work together towards greater levels of negotiation and understanding. She has confronted the difficulty that many people with learning difficulties have in communicating their ideas and wants through speech and the ways in which this disadvantages them in the process of negotiation. Her approach is to guide staff to work at their listening skills, as in this sample checklist:

- Do you sit positioned away from, or turn away from people while they are speaking?
- Do you frown, yawn, or grimace in a distracting way while someone is speaking?

- Do you use words people cannot understand?
- Do you interrupt people in mid-sentence? (Mosley, 1994, p. 25)

If staff are no longer going to speak on behalf of their clients with learning disabilities but are to listen to their forms of self-expression, then this requires a form of gentle listening that nurtures rather than controls.

One of the most difficult aspects of self-empowerment involves dealing with emotions and learning to both control them and to express them with confidence. Speake and John (1994) perceive the process of helping people with learning disabilities cope with their emotional expression as a key route into increasing their personal effectiveness as adults in the community. Past expectations were often that they were too emotionally immature to manage their own care needs or to make informed decisions. An illustration of the extent to which these assumptions have been changed can be seen in recent publications like that of Townsley and Macadam (1996), which demonstrates the ways in which people with learning difficulties can become involved in recruiting the staff who will be responsible for their care. The importance of user involvement in this process is seen as an integral part of genuine empowerment, which can change the context of daily interactions and shift the balance of power relationships.

Camerson and Blunden (1996) reinforce the need for client consultation in their focus upon quality assurance relating to the purchasing of services for people with learning disabilities, challenging behaviors, and mental health needs. In their reflections on assessing the quality of services, they include the assessment of users who ask for provision, which will offer

> Help to live life the way I want to . . .
> Help to stop me hurting others . . .
> Fun and positive relationships . . .
> Speaking up and being listened to . . .
> (Cameron & Blunden, 1996, p. 26)

Part of the negotiation process includes an individualized care plan that is built around the distinctive needs of each person (Murphy & Watters, 1996). These needs may be complex where there is a combination of learning difficulty and mental illness (James et al., 1996). In some instances, the person with learning difficulties has been charged with offending against the law and may need guidance on how to cope in court. In order to help someone with multiple needs, the use of both professional advocacy and self-advocacy is often essential.

SELF-ADVOCACY: LEARNING TO SPEAK OUT

There has been a powerful and sustained move in the United States and the United Kingdom to support the self-advocacy of people with learning difficulties, which is now well established and valued. It is mainly concerned with encouraging people to express their own needs and to participate in debates that involve both nondisabled and disabled people. It has become an intensely political area, linked as it is to civil rights issues and campaigns against discriminatory practices. There has also been a certain degree of skepticism about the extent to which staff act in an empowering way with clients whose decisions they may have a vested interest in influencing.

At both a macro-level in the wider political arena, and at a micro-level within institutional dynamics, self-advocacy can be seen to offer a source of tension and a site of potential struggle. Ways of influencing the behaviors and belief systems of vulnerable people can be subtle and invidious, leading to a very restricted form of self-advocacy. Often there are only a few people with learning difficulties who feel able to participate in political activities or even to play a prominent role in the running of their day center or social club. Much depends upon their level of confidence and security and the degree to which they feel supported by staff and family. To speak out about views and feelings related to civil rights and service providers risks possible recrimination and may create distress rather than a resolution of difficulties. Mittler (1996) recognizes the need for lengthy preparation and confidence-building to support effective self advocacy.

A less threatening form of self-advocacy is provided in the area of disability arts. This is a fringe activity, usually in drama, music, ballet, poetry, art, or photography, in which people with physical and learning disabilities have opportunities to perform and present their work in ways that may be denied them in the mainstream arts arena.

THE USE OF POETRY TO EXPRESS SELF

In the American journal *The Disability Rag,* Wade (1994) describes disability cultural art as:

> Identity. Art that tells who we are, where we come from, where we're going, how we got here. Art that expresses the dreams and realities of a people. Of survivors. (p. 29)

This image is powerful and strong, illustrating the force of disability culture. It is an expression of that territory that professional carers and trainers cannot enter. Gaspari (1995) provokes his readers by suggesting that disabled people need a ghetto. His assertion is that where discrimination is deeply ingrained in a society, the ghetto offers security and sanctuary to build up solidarity. A ghetto of disabled people would, in any event, be richly diverse if it were to reflect the range of people who constitute this heterogeneous group (Williams, 1992). For some critics, the area of disability arts may be seen as just one more artificial structure designed to display a social movement that is now seen as disability politics (Campbell & Oliver, 1996). Perhaps it is unhelpful to agonize over whether there ought to be such a thing as disability culture, and better to assess the extent to which it can serve as an empowering force for collective and individual identity.

One of the critical factors within the disability arts world is that any new magazine, play, musical group, arts organization, or performance-related venture has to compete in a ruthless, massively oversubscribed market where very few will finally succeed. It is notable that there have been several disability arts, culture, and politics journals launched in the UK in the last few years that have only lasted for a short period before having to close through lack of funds. One of the longest lasting was the *Disability Arts Magazine,* which described regional activities for disabled people, included those with learning disabilities. In England, Scotland, and Ireland, examples were found of people being supported in music and drama to find expression to their feelings and to prove their capabilities (Harris, 1992; Silverwood, 1992; Graham, 1994). The value of disability arts as an empowering process was demonstrated in many instances of progress and fulfilment through group participation. While it might be argued that disabled people should ideally be participating in mainstream arts programs, the reality is that fierce competition for inclusion is likely to limit them to either minimal participation or a stereotyped role in which their scope for development is severely constrained.

Poetry might be seen as a particularly powerful and liberating form of self-expression. As an example of a self-help arts organization, a poetry group for survivors of the mental health system is a useful model of self-empowerment. The case study example was formed in the United Kingdom in 1991 by four poets who had all experienced the mental health system, each of whom had a unique voice to communicate to the world. This organization has been extremely successful where many other fringe arts groups have failed. Registered now as a charity, it seeks funds from various benefactors who support fringe arts ventures. Poetry has always been a poor relation of other arts areas such as music and drama. It is seen as a minority interest and, as such, of only marginal cultural value. However, in the psychiatric world, poetry has long been regarded as a rich resource to be used for catharsis, expression of anger and emotional frustration, and to provide material for psychoanalytical reflection. The poetry group that was formed in 1991 rejected a narrow labelling of poetry for catharsis and devised workshops to develop skills of presentation and performance as well as creating regular evenings where established poets could present their work. Their movement was both political and artistic. It enabled those who felt they had been oppressed by the system to vent their feelings in verse and free-flowing imagery while also striving to reach a high level of artistic integrity.

The range of people attending workshops and participating in performances is considerable. It includes the university-educated as well as those who attended special schools for children with learning disabilities. This diversity demonstrates that psychiatric survivors are indeed a substantial part of the disability movement, reflecting many different levels of experience (Chamberlain, 1995). It also indicates why there may be tensions among a group that reflects this range of perspectives.

TENSIONS IN DISABILITY ARTS GROUPS

The case study example of a performance- and workshop-based poetry group offers a valuable illustration of the complex demands that make for a potentially stressful situation. The group can be seen to have a dual purpose. At one level, it serves to support vulnerable people and to empower them through self-expression. At another level, it is competing in a fierce market where many small arts groups will go under. There is a need to be efficient, businesslike, and enterprising. This can rest uneasily with the additional need to be supportive, understanding, and caring. There are two sets of survival strategies that coexist here: to keep the organization solvent and thriving, and to nurture and empower a wide range of members.

This is an example of a group that is run by disabled people, for disabled people. As such, it is in the forefront of new initiatives to empower people who are used to experiencing professional care rather than being able to negotiate developments in a democratic forum. Committees include a wide diversity of members, from former business executives who had nervous breakdowns to people who have never been in paid employment and who attended special schooling. This range of experience inevitably means that some people will have developed advanced skills of debate and decision-making while others are confused and lacking in confidence. The committees tend to take a long time to complete their business and require considerable listening skills, sensitivity, and tact. It is not uncommon for one member to make offensive comments to another, through frustration or a lack of social skills, which gives rise to misunderstandings. These meetings are both potentially oppressive and channels of energy for collective growth. The struggle between individual and collective identity is always a central issue. Both are seen as important but can sometimes pull against one another, especially if one individual is demanding of a level of support that impedes the progression of the group endeavors. Genuine empowerment is inevitably difficult, complex, and time-consuming to develop and sustain.

PRODUCING A PORTFOLIO

A group like the poetry arts organization just described tends to support those people with learning disabilities who are able to use verbal language to express themselves. There are also many other people whose lack of a conventional voice leaves them reliant on nonverbal expression and visual representation. Within the hierarchies of the disability movement, it is this group of people with profound and multiple disabilities who are most vulnerable to exploitation and abuse. Empowerment, for them, involves finding ways in which their personal needs and preferences are clearly articulated without in any way diminishing their human dignity.

When someone with profound disabilities requires intensive levels of physical care—including being washed, fed, taken to the toilet, and put to bed—they are dependent upon the sensitivity and empathy of their carer. In some instances, this person may be a parent, partner, or member of the family, but within the "care in the community" initiative it is increasingly likely to be a stranger who is paid to provide these services. In a 24-hour care program, this may involve several changes of personnel; in residential care, there may be regular replacements of short-term care staff. For people with profound learning disabilities, this can involve a stressful process of coping with clumsy handling and inappropriate support, which is inevitable when staff are working on a trial-and-error basis.

Written case notes in a file are obviously useful to guide professional carers in working with clients who lack verbal language or have minimal means of expression. These notes can be seen as a basic framework on which to base an assessment of personal needs. However, they are cold and impersonal, providing only medical and psychological evaluations, details of social circumstances, and family connections, which place the person at the center but as seen by the professional gaze. This tends to focus upon specific difficulties and problems rather than upon personal qualities and valued aspects. It tells the carer what to do but may give them little encouragement to empower the client. The imbalance of the power relationship acts against this.

A multimedia performance group in the United Kingdom has devised a novel system of both creating artistic processes and providing survival strategies. They work in conjunction with the person with profound learning disabilities and their key worker to compile a visual portfolio profile. By filming videos, taking photographs, and building up a media file on the computer, a composite picture of the individual concerned is created. It does not just focus on the practicalities, like how to lift them in and out of their wheelchair or how to feed them most effectively (although these issues are still included). The purpose of this multimedia framework is to record and report the individual's widest possible range of interests and concerns. For example, a young man who has spent years in a large institution and who spends his days facing a window in the ward, looking outside from his wheelchair, was regarded by many staff as unaware of his surroundings. Working closely with him and his key worker, the multimedia project found that he had created a quiet space for himself and had all kinds of interests and memories. They built a visual sequence for him, from a series of photos in which he looked from the window to see trains, trees, close-ups of grass, and other memories from the past. His profile on the computer included visual reminders of his earlier life, his day-to-day activities, and the people who were part of his life.

Another profile was that of a woman who wanted to move into a larger room in her community residential home. The computer screen enabled the key-worker and this woman to explore the location of a variety of objects, such as chairs, waste-bins, television, handbag, and cupboard to different places within the room. It was a process of actively involving the person with learning disabilities in the planning of their living environment in a way that was accessible to them.

At their most innovative and powerful, disability arts can offer a more empowering energy than the overt force of political activism. Groups like this one are concerned with flexible and creative means of communication. They want to help people with learning disabilities to tell their own story, challenging the idea that they will have nothing to say. Through multimedia profiling, they display people as individuals with a past, present, and future. The focus is person-centered and interactive, filling in a picture that brings the multidimensional aspects to life. There are areas like those of emotional needs, personal possessions, and likes and dislikes, which will only be illustrated by using multimedia filing rather than the conventional approaches. This empowering and creative development is of direct practical value for service planning and its technological focus is apt for the growth toward the 21st century.

THE VALUE OF CREATIVE GROWTH

Writing in a disability arts journal, Penny Boot says that,

> As creative artists, we are almost obliged to look to an inner landscape and bring to the surface those experiences that are *not* comfortable, acceptable or to be neatly labelledinto any standard social model box. (1996, p. 1)

In this statement she is revealing the power of the personal as political. There is considerable pressure from within the disability movement to work together as a collective to demonstrate solidarity and a common cause. This emphasis upon cohesion and civil rights antidiscrimination campaigning sits uneasily with personal platforms. Boot recognizes this when she says that feelings will not fit neatly into a "standard social model box." Yet creativity has to include personal perspectives and inner life if it is to support growth and fulfilment.

People with learning disabilities are so often treated as deficient in basic skills and in need of training. There tends to be an emphasis on teaching them to dress, feed themselves, and cope with day-to-day simple tasks or to read and write and manage basic numeracy. This is premised on the traditional model of skills hierarchies, which assumes that basic living skills need to be learned before an individual can move on to more creative aspects of learning and living. For some people with learning disabilities, this limits them to a very constrained way of life that is composed largely of dull, repetitive tasks.

Pearson & Aloysius (1994) proved that children with severe learning disabilities were able to gain considerable value from visiting museums and art galleries. They observed and recorded the rich learning experience this opportunity offered. The children delighted in artifacts and pictures for their own sake and displayed excitement and enthusiasm in the experience. In her earlier investigation into the value of art appreciation for children with severe learning disabilities (Aloysius, 1990), Chitra Aloysius demonstrated the creative growth that aesthetic experience offered to all learners, regardless of intellectual ability.

Poetry, drama, music, dance, and filmmaking are all sources of potential empowerment through creative growth. For people with learning disabilities, their learning experiences are often of repeated failure to cope with basic skills and reaffirmation of their weaknesses. This is an oppressively disempowering process, fostering low self-image and loss of confidence. Where disability arts and a flexible, open approach to aesthetic education can be forcefully empowering is in offering experiences of self-expression that are so positive, proud, assertive, and successful. Expressing feelings, enjoying music, art, and drama, and working collaboratively to create new performances or presentations is empowering in the most subtle and profound sense. It can be energizing and exciting, opening up potential rather than closing off possibilities based on limited criteria for judging intellectual capability.

CONCLUSION: RELOCATING THE DISCOURSES OF POWER

This chapter has explored ways in which self-help groups of people working within the broad area of disability arts can empower themselves through the process of creative growth and self-expression. This includes people with learning disabilities and additional mental health problems as well as those with profound and complex needs. The use of imaginative and affirmative forms of exploring personal qualities and confirming a positive identity acts as a life-enhancing force for asserting self-worth and human dignity. Groups run by disabled people for disabled people are structured to provide mutual support, empathy, and encouragement.

Survival skills are complex and elusive. They involve a range of strategies for coping in a hostile world where competition and a market culture create tensions and economic stress. People with learning disabilities need more than just basic skills. They require that same degree of creative growth that all human beings need in order to help them develop a positive identity and connect to others. Expression for some is in poetry; for others it is in art, visual imagery, or music. Language and communication has to be understood in its widest sense, as self-expression that is personal and profound. In relation to people whose learning disabilities are complex, their communication may take the form of eye movement or body language rather than speech. To "hear" them requires intense listening skills.

In a recent explanation of the use of language relating to disability, I emphasized the need to relocate the discourses of power and to learn to listen to disempowered "voices," however unfamiliar their expression (Corbett, 1996). The disability movement in the United States and the United Kingdom has challenged the dominant discourses from medicine, psychology, and education. It has rejected their use of jargon and labeling of disabled people, neatly categorized and stereotyped into "cases" based on their conditions and classification rather than on their personal identities, qualities of character, and interests. The professional discourse is powerful for it defines, diagnoses and specifies treatment. This language alienates many disabled people, making them feel disempowered and vulnerable.

Disability arts groups can support self-expression and provide space for reflection, creative growth, and development. However, they may be unable to overcome the damage that years of poor self-esteem has engendered. The poet, James Turner (1992), expresses the pain of disempowerment in his poem "Who Stole Your Mind?" in which he says,

> Who stole your mind when you were still a child?
> Who built a fence around it, locked the gate,
> Mislaid the key, then looked at you and smiled
> A loving smile? And why? Thus domiciled
> And tamed, your thoughts—confused—would soon stagnate
> And sicken pale as covered grass. So mild,
> Obedient, you became. Your charm beguiled
> Us, hid your sadness, fear, and (later) hate. (p. 101)

The "tamed" mind is hard to enliven. For many people with learning disabilities, especially those with additional mental health problems, there is a powerful impetus to stay inside the prison of their containment because it feels safe. Empowerment is frightening. It requires courage and strong support networks. Creativity in arts groups can offer a valuable start. However, the limits of any efforts to empower are determined by the extent to which that individual has been encouraged to take on a victim role, a passive dependency, and a compliant modeling of what others define as appropriate behaviors.

REFERENCES

Aloysius, C. (1990). *Art galleries and special schools*. Unpublished master's dissertaion, University of East London.

Baxter, C., Poonia, K., Ward, L., & Nadirshaw, Z. (1990). *Double discrimination: Issues & services for people with learning difficulties from black & ethnic minority communities*. London: King's Fund.

Boot, P. (1996). Editorial. *DAIL (Disability Arts in London) Magazine, 113*, (May), 1–2.

Brown, H. (1996). Ordinary women: Issues for women with learning disabilities. *British Journal of Learning Disabilities, 24*(2), 47–51.

Cambridge, P. (1996). Assessing and meeting needs in HIV and learning disability, *British Journal of Learning Disabilities 24*(2), 52–57.

Cameron, A., & Blunden, R. (1996). Quality Assurance. In J. Harris (Ed.), *Purchasing services for people with learning disabilities, challenging behaviour and mental health needs*. Kidderminster: BILD.

Campbell, J., & Oliver, M. (1996). *Disability politics: Understanding our past, changing our future*. London: Routledge.

Chamberlain, J. (1995). Psychiatric survivors: Are we part of the disability movement? *The Disability Rag*, March/April, 1–5.

Corbett, A., Cottis, T., & Morris, S. (1996). *Witnessing, nurturing, protesting: Therapeutic responses to sexual abuse of people with learning difficulties*. London: David Fulton.

Corbett, J. (1996). *Bad-mouthing: The language of special needs*. London: Falmer Press.

Davidson-Paine, C., & Corbett, J. (1995). A double coming out: Gay men with learning disabilities. *British Journal of Learning Disabilities, 23*(4), 147–151.

Gaspari, R. (1995). We need a ghetto. *The Disability Rag*, May/June, 16–20.

Graham, C. (1994). Light opera in Scotland. *Disability Arts Magazine, 4*(4), 38.

Harris, L. (1992). Disability arts in the Republic of Ireland. *Disability Arts Magazine, 2*(3), 27–29.

James, D., Mukherjee, T., & Smith, C. (1996). Schizophrenia and learning disability. *British Journal of Learning Disabilities, 24*(3), 90–94.

Mittler, P. (1996). Laying the foundations for self-advocacy: The role of home and school. In J. Coupe O'Kane & J. Goldbert (Eds.), *Whose choice?* London: David Fulton.

Mosley, J. (1994). *You choose*. Wisbech: LDA.

Murphy, G., & Watters, C. (1996). Purchasing for people with learning disabilities, challenging behaviour and mental heath needs. In J. Harris (Ed.), *Purchasing services for people with learning disabilities, challenging behaviour and mental health needs*. Kidderminster: BILD.

Pearson, A., & Aloysius, C. (1994). *Museums and children with learning difficulties: The big foot*. London: British Museum Press.

Silverwood, A. (1992). In the North West. *Disability Arts Magazine, 2*(4), 49–51.

Speake, B., & John, H. (1994). Increasing the personal effectiveness of adults in the community. In J. Coupe O'Kane & B. Smith (Eds.), *Taking control: Enabling people with learning difficulties*. London: David Fulton.

Townsley, R., & Macadam, M. (1996). *Choosing staff: Involving people with learning difficulties in staff recruitment*. Bristol: The Policy Press.

Turner, J. (1992). Who stole your minds? In *"Survivors" Poetry From dark to light* (p. 101). London: Survivors' Press.

Wade, C. (1994). Creating a disability aesthetic in the arts. *The Disability Rag*, November/December, 29–31.

Williams, S. (1992). Theatre and disability conference. *Disability Arts Magazine, 2*(3), 38–41.

PART III

The Community

CHAPTER 10

Welcoming Immigrants With Disabilities: The Israeli Experience

STANLEY S. HERR
University of Maryland School of Law

Although immigration presents legal and public policy questions of global impact, its implications for the disability community have received scant attention. This chapter presents a case study of Israel's singular experience in opening its doors to immigrants with disabilities. It stands as a generous and humane endeavor, posing a sharp contrast to the laws and policies of the United States and many other nations. The U.S. government has long-erected barriers to entry for immigrants who disclosed their disabilities or presented visible disabilities. American immigration policies, for example, required the exclusion of immigrants with mental retardation (Herr, 1983). Even today, an alien can be excluded from the United States if he or she has "a physical or mental disorder and behavior associated with the disorder that may pose, or has posed, a threat to the property, safety, or welfare of the alien or others" (Immigration and Nationality Act, 1997). Advocates have also invoked the Americans with Disabilities Act of 1990 to challenge a lack of reasonable accommodations in citizenship testing procedures. In recent years, immigrants to the United States with HIV have become the latest group to bear the brunt of exclusionary immigration policy, treated as having a "communicable disease of public health significance" (Immigration and Nationality Act, 1997; Kidder, 1996). But their difficulties reflect the broader problem of an immigration law that served as "a preserve for prejudices about race, disability, and sexual orientation no longer considered polite in domestic discourse" (Margulies, 1994, p. 555).

Against this point of comparison, Israel's policy stands out as exceptionally generous and hospitable to persons with disabilities. Israel's open-door policy to Jewish immigrants includes immigrants with all types of mental and physical disabilities. This policy is a distinctive national feature and stands in sharp contrast to widespread exclusionary practices against such persons in other countries.

This preliminary study analyzes the unique Israeli experience in accepting and assimilating immigrants with disabilities. It also identifies some of the accomplishments made and challenges posed in the recent waves of immigrants from the former Soviet Union and Ethiopia. It concludes with recommendations for planning to foster the successful assimilation of immigrants with disabilities in their new homeland.

Despite the central importance of immigration to Israel and the continuing influx of immigrants with disabilities from various regions, no legal literature exists on this topic. Although one Hebrew-language study deals with disabilities and some English-language articles examine the psychological and mental health aspects of former-Soviet immigration and absorption (Leshem & Sor, 1994), the legal and public policy implications of disability and immigration deserve exploration. This need for research reflects both the underdevelopment of disability studies in general and of human rights research on Israelis with disabilities in particular (Herr, 1992). As Israel struggles to cope with massive waves of newcomers, Israeli society and its immigrant families are beginning to pay closer attention to the needs of immigrants with disabilities. With the slowing Jewish exodus from the former Soviet Union and the virtually complete evacuation of ethnic Jews from Ethiopia (Kaplan & Rosen, 1994), it is both possible and essential to assess how these newcomers with disabilities have fared in the immigration and post-immigration processes.

HISTORICAL AND DEMOGRAPHIC OVERVIEW

Israel's history and mission is intertwined with immigration and rescue. After World War II, some survivors of Nazi oppression—many with broken bodies, minds, and spirits—managed to enter the British-controlled Palestine Mandate. More of these refugees migrated to Israel after it became a state in 1948. Although the West German government made reparations to them in the form of monthly pensions, these payments were cash benefits and were not earmarked specifically for rehabilitation services.

Subsequent waves of Jews, expelled from Arab countries such as Yemen and Iraq, resisted Israeli attempts at disability identification, evaluation, and treatment processes. They disliked the labeling and the perceived social stigma of having a family member regarded as disabled (Herr, 1992; Shacher, 1985).

Since its founding in 1948, Israel has received over 2.3 million immigrants. Over 28% of them were natives of the former Soviet Union, and many of them arrived in the early 1990s. At its peak in 1990–1991, the rate of arrival had reached some 35,000 individuals a month (Leshem & Sor, 1994).

The Legal Process, Open-Door Policy, and Its Effects

Israeli law essentially provides an open-door policy to Jews with disabilities. Like other Jews, these immigrants enter Israel under the Law of Return. The Law of

Return (Amendment No. 2, 1970) provides that any Jew (i.e., a person born of a Jewish mother or a convert to Judaism [§4B] who is not a member of another religion) can enter and receive citizenship in Israel. This law does not distinguish between those with and those without disabilities, and thus attracts immigrants of all abilities.

The positive image Israel's health system enjoys abroad serves as an additional motivation for a number of disabled elderly persons. When faced with the option of going to the United States or Israel, some of these persons with medical problems (especially cancer) may have chosen Israel because of its promise of free medical care for immigrants.

The price of this open-door policy may have macroeconomic and other social effects that have not yet been fully assessed or even felt. Statistics suggest that younger, more affluent, and less disabled former Soviet citizens are opting for the United States. In 1988, 90% of those Jews receiving Israeli visas dropped out of that immigration process and went to Western countries. By 1993, half of those emigres still went to the West. According to Hebrew University specialist Elazar Leshem, some 25% of the immigrants, or *olim* (Jews immigrating to Israel; the singular form is *oleh*), have a family member with a disability. In contrast to the general Israeli population (hereinafter referred to as veteran Israelis), the Russian *aliyah* constitutes a more elderly population, and 5% of them receive National Insurance Institute disability benefits (Leshem, 1994). These findings reveal that immigration policies may lead to more persons with disabilities in an aging population.

The Jewish Agency (Status) Law charges the Jewish Agency with coordinating governmental and nongovernmental efforts in "gathering in the exiles," assisting "immigration to [Israel] of the masses of the people," and conducting absorption projects. In this capacity, the Jewish Agency exercises quasi-governmental functions, such as the promotion of immigration and absorption. Although the Jewish Agency has been held to be a voluntary agency, its denial of benefits and aid to a potential *oleh* is not justiciable.

The Nationality Law (1952) and its amendments imposes restrictions on entry and citizenship. For instance, the non-Jewish parents of an *oleh*'s non-Jewish spouse might seek to apply for entry under this law. Benefits would be limited (the so-called "absorption basket" would not be available) and discretion would be exercised in determining entry based on humanitarian (e.g., family unification) or other special circumstances (e.g., attachment to or "love of Israel").

Israeli case law has neither specifically addressed disability factors in immigration nor hindered the entry of persons with disabilities. Judicial controversies have centered on the question of who is a Jew under the Law of Return. The law does not adopt Halachic definitions (the religious code that recognizes the mother's religion as the determinative factor), because children of a non-Jewish mother married to a Jewish spouse are granted Law of Return status on Sholomo Aveneri's theory that they are in solidarity with the Jewish people. Thus, the Law of Return (Amendment No. 2, 1970) also vests citizenship to anyone who is a child, grandchild, or spouse of a Jew, or the spouse of a child or grand-child of a Jew (§ 4 A.[a]). Similarly, a Jew who converts from Judaism forfeits this status, as he or she has voluntarily separated from the Jewish people. Cases have established that entries by non-Jews are subject to the complete discretion of the Ministry of the Interior. However, the courts have also denied entry to Jewish in-dividuals with records of dangerous criminal activity, and to so-called "messianic Jews" (*Lansky v. Minister of the Interior,* 1972).

Some 12,000 non-Jews enter Israel every year to become citizens. Like the Jewish immigrants, disability per se is not grounds for denying them entry. How-ever, since immigration is a privilege and not a right under the Law of Entry (in contrast to the Law of Return), officials need not offer any reason for denying cit-izenship to non-Jews, and presumably a disabled person could be denied citizen-ship without knowing whether disability played a factor in the decision.

Advocacy groups are not aware of individuals making legal claims of discrim-ination based on disability in any phase of immigration and absorption activity. For instance, the Association for Civil Rights in Israel (ACRI) has not been ap-proached by complainants citing problems with disabilities or with conditions of public health significance seeking redress. Nor has ACRI encountered any judi-cial case decided on the basis of the Law of Return's public health exception. Similarly, very few administrative proceedings arise in which a prospective en-trant is challenged due to a public health risk or a disability, such as tuberculosis or serious mental illness.

ACRI does, however, report one positive case involving a new immigrant liv-ing in northern Israel who was totally disabled and who sought home-based care. No one was willing to treat him, but after an administrative appeal and with a fa-vorable atmosphere for resolution, the Welfare Ministry agreed to obtain serv-ices for him.

Immigrants with disabilities may often be overlooked in the crush of new ar-rivals. In 1990 and 1991, 375,617 immigrants entered the country. This total in-cluded 341,792 from Europe, 24,719 from Africa, 7,338 from North America, and 1,562 from Asia (Weinraub, 1993). Since 1989, immigrants from the former Soviet Union alone amounted to over 500,000 (Israel Foreign Ministry, 1994), 66,000 of whom (13%) were over the age of 65. Israel has seen waves of immi-grants since its founding but never of this magnitude.

This mass influx of people in such a short time has profoundly challenged the Israeli government and society. Critics such as Robert Golan, leader of the Soviet Olim Association for the Disabled, condemned delays and the lack of govern-ment preparedness in meeting the particular needs of disabled immigrants (Fried, 1993).

To better understand the difficulties and dilemmas facing immigrants with disabilities, it is necessary to examine the process by which they enter Israel, the problems associated with their absorption, and to explore some possible reme-dies. Israel's population, now numbering 5.4 million (Haberman & Hedges, 1993), strains existing Israeli disability services, health care, and employment resources. The new arrivals from the former Soviet Union include disproportionately large numbers of elderly, disabled, and seriously ill migrants when compared to veteran Israelis.

Many immigrants with disabilities face poverty, joblessness, and despair. The Sarashevski family illustrates some of the problems confronting immigrants with disabilities. Vitali Sarashevski, with his wife and two children, left the former Soviet Union in the early 1990s to find a better life in Israel. Vitali, an aircraft engineer disabled since childhood, could barely walk. As a result of a car accident, his wife is also disabled. Neither Vitali nor his wife were able to find a job. They relied on the Israeli government to help them provide for their family, but the "absorption basket" of benefits did not offer them supplemental help based on their disability. Instead, the Israeli support system provided for Vitali and his family. In the past, when he asked for more money to help feed his family a clerk at the unemployment office coldly told him, "we don't need handicapped people in Israel . . . we need children." Vitali did not receive an unemployment check one month because he was not physically able to walk to the unemployment office to present himself eight separate times per month as required by regulations (Fried, 1993). The Sarashevskis, like many other immigrants with disabilities, struggled to cope with scarce resources and abundant red tape.

The Ethiopian newcomers, in contrast to Russians like Sarashevski, proved healthier and experienced proportionately fewer disabilities than other immigrant groups. This phenomenon is attributed to circumstances in Ethiopia that limited disabled persons from surviving, or at least from traveling. Commenting on Operation Moses, the 1984–1985 airlift from Sudan, Ethiopians who reached Israel reported that they left some elderly or other frail family members behind because they could not have managed the long trek to staging areas.

Compared to immigration policies for Jews who are considered "endangered," Jews from Western countries may be viewed more selectively by Jewish Agency officials. Those officials may seek to discourage a sick or disabled person from coming as an *oleh* on the grounds that the pre-existing condition may make health insurance difficult to obtain or that Israel's publicly funded welfare and health services are already overburdened. Although the Jewish Agency as a private organization can withhold loans or aid in the pre-immigration stage, the Law of Return precludes a Jew with a disability from being denied entry by Ministry of Interior officials.

Pre-*Aliyah* Process and Disability

The immigration process does not involve any formal screening for disabilities. Nor does disability status appear to play a significant role in the pre-*aliyah* contacts with prospective immigrants or their ability to obtain permission to leave their former countries. Due to persecution, endangered status, or political constraints on exiting certain countries, Jewish refugees had to navigate through the bureaucracies of both Israel and their former countries.

Under the Soviet regime, the prospective emigrant faced a three-step obstacle course to gaining an exit visa to Israel. He or she first needed an invitation from a close relative who lived in Israel. The Soviet Ministry of Interior then decided whether or not to issue a passport for external travel. The authorities could deny such exit requests on the basis of the applicant's having "poor relatives" who would be left behind or because the applicant had knowledge of vaguely defined "state secrets." Finally, the applicant would have to travel to Moscow for a personal interview with Israeli consular officials to obtain a visa.

The dissolution of the Soviet Union led to more liberalized and convenient exit processes, with the opening of Israeli embassies in ten newly formed countries of the Commonwealth of Independent States, as well as consular offices in St. Petersburg and Odessa. Now, a visa applicant no longer has to travel vast distances to reach Moscow and visas are now generally granted on the same day as the personal interview. Since April 1993, the Russian government has dropped the requirement of an invitation from a relative. Most significant for this study, according to an official in Israel's Washington embassy, is that disability status is not a factor in the permission-to-emigrate process. The official knew of no obstacles placed in the way of families or individuals with disabilities. Although he conceded that some Jewish Agency officials might informally discourage some older persons from undertaking the rigors of migration, he concluded that a family with a disabled child would pose no problem, and would be well received in Israel.

With respect to barriers imposed from the Russian side, the Israeli official was not aware of any emigrant being denied permission to leave on the basis of the "poor relatives" grounds and a claim that a relative with a disability was being abandoned. When they do arise, such cases are raised by private citizens seeking to settle old scores rather than by government officials fearing custodial obligations being thrust upon them.

Although the National Conference on Soviet Jewry expects some 60,000 to 70,000 persons to depart for Israel over the course of a year, turmoil in the former Soviet Union may increase the flow of migrants. In fact, 68,000 of Israel's 82,000 immigrants in the Jewish year ending in September 1995 were from the former Soviet Union (Israel Foreign Ministry, 1995b). No specific information is available on the percentage of people with disabilities currently in the "immigration pipeline." According to Dr. Murray Feshbach, a demographer at the Georgetown University Center for Population Research and a specialist on the former Soviet Union, Soviet immigrants were once disproportionately elderly as a group, but many have left by now (Feshbach & Friendly, 1992). This suggests that the precipitating factor in a Russian's decision to leave tends to be deterioration of conditions at home rather than the allure of better health and disability services abroad.

The Ethiopian migration, in contrast to that from the former Soviet Union, has yielded a younger group with a different constellation of health, educational, and disability service needs. Of the nearly 45,000 Ethiopian Jewish immigrants from 1972 to 1993, 46% were aged 18 and under, 36% were aged 19–44, 11% were 45–64, and 7% were aged 65 and older (Kaplan & Rosen, 1994, p. 70). As of January 1996, the Ministry of Absorption estimated that some 56,000 Ethiopian Jews lived in Israel (Israel Foreign Ministry, 1996).

The process involved the prospective immigrant making contact with the Israeli Consul, as this individual would fax the application to the Jewish Agency in Israel. That office then transmitted these materials to the Interior Ministry, which determined the authenticity of the would-be *oleh*'s claim of Jewish status under the Law of Return. It is estimated that 300 to 400 Bet Israel (Falashas) Jews remain in Ethiopia; another 25,000 Ethiopian "Falashmuras" are descended from families who converted to Judaism in the past. The fate of these individuals is hotly debated in Israel. Former Absorption Minister Tsaban had supported the cause of liberalized entry, and the Israeli cabinet has adopted the Tsaban Committee's recommendation that some Falashmuras should be allowed to come to Israel on humanitarian grounds of family reunification (Kaplan & Rosen, 1994). From August 1993 to June 1995, some 2050 Ethiopians arrived in Israel, 60% under the Law of Return and the rest under the Law of Entry (Israel Foreign Ministry, 1995a).

Operation Solomon brought 14,400 Ethiopians to Israel in May 1991, and nearly 6,000 others have since followed. It is estimated that less than 1% of the total Ethiopian migration (200–250 persons) are HIV-positive. While potential migrants must wait in Addis Ababa to have their papers processed, the Joint Distribution Committee (JDC) provides them with intensive public health education, including illustrated booklets in Amharic on methods of preventing the spread of HIV/AIDS, such as safe sex.

Although no precise data exists, JDC officials believe that few Ethiopians arrive in Israel with traditional physical or mental disabilities. Nevertheless, interest in disabled Ethiopians has begun to stir. Ellen Goldberg, Area Head for Ethiopian Absorption in JDC's Israel Office, described it as "a hot topic" that has generated a pilot survey. After two Ethiopian children with serious disabilities were discovered and treated at Alyn Hospital in central Israel two years after their entry in the country, the hospital decided to reach out to others who remained untreated. To identify additional disabled Ethiopians, hospital officials sent notices in Hebrew and Amharic to the directors of caravan sites (temporary home parks) that the hospital was willing to receive referrals from and to consult with interested persons. In May 1993, hospital staff discussed specific cases uncovered in a survey at one mobile home site, Bet Ha'sur. Of the 1,620 Ethiopians and 6,880 Russians at the site, 43 were identified as seriously disabled, including 13 adults with mental retardation, 8 children with mental retardation, 19 adults with physical disabilities, and 3 children with physical disabilities. Social workers also diagnosed a "high proportion" of persons with mental illnesses. JDC staff assumed that this 2% incidence of severe disability was encountered in the entire sheltered population of immigrants (which then included 12,000 people in caravan sites and 1,500 in hotels).

Although the Law of Return permits individuals posing public health risks to be barred from entry, this exception has not been applied to Ethiopians or other endangered Jews. For example, a couple that received permission to immigrate consisted of a 70+-year-old man with tuberculosis and his 40+-year-old pregnant wife. In such cases, JDC workers in the field fax the details of the case to Israel where advance preparations will be made to receive the patient.

Unlike Jews from Russia and Ethiopia, immigrants from the West may be subjected to greater scrutiny and a type of informal, unofficial screening. The Israeli public and some government officials are wary of potential immigrants who are mentally unstable, whose families may be seeking to "unload" them on Israeli authorities, or who may be seeking immigrant status as a subterfuge for short-term entry for medical treatment. As previously noted, the Jewish Agency will not approve *aliyah* in such instances. For example, if an individual is receiving dialysis treatment under England's free national health service but otherwise lacks the means for payment of such treatment, the agency would discourage him or her from migrating. Western applicants are asked to sign a declaration disclosing whether they are HIV-positive, have tuberculosis, or have any other specified condition. In theory, a false negative reply could be grounds for deportation. In practice, civil libertarians know of no such cases and Health Ministry officials acknowledge that the self-reporting declaration is not an effective screen.

In the final days of the Shamir government, the Israeli ministries of the Interior, Health, and Absorption floated a controversial proposal to test potential *olim* from the West for AIDS. If the Ministry of Health declares any disease or condition a dangerous communicable disease, its director-general has broad powers to regulate it. In November 1987, AIDS was given this label in the official gazette of government actions. Still, the director-general proceeded with caution in taking specific measures, concerned both with protecting civil liberties and with avoiding censure from the World Health Organization. In 1991, a new director-general, determined to limit the number of HIV-positive cases in Israel, considered imposing restrictions on immigrants, students, and long-stay foreign workers. In January 1992, however, the Knesset Absorption Committee of Israel Parliament reacted negatively and strenuously to any proposal that would test *olim* from Western countries or in any way interfere with the Russian or Ethiopian *aliyahs*. According to Yora Kranot of the Ministry of Health, the Absorption Committee's parliamentary members shouted at government officials, arguing that every effort should be made to bring immigrants to Israel. This uproar and subsequent protest in the media and by American Jewish organizations blocked the adoption of new restrictions.

The AIDS controversy posed a politically delicate dilemma for the Israeli government. On the one hand, relevant ministries are charged with protecting the Israeli people. They act under broad public health laws that date from the British Palestinian Mandate as well as the Israeli Penal Code, amended in 1977, that made the carrier punishable for the negligent or malicious spread of a communicable disease. On the other hand, these officials are mindful of the privacy, human rights, and *aliyah* promotion considerations that run contrary to mandatory testing. The Zionist imperative is so strong that government officials feel they must save the Ethiopians even if the immigrants include "sick people." According to one official, "you even forget it if they have TB."

Because the United States and some Western European countries have higher rates of AIDS than Israel, and because testing facilities exist in the West but not in the lands where the endangered Jews of Africa and the East live, the Ministry of Health continues to study this problem. Complaints in the Knesset, the media, and from other critics have stopped proposals to restrict immigrants.

If measures to restrict the entry of HIV-positive immigrants should arise, ACRI has declared that it will take legal action to invalidate those restrictions. ACRI holds that AIDS, or HIV, is not per se a contagious disease because, in the words of its spokesman, "it is not passed through the air." According to this view, such a proposal would be illegal under the Law of Return.

POST-IMMIGRATION SUPPORT AND INTEGRATION

Theory of Direct Absorption

Immigrants with disabilities may experience difficulties in entering the Israeli mainstream. Under the theory of direct absorption, immigrants proceed directly from the airport to an independent living situation. At the airport, they receive money, written materials, and the opportunity to telephone relatives to arrange family support. Those with no relatives are placed in temporary housing like hotels or shelters. On the following day, the new arrivals appear at the local office of the Ministry of Absorption where the determination is made whether a member of the family has a disability or major illness. There are a number of incentives to self-identification since, as one ministry official described it, this status is "a catalyst to an apartment solution." Between 6,000 and 7,000 public housing units are available for new migrants, and persons with disabilities received top priority in the assignment process. Workers in local offices also make referrals to welfare, health, and other local social services and are responsible for coordinating these forms of support. The Absorption Ministry provides a few direct services workers, but many lack specialized training and its welfare department has only one social worker.

Regulations by the Ministry of Labour and Social Affairs also outlined how immigrants with disabled should be absorbed. Disabled immigrants who do not need special services and facilities "should be integrated into the normative local networks to which they have been directly absorbed" (State of Israel Ministry of Labour and Social Affairs, 1990, p. 26). Those who need special rehabilitation services are to be integrated into existing services for Israelis with disabilities, but the Ministry recognized the need for "expanding the infrastructure and building new facilities for the disabled population" (State of Israel Ministry of Labour and Social Affairs, 1990, p. 26). The thrust of these regulations, however, emphasized making community-based services accessable to immigrants who are blind, deaf, retarded, or otherwise disabled. Those enumerated services included diagnostic centers, training day-care centers, therapeutic day-care centers, and supported services at home for immigrants with mental retardation as well as a variety of rehabilitative services for deaf and blind immigrants.

Although direct absorption is perceived as working well for two-thirds of the immigrants, such absorptions are not as effective for the remainder who are disabled, elderly, or over age 50 and unable to find work. Absorption Ministry officials recognize the need to build a system for the hard-to-assimilate minority who need special programs. These immigrants need help in applying for and receiving apartments, in finding work, in applying for welfare, and in obtaining rehabilitation services. With the candid admission that "direct absorption is not well-suited" for this segment of new Israelis, ministry officials recognize the tremendous need to retrain local office workers with "multidisciplinary perspectives" so that they may assist migrant individuals in gaining various disability and related services. They report a process of restructuring their day-to-day operations to improve coordination and remedy these problems.

Some government policy initiatives recognize the need for programs and preferences for disabled populations. Few are directed to the needs of immigrants with disabilities. These include special instructions from the Ministry of Labour and Social Affairs, promulgated in July 1992, to define the rights and treatment of disabled immigrants. These instructions to its employees include policy statements and call for integration of new Israelis with veteran Israelis in disability services in welfare and employment fields. They also initiate transitional services to bridge cultural or linguistic gaps for some groups and reserve certain services for the newcomers. Other policies provide linguistic translations or interpreter assistance for the exams and assessments of new migrants, with short-term separation from veteran Israelis for assessment and treatment purposes.

Scattered pilot projects also offer some special programs for persons with disabilities. Examples of these pilot or special projects include:

- Treasury Ministry funding for reserved places in mental retardation institutions, sheltered workshops, and day centers for new immigrants;
- housing for the elderly, with a 50-unit project in Ashkelon and 1,000 units in a planned retirement village; and
- placements in a school for the deaf in Jerusalem as well as support and

Hebrew sign-language training for 300–400 deaf immigrants of predominately Russian background.

Private agencies have an array of proposals and modest initiatives underway. For instance, the JDC is assisting deaf Russian women to market their tailoring or handicrafts. JDC and other nonprofit organizations are also starting self-help groups for new immigrants with disabilities such as orientation classes in Beer-sheva for parents and others coping with the effects of disabilities and the difficulties of their new lives in Israel. Dr. Alex Kozulin, a Russian-born psychiatrist working with the renowned learning theorist Reuven Fuerstein, is involved in the assessment of 300 immigrant children with special needs (Kozulin, 1993). Finally, AKIM Jerusalem (a nonprofit agency delivering mental retardation services) proposed a diagnostic center for Russian and other immigrants with developmental disabilities. This would ensure a full evaluation of the individual with disability and provide family counselling and guidance as to placement options (AKIM, 1990a).

Special education appears to be a bright spot in the services available to migrant children. Compared to the low standard of such education in the former Soviet Union and its virtual absence in Ethiopia, these disabled children (to age 21) receive tremendously improved treatment and education.

The potential pitfalls facing newcomers with disabilities are manifold. To be a foreigner starting over in a new country poses a challenge in itself. But the crisis of being absorbed with a "dual disability" in a new society, of coping with both a pre-existing physical or mental disability in addition to immigrant status, is substantially harder. The migrant with a disability faces not only the usual difficulties in overcoming language and cultural barriers, but also bureaucratic obstacles when seeking disability services that are already in short supply. Due to cultural differences, Russian immigrants, for instance, may not wish to talk about social problems in front of children, or they may strongly fear and oppose institutionalization. Their suspicion of authority and the harsh reputation of Russia's institutions may cause them to view sending a family member to an institution as tantamount to lifelong banishment. Other cultural differences and insensitive testing procedure may result in the over-identification of Ethiopian or Sephardi children as disabled.

Families with disabled members may confront other difficulties in accessing disability services. They may be physically isolated in development towns far removed from sophisticated services (AKIM, 1996). Another difficulty is that immigrants are more capable of claiming monetary benefits that are entitlements than of obtaining community-based services that are discretionary.

The crisis of absorption for disabled migrants may be particularly acute in the second year, after the initial optimism wanes and as social problems become more apparent. In Tel Aviv, the sight of homeless immigrants has generated concern for, and media attention to, homelessness as a social problem. Migrants have also recorded high rates of medical service usage, particularly the cancer victims of Chernobyl, with 45% of all Russians classified by a *Histradut* report as high users of medical services. Unless migrants with disabilities receive targeted and continuing aid, they may join the ranks of Israel's growing underclass (Lo-Lordo, 1998.)

Critiques of Israel's efforts, however, must be tempered by a recognition of the relative liberality of those efforts compared to nations of far greater wealth. For example, the United States, in a time of unparalleled prosperity and peace, has chosen to drastically reduce the aid it offers its legal migrants. Expressions of xenophobia and political unpopularity have led to harsh cutbacks in aid for legal aliens. Under the guise of welfare reform , 930,000 legal aliens were stripped of food stamps (Vobejda & Jeter, 1997), Supplemental Security Income (SSI), and related benefits under the Personal Responsibility and Work Opportunity Reconciliation Act of 1996. Although Congress, in response to tales of suffering, restored SSI eligibility for certain qualified aliens who were disabled and lawfully residing in the United States on August 26, 1996 (Immigration and Nationality Act, 1996), federal food stamps still remain out of reach. Thirteen states moved to stave off hunger by using their own funds to keep nutrition benefits intact for their legal immigrants. In 1998, the Clinton administration proposed and Congress restored food stamps to many legal immigrants with disabilities. Thus, the administration's budget presented to Congress sought $2.5 billion to provide food stamps over the next five years to hundreds of thousands of legal immigrants (Dao, 1998). A senior official noted that with a strong economy and fiscal discipline, "we can be a little more generous now" (Goldstein & Harris, 1998). In contrast, Israel has always tried to provide its newcomers with a generous basket of aid.

CONCLUSION

Although in places valiant efforts are being made, immigrants with disabilities must overcome many obstacles before they can fully participate in Israeli society. It often takes newcomers several years to recognize the need for, and ultimately find, disability services appropriate for a family member with a mild or moderate disability. For a family that must care for a disabled individual, the family may become dysfunctional if it is unable to quickly obtain adequate care-giving support.

Israel needs a systemic plan to help immigrants with disabilities adjust to and succeed in their new home. The plan's elements should include:

- Training immigration officials to identify individuals with disabilities and make appropriate early referrals for support and assistance;
- Training and hiring Russian- and Amharic-speaking social workers to help their compatriots with disabilities and counsel them on available services;
- Training physicians and other health-care providers to screen newly arrived immigrants for disabilities, and conduct or make referrals for appropriate assessments and treatment;

- Providing access to advocacy services, such as the Israel Human Rights Center for People with Disabilities (Bizchut), ACRI, and other agencies;
- Launching a media campaign to raise public awareness of the needs, rights, and resource centers for immigrants with disabilities, and educating such immigrants and their families on the value of accepting specialized services;
- Reducing unnecessary red tape, such as special applications for Social Security for those with full or partial disabilities (that would require less frequent reevaluation for benefits);
- Developing individualized adapted learning plans for adults with disabilities, including the use of computers to aid in teaching Hebrew and other forms of intensive help for immigrants with disabilities who cannot go to classrooms or who may learn at different rates;
- Sensitizing school personnel to recognize learning needs of immigrants with disabilities and to correctly classify those students whose needs arise from disabilities rather than from simple cultural differences;
- Protecting immigrants with disabilities from excessive or exploitative rents so that they can have affordable housing and meet other expenses from the "absorption basket" subsidies;
- Placing immigrants who need specialist services and therapies in urban population centers rather than in remote areas far from essential services and facilities;
- Providing special transportation services adapted to persons with disabilities who cannot use generic transportation services;
- Improving existing laws and their implementation to better meet the needs of all Israelis with disabilities; and
- Enacting the recommendations of the Shnit Committee to revise developmental disabilities law and to secure full passage of an antidiscrimination law governing employment, public services, and public accommodations, now before the Knesset in 1998 (The Equal Rights for People with Disabilites Law covering employment, enacted in February 1998, is due to come into effect in January 1999).

The achievement of these fundamental goals will require that immigrants with disabilities and their families turn to the political process in Israel. These individuals could join with veteran Israelis in an umbrella advocacy organization for people with disabilities. Such an organization could have considerable influence if it could elect members to Israel's parliament, given the narrow margins on which a governing coalition hinges in the Knesset. In the meantime, immigrants can look to existing disability organizations, as well as organizations promoting the interests of immigrants, for political support and mobilization.

Experts on absorption sum up the settled political understandings on disabled immigrants in these terms: "it is all part of the deal." Whether as family members or as single persons, immigrants with disabilities are free to enter. As a result of its Zionist commitments, Israel confers a constitutional right to every Jew to become an Israeli citizen. The inclusiveness of this pledge is a testament to the strength and vision of the Israeli political leadership. It is a human rights approach consistent with the egalitarian premises of the United Nations Declaration on the Rights of Disabled Persons in 1975.

The Israeli experience with disabled migrants is also framed by its distinctive history and ongoing conflicts. It is part of Israel's mission to embrace Jewish immigrants. In emphasizing the geopolitical motives for this unrestricted immigration, Yale history professor Paul Kennedy noted that "even the Israel-Palestinian quarrel has become an issue of demography, with the influx of Soviet Jews intended to counter the greater fertility of the Palestinians" (Kennedy, 1993).

Yet this policy of unrestricted right of entry is not without costs. In the view of some specialists, it may well prove a "time bomb" as the demographics of aging and an increasingly disabled population place high demands on health and welfare services. Furthermore, unless Israeli society can create new jobs and improve the quality of life for its immigrants, the "crisis of absorption" could aggravate mental health problems and lead to the further deterioration in the overall health and well-being of these newcomers. And as the three-year period for the migrant's subsidies draws to a close, new stresses could destabilize families that have members with disabilities. This consequence can and must be avoided. By reorganizing and attending to the special needs of these immigrants and their families, Israel can fulfill its highest purpose—to offer a homeland where each individual can enjoy a life of dignity and freedom.

It can also offer an inspiring example to other nations. At a time of heightened international interest in immigration policy and domestic calls for greater restrictions on aliens (Popeo, 1998; Miller, 1994; Haberman, 1994), Israel's embrace of immigrants with disabilities stands out as both compassionate and courageous. In a world in which the 500 million people with mental, physical, or sensory impairment suffer discrimination and disproportionate poverty, this huge minority looks for societies that model inclusion. While the United Nations proclaims that this group "possess[es] an enormous reservoir of talent and energy that must be tapped" (Annan, 1997), individuals with disabilities wait for countries to act consistently with that belief. The Israeli experience is a step in that direction that deserves further study and emulation.

ACKNOWLEDGMENTS

The author gratefully acknowledges the support of a summer research fellowship from the University of Maryland School of Law, the research assistance of Joshua Udler and Jonathan Grossman, and the encouragement of Dean Donald G. Gifford. Thanks are especially due to the many specialists who agreed to be interviewed for the study, including Ariela Auphir, Attorney, Bizchut (Israel Human Rights Center for People with Disabilities); Ruth Bello, Coordinator, Association of Soviet Immigrants in Israel; Ami Bergman, Area Director for Turkey and Egypt, JDC; Ram Ca'aan, Professor, School of Social Work, University of Pennsylvania, Philadelphia; Aron Fine, Director, Observation Institute; Pesach Gitelman, then Head of Department for Handicapped and Social Work, JDC; Ellen Goldberg, Area Head for Ethiopian Absorption, JDC; Neta Ziv, Director of Litigation, ACRI; Dorit Karlin, Assistant to Minister of Absorption Tsaban; Yorn Kranot, Legal Adviser, Ministry of Health; Elazar Leshem, Adjunct Lecturer, Hebrew University & Tel Aviv University Social Work Schools (formerly Deputy General-Director, Ministry of Absorption); Miriam Levinger, Lecturer, Tel Aviv University Shapell School; Basil Porter, Director, Child Development Center, Siroka Hospital, Beersheva; Arik Rimmerman, Dean, Faculty of Social Welfare and Health Studies, Haifa University; Sarah Sadounik, Director, Residential Services; Amir Schwartz, Head Social Worker, Mental Retardation Service; Chaya Schwartz, Lecturer, School of Social Work Bar-Ilan University; Dan Shnit, Professor, Tel Aviv University Shapell School of Social Work; Joshua Shoffman, Legal Director, ACRI; Ari Stanger, Legal Adviser, Ministry of Health; Eran Tauss, Adviser to Ministry of Absorption Tsaban. I also owe appreciation to the Tel Aviv University's Bob Shapell School of Social Work and the Association for Civil Rights in Israel for their co-sponsorship of my seminar on disability advocacy, which enabled me to travel to Israel and to counduct these interviews.

REFERENCES

AKIM (Israeli Association for the Rehabilitation of the Mentally Handicapped, Jerusalem). (1990a). *Diagnostic Center for the Evaluation and Observation of the New Immigrant with Developmental Disability.* Unpublished proposal.

AKIM (Israeli Association for the Rehabilitation of the Mentally Handicapped, Jerusalem). (1990b). *The Russian immigrant with developmental disability: Stages towards a solution.* Unpublished proposal.

Americans with Disabilities Act of 1990, 42 U.S.C. §§ 12101-12213 (1994).

Annan, K. (1998, December 3). *Secretary-General's message on International Day of Disabled Persons cites discrimination against "world's largest minority."*

Dao, J. (1998, Feb. 2). Aliens would get food stamps back in Clinton budget. *New York Times,* A1.

Feshbach, M., & Friendly, A. (1992). *Ecocide in the USSR: Health and nature under seige.* New York: Basic Books.

Fried, S. (1993, Jan. 19). Handicapped immigrants hobbled by the absence of special assistance. *The Jerusalem Post,* 5.

Goldstein, A., & Harris, J. (1998, Jan. 3). Clinton to ask for expansion of social aid; Budget proposals would affect food stamps, Medicare benefits. *Washington Post,* A1.

Haberman, C. (1994, Oct. 6). "Lost Tribe" has Israelis pondering Law of Return. *New York Times,* A3.

Haberman, C., & Hedges, C. (1993, Sept. 18). Key to Israel-P.L.O pact is seen in economic ties, *New York Times,* A1.

Herr, S. (1983). *Rights and advocacy for retarded people.* Lexington, MA: Lexington Books.

Herr, S. (1992). Human rights and mental disability: Perspectives on Israel. *Israel Law Review, 26,* 142–194.

Immigration and Nationality Act. (1997). 8 U.S.C. § 1182 (a) (1) (A) (iii) (I) (Supp. 1997).

Immigration and Nationality Act. (1996). 8 U.S.C. § 1612 (a) (2) (f).

Israel Foreign Ministry. (1994). 500,000 immigrants from former Soviet Union since 1989. Information Division, Jerusalem, June 2, 1994. Available: http://www.israel-mfa.gov.il.

Israel Foreign Ministry. (1995a). Ministry of Absorption. Israel continuing to absorb thousands of Ethiopians. Information Division, Jerusalem, June 20, 1995. Available: http://www.israel-mfa.gov.il.

Israel Foreign Ministry. (1995b). Jewish Agency. Alliyah up 9% over the last year. Information Division, Jerusalem, September 28, 1995. Available: http://www.israel-mfa.gov.il.

Israel Foreign Ministry. (1996). Ministry of Absorption. The absorption of Ethiopian immigrants in Israel: The present situation and future objectives. Information Division, Jerusalem, January 1996. Available: http://www.israel-mfa.gov.il.

Israel Penal Code §218 (1977).

Jewish Agency (Status) Law. (1952). Laws of the State of Israel 3 §§ 1, 3–5.

Kaplan, S., & Rosen, C. (1994). Ethiopian Jews in Israel. In D. Singer & R. R. Selden, (Eds.), *American Jewish Yearbook, 94.* 59.

Kennedy, P. (1993). *Preparing for the twenty-first century.* New York: Random House.

Kidder, R. (1996). Administrative discretion gone awry: The reintroduction of the public charge exclusion for HIV-positive refugees and asylees. *Yale Law Journal, 106,* 389–422.

Kozulin, A. (1993). Psychological and learning problems of immigrant children from the former Soviet Union. *Journal of Jewish Communal Service, 70,* 64–72.

Lansky v. Minister of the Interior, 26(2) P.D. 337 (1972) (Isr.).

The Law of Return, Laws of the State of Israel 4:114, 5710–1950.

The Law of Return (Amendment No. 2), Sefer-Ha-Chukkin No. 586:34, 5730–1970.

Leshem, E. (1994). *The Russian aliyah during the 1990s.* Jerusalem: Henrietta Szold Institute.

Leshem, E., & Sor, D. (Eds.). (1994). *Immigration and absorption of former-Soviet Union Jewry: Selected bibliography and abstracts 1990–1993.* Jerusalem: Henrietta Szold Institute and the Hebrew University of Jerusalem.

LoLordo, A. (1998, Jan. 15). David Levy's Israel is out of work, poorer: Ex-foreign minister is rooted in places prosperity spurned. *Baltimore Sun,* A1.

Margulies, P. (1994). Asylum, intersectionality, and AIDS: Women with HIV as a persecuted social group. *Georgetown Immigration Law Journal 8,* 521–555.

Miller, M. (Ed.). (1994). *Strategies for immigration control: An international comparison.* Thousand Oaks, CA: Sage Periodicals Press.

Nationality Law, Laws of the State of Israel 6:50, 5712–1952.

Personal Responsibility and Work Opportunity Reconciliation Act of 1996, 8 U.S.C. § 1183 (a).

Popeo, D. (1998, Jan. 21). Illegal immigration and American lawyerland [paid opinion piece]. *New York Times,* A21.

Shacher, Y. (1985). Culture, insanity, and the right to be wrong. *Israel Yearbook on Human Rights, 15,* 204–223.

Shnit Committee. (1993). *Report to the Minister of Labour & Social Affairs on Revision of Mental Retardation and Other Developmental Disabilities Laws* (in Hebrew).

State of Israel Ministry of Labour and Social Affairs, Bulletin of the Director General. (1990, Dec. 30). *Regulations and announcements: Direct immigrant absorption by municipal authorities.* Jerusalem.

United Nations Declarations on the Rights of Disabled Persons (1975). G.A. Res. 3447, 30 U.N. GAOR, Supp, (No. 34) 92, U.N. Doc. A/10034.

Vobejda, B., & Jeter, J. (1997, Aug. 22). Though welfare rolls are down, true test of reform is just starting, experts say. *Washington Post,* A13.

Weinraub, Y. (1993). *The Jewish Agency and Aliyah: An Update.* Jewish Agency Pamphlet.

An International Perspective on School-To-Work Systems and the Participation of Persons With Disabilities

JAMES M. BROWN
University of Minnesota

JAN N. STREUMER
University of Twente
Enschede, The Netherlands

The School-to-Work Opportunity Act of 1994 (P.L. 103-239; hereafter, STWOA), which was signed into law in the U.S. on May 4, 1994, calls for major restructuring and significant systemic changes. These changes are intended to facilitate the creation of a universally available, high-quality, school-to-work transition system that enables all students in the U.S. to successfully enter and function within work settings. The STWOA makes special reference to the conviction that all students have equal opportunity to participate in systems advocated by the STWOA. In addition, the participation of youth with disabilities in various programs of the act must be guided by the already-established transition service requirements of Part B of the Individuals with Disabilities Education Act (IDEA; Pub. L. No. 101-476) (National Transition Network, 1994).

The lack of a comprehensive and effective school-to-work transition system in the United States has had a serious impact on many students. It also means significant costs to business and our economy as a whole. A skill-deficient workforce hampers the nation's economic growth, productivity, and ability to compete in an international economy. In recognition of these problems, "school-to-work transition" has become the catchphrase for American education in the 1990s (Charner, 1996a, p. 1). Recent efforts to effectively address the STWOA in terms of its implications for individuals with disabilities have precipitated an interest in the nature of effective school-to-work-related reform efforts within the U.S. as

well as in other countries throughout the world. This chapter examines factors
believed to impact school-to-work initiatives internationally. It also examines research data from the Netherlands that give a unique perspective on the evolution
and current status of school-to-work transition reform efforts in a European context. Before beginning this discussion, the following section sprovide a general
definition of the school-to-work concept.

DEFINITION OF SCHOOL-TO-WORK

School-to-work initiatives represent multistakeholder partnerships comprised of
schools (pre-kindergarten through university), families, business and industry,
government, and community-based organizations. Within schools, attention is
on all students, all subject areas of the curriculum, and all staff. STWOA specifies
that school-to-work systems should provide three types of learning opportunities: (a) school-based learning, (b) work-based learning, and (c) connecting activities. This chapter focuses on the work-based component of school-to-work systems and the implications of that component for persons with disabilities within
the U.S. and selected European settings.

By design, the STWOA views work settings as environments within which academic and occupational learning experiences are effectively integrated. This flexibility affords all students, including students with disabilities, multiple options
and opportunities for learning in applied community-based settings (National
Transition Network, 1994, p. 6).

The STWOA encourages multipartnership stakeholders to actively engage in
discussions regarding the interrelationship of the STWOA to the transition service provisions of IDEA (National Transition Network, 1994). This interaction
between two major federal legislative initiatives provides a clear motivation to
examine school-to-work issues and practices both within the U.S. and elsewhere.
The remainder of this chapter will seek to identify and examine some of those
major school-to-work issues and practices.

ONGOING CHANGES IN THE WORK FORCE

School-to-work efforts are not limited exclusively to educators, nor to the U.S.
School-to-work initiatives are complex endeavors that are tied to economic, political, and social issues, many of which are international in nature. Tomervik
(1994) recently noted that powerful changes related to population demographics, technological growth, and the global nature of today's international economy have made it essential for many components of our society to reexamine
the policies, programs, and practices that are impacted by these changes. Business and education leaders have been facing the unavoidable challenge of ac-

commodating changes in the economy, the work place, and the work force for over a decade (Johnston & Packer, 1987). Tomervik (1994) also reported that these changes have fostered the development of a new organizational development focus within businesses that has been discussed by numerous other researchers (Cox & Nkomo, 1990; Jamieson & O'Mara, 1991; Loden & Rosener, 1991; Thomas, 1990, 1991). These emerging efforts focused on accommodating the increasing diversity encountered within work settings range from "system wide management approaches to short-term training activities focused on acknowledging, appreciating, valuing, and managing work force diversity" (Tomervik, 1994, p. 2). A wide variety of researchers have suggested that the nature of the workforce is one of the greatest challenges impacting today's workplace (Copeland, 1988a, 1988b, 1988c; Dreyfuss, 1990; Geber, 1990a, 1990b; Harris & Moran, 1987; Sekaran & Leong, 1992; Tomervik, 1994; Townley, 1991). Thus, the school-to-work movement and its implications for the effective accommodation of workers with disabilities is the primary concept that this chapter addresses.

IMPLICATIONS OF INTERNATIONAL TRENDS FOR SCHOOL-TO-WORK INITIATIVES

Several so-called megatrends have a major impact on work settings and the way work is organized (Streumer & Feteris, 1994). A key question for vocational educators and trainers is whether persons with disabilities can be prepared, not only for today's jobs, but also for tomorrow's. Vocational education and training programs should strive for methods of creating flexible employees, as this is seen as a mechanism to improve the quantity and quality of the labor market in terms of demand and supply (Nijhof & Streumer, 1994).

When discussing the changing U.S. economy, Stern, Bailey, and Merritt (1996) concluded that traditional forms of education do not provide the best preparation for this emerging economy. Vocational education has tended to become too focused on specific skills and occupations that are likely to change in the future. Traditional academic education programs by themselves are also deemed to be inadequate because they does not equip students to apply their abstract knowledge effectively in work settings or to learn effectively in practical problem solving contexts (p. iii). Stern et al. (1996) reported that industrialized countries in Europe, Asia, and Australia also are pursuing school-to-work-related reform initiatives similar to those under way in many American communities. Thus, they are seeking to overcome traditional distinctions between vocational and academic curricula and to combine the two with work-based learning in integrated programs of study that prepare students both for careers and for college or university education programs (p. vii).

Stern et al. (1996) suggested that recent policies in many industrialized countries have begun focusing increasingly on four principles: (a) new curricula should integrate academic and vocational concepts; (b) occupational and educational performance standards should be closely related; (c) work-based learning should be provided for all students; and (d) employers and educators (both academic and vocational) must share responsibility for revised educational systems. The first principle (integration of academic and vocational curricula) is considered crucial within the United States, because it affects the other two principles. When developing new policies to promote skill standards and work-based learning, it is crucial to ask if they are being developed in a way that promotes continued divisions between vocational and academic education or, in contrast, promotes education more appropriate for learning-intensive work (p. 7). Stern et al. (1996) also concluded that all work is becoming more "learning-intensive" and that all workers need to be able to continuously learn, in order to better cope with rapid changes in jobs and workplaces. Finally, they discussed the need to integrate vocational and academic education and the need for education programs to promote "high-level thinking skills for all students, not just for the elite as in the past" (p. 12).

The following integration approaches were listed by Stern et al. in their discussion of international trends in vocational education and training:

1. Japan: A new "integrated" vocational academic high school course was initiated in 1994 (p. 13).

2. France: An array of secondary diplomas are provided: general, technical, and vocational. The vocational diploma gives graduates of two-year vocational programs the option to receive upper secondary diploma after additional two years (p. 13).

3. Norway: A comprehensive reform of upper secondary education was implemented in 1994. The three year sequence consists of a common core curriculum the first year, specialization in the next two years, with work-based learning also being provided during the third year (p. 14).

4. Germany: "Imparting a high level of theoretical and academic knowledge is an important goal of the German dual system" (p. 15). A growing number of individuals in Germany are entering university programs after successfully completing their apprenticeships.

5. Great Britain: There is an ongoing effort to "remove remaining barriers to equal status between so called academic and vocational routes."

6. United States: While the social demand for higher education in other industrialized countries is giving rise to policies that attempt to preserve vocational education by linking it to the university, the pressure for universal access to higher education is even greater in the United States. The U.S. has a high proportion of persons who complete bachelor's degrees or higher of all Organization for Economic Cooperation and Development countries—only Canada is higher (p. 17).

GENERAL CONCLUSIONS REGARDING INTERNATIONAL VOCATIONAL EDUCATION AND TRAINING TRENDS

In some countries, Stern et al. (1996) report, the merging of vocational and academic streams has been occurring through upgrading the academic content of studies within vocational institutions or programs. In France and Sweden, vocational education takes place mainly in schools—unlike Germany, where employers themselves do most of the training (p. 48). By contrast, Great Britain and Japan have recently created new curricular options that are not confined to vocational institutions (p. 48). In all these countries, one explicit purpose of linking vocational with academic education is to make it easier for vocational graduates to continue their education at a university or postsecondary institutions. Conversely, those who proceed directly to higher education have the option to change their minds and enter the workforce (p. 48). Clearly, efforts to prepare individuals for work, pursue continued learning, and enhance individuals' ability to move easily between work and learning settings are increasingly viewed as being important for all members of numerous societies throughout the world. The United States does not, in fact, have the least effective school-to-work system in the industrialized world, but it does not have the most effective either (p. 48).

Stern et al. (1996) believed that the main cause for school-to-work-related optimism in the United States is that the reforms recently emerging in some American schools and communities (combining an occupational and academic curriculum with work-based learning and high standards for all students) are likely to provide the best preparation for young people entering an economy where learning and work are increasingly intertwined. The fact that most other industrialized countries either have been moving in this direction for some time or are now beginning to do so corroborates the appropriateness of these efforts (pp. 48 and 49).

SKILL STANDARDS AND THEIR RELATIONSHIP TO SCHOOL-TO-WORK EDUCATION AND TRAINING

Stern et al. (1996) report that skill standards also play a major role in school-to-work-related vocational education and training efforts in the following countries:

1. Australia has developed a system for competency-based training and assessment for its Vocational Certificate Training System (VCTS). The VCTS focuses on two kinds of competencies: "key competencies," which show resemblance to SCANS skills in the United States; and "functional competencies," which deal with employment-related skills in workforce preparation. The key

competencies have already been incorporated into the curricula of many upper secondary schools (pp. 21–22).

2. England and Scotland have two parallel educational streams, one vocational and one academic. Both countries now use the General National Vocational Qualifications (GNVQs). Critics say they are too task-based, even though GNVQs are aimed at integrating academic and vocational education (pp. 23–24).

3. In Germany, increasing numbers of individuals who attain GNVQs also are subsequently applying for admission to university programs, in the belief that having both types of training is more beneficial having just one. Germany has a growing number of employers who used to hire new workers primarily from apprenticeship programs that are now increasingly hiring university graduates. Correspondingly, Germany has introduced a number of related policy reforms, including a reduction in the number of occupational titles, and changes that increase students' ability to move between the apprenticeship and university systems: "Increasingly, young Germans are also entering universities after completing apprenticeships" (p. 28).

4. Denmark has focused on the goal of educational mobility, while also maintaining distinct vocational and academic secondary credentials; "the Danish system increasingly permits students to cross back and forth between the two pathways" (p. 27).

Overall, a number of countries are developing vocational credentials that can serve as stepping stones to Universities.

INTERNATIONAL WORK-BASED LEARNING AND SCHOOL-TO-WORK-RELATED EDUCATION AND TRAINING TRENDS

There are two general types of work-based learning opportunities that are relevant to school-to-work-related education and training: traditional apprenticeships and relevant work experience that enhances work-related schooling and training. The following conclusions by Stern et al. (1996) summarize some of the work-based learning trends identified in various countries:

1. Netherlands, United Kingdom, Australia, and Spain are all trying new "modern" apprenticeships (p. 32).

2. Within the United States, cooperative learning is still most the common form of school/work-based learning and is often still tied to vocational programs.

3. In Australia, work-based learning is trying to be tied to academic subjects.

4. One major problem many countries have with work-based learning programs is the lack of effective coordination between employers and edu-

cation/training representatives. Even in Germany, there is a lack of effective direct, ongoing coordination between schools and firms that compose dual training system (p. 34).

PARTNERSHIPS AND SCHOOL-TO-WORK-RELATED EDUCATION AND TRAINING IN EUROPE

Stern et al. (1996, p. 39) noted the importance of effective partnerships between educators and employers in Western Europe. The apparent success of school-to-work efforts in German-speaking countries seems to reflect the exceptional degree of responsibility that employers have accepted in the effort, as well as the close collaboration that has occurred between participating employers and educators. In other European nations, employers traditionally have not participated in the education and training of young people to the same degree as in German-speaking countries, but the tradition of centralized decision-making between government and the social partners does exist. Many English-speaking European countries seem to lack any tradition of major employers' participation within educational initiatives, and traditions of strong centralized decision making between government and social partners also appear to be missing.

Hasan (1994) suggested that "the major problem is with the general public perception and status of vocational training and the careers it leads to" (p. 17). Hasan also believed that major deficiencies exist in European school-to-work processes. These deficiencies were believed to be so significant, especially for the disadvantaged, that school-to-work represents a major problem area and should be assigned a high priority (p. 18).

SCHOOL-TO-WORK FOR INDIVIDUALS WITH DISABILITIES IN THE U.S. AND WESTERN EUROPE

United States

Within the U.S., school-to-work models typically have stressed work as a final outcome in transition models. Emphasis is on "integration, both during the school years and afterward, in employment and community-living circumstances. . . . Transition in the U.S. is probably best viewed as a bridge from education to business and industry, with various social service agencies and options flowing by beneath" (Sailor, 1989, p. 19). This approach often suffers from problems associated with the challenges related to coordination of the various agencies' functions and policies.

Sailor (1989) listed the following components as being representative of school-to-work systems within the U.S.:

1. Integrated education and zero rejection; students with disabilities tend to be integrated into public schools (p. 20).

2. Individualized Transition Plans (ITPs); service providers, parents, and disabled individuals meet for conferences where they develop/agree upon written individualized plan with school-to-work components (p. 23).

3. Vocational preparation is addressed within the school-to-work components of the individualized plans (p. 25).

4. Community and vocational placement strategies are related to information produced by assessing each individuals' domestic environments, recreational opportunities, domestic living sites, and transportation needs and resources (p. 26).

Switzerland

Ethnic and linguistic diversity throughout Switzerland makes it difficult to categorize school-to-work efforts in that country. In the recent past, Switzerland has had a record of providing a range of school-to-work services for persons with disabilities, but in separate, protective settings. During the 1980s Switzerland was trying to integrate many of its school-to-work services related to schooling and postschool, adult life.

> The social insurance scheme in Switzerland has strong historical links to the existing network of sheltered workshops, both as training facilities and as terminal placements. As a result, even individuals with relatively mild disabilities find sheltered employment to be the only option I many cases, because acceptance of a regular job in an integrated setting would jeopardize benefits. (Sailor, 1989, p. 29)

United Kingdom

England and Wales have tended to approach school-to-work from a philosophical view, related to those countries' severe labor problems and very high rates of unemployment. Guiding influence in the United Kingdom is the "1978 Warnock Report on Special Education" (Sailor, 1989, p. 30): "This report introduced a concept called 'significant living without work' and suggested that some disabled people might be assisted to create a lifestyle that is characterized by finding meaning in areas other than compensated employment" (p. 31). The Warnock Report was the forerunner to the 1981 Disability Act in the United Kingdom. Opposition to the concept of significant living without work has emerged, but work is still devalued in most plans. Currently, transition planning in the United Kingdom is being tied more to the community colleges and universities through the Further Education Unit (FEU) (Sailor, 1989, p. 33). Current directions in the UK for transition programs appear to include the expansion of the FEU model to include persons with more severe disabilities, eventually approximating a zero rejection model, with strong public pressure supported by the Department of Education and Science to increasingly integrate numbers of students with disabilities into the compulsory education system (p. 36).

France

A number of social experiments have been conducted within different regions of France. "Children with disabilities, including those from specialized institutions, may be integrated into regular schools when there is agreement to do so among the teachers and administrators at the school site" (Sailor, 1989, p. 43). These experiments have established a contexts in France that could facilitate the implementation of future school-to-work efforts for persons with disabilities.

Italy

School-to-work efforts are quite extensive in Italy, and much school-to-work-related experimentation is being conducted. The country's municipal health authority provides funding for various experimental approaches to school-to-work initiatives. When the linkage between integrated school programs, job preparation programs, residential and community living support programs, job placement functions, and coordination and follow-up are finally developed, school-to-work programs in Italy may serve as a conceptually complete model, likely to be worthy of replication in other countries (pp. 46–57).

The Netherlands

The Netherlands spends more per capita for individuals with disabilities than other European countries, but services are very segregated. While virtually all of these protective services, including education, are self-contained and separate, often clustered by nature of the disability, it is clear that this occurred because of a desire to provide a better system for individuals with disabilities. Individuals with disabilities in the Netherlands desire to be more full integrated into society, especially in employment and education settings. School-to-work efforts in the Netherlands are viewed as being an effort to plan individuals' transition between very different settings. Personnel at The Hague are interested in integrating and improving services, but it is felt that doing so might put individuals with disabilities at a disadvantage, compared to the current system. Sailor (1989) stated that California and Missouri, which built large complexes of segregated schools during the 1960s and 1970s for persons with disabilities, did find it difficult to reintegrate those persons into regular schools (pp. 37–41).

SCHOOL-TO-WORK TRANSITION FOR PERSONS
WITH DISABILITIES IN THE NETHERLANDS

The research findings discussed in this section of the chapter are focused on persons with physical and mental disabilities. The target group was limited specifically to people with a physical, hearing, or visual impairments (also known as "physical disabilities" in Europe) and those with mild mental retardation. The aim of school-to-work initiatives is to acquire a life in work, which occurs when persons with disabilities are engaged in paid or unpaid unemployment. To achieve this goal, it will be important that persons with disabilities be integrated into society's work settings as early as is feasible and appropriate. The Organization for Economic Cooperation and Development, Center for Educational Research and Development (OECD, 1994) described three phases during which this integration should occur if successful integration into work is to be achieved.

School Time

School time is defined as the number of years that students with disabilities have to attend school. Education is compulsory for all children in the Netherlands between the ages of 5 and 17; after age 16 education is compulsory for two days per week. Education for students with disabilities is based on three principles: educability, equal opportunities, and integration. There are few persons with disabilities who are excluded from recognizable educational settings in the Netherlands. For the past 20 years or so it has been generally accepted that almost everyone is educable. The right to equal opportunities implies that the educational system is open to everyone of school age. The aims of education are the same for all pupils (European Commission, 1997). In the Netherlands, more and more pupils are attending regular schools as a result of this principle, but special education also continues to play an important role. By attending regular education, persons with disabilities automatically come more into contact with the demands of daily life.

Transitional Period Including Vocational Preparation
and the First Period of a Life in Work

The transitional period follows on from compulsory education. The age at which persons with disabilities in the Netherlands finish their school time varies greatly from one individual to another, depending on the severity and the nature of the disability. During the transitional period each individual follows his or her own way; every individual is considered unique, as are all persons' school-to-work transitional experiences. Consequently, there is no clear-cut, phased plan for this period. Vocational preparation of persons with disabilities takes place mainly in

Regional Training Centers for Secondary Vocational Education (ROCs). In these ROCs, training is provided at four levels, on the basis of a new national qualification structure. The four levels are: elementary training; basic vocational training; vocational skills training; and middle management and specialist training. Two learning pathways may be followed: the apprenticeship pathway and the full-time, regular vocational education at secondary level pathway. The distinctive features of the ROCs are that the training courses are flexibly structured; have a modular form; individual supervision of students is considered important; and modern, technological methods of training are used.

Work Integration

There are many institutions engaged in the integration of persons with disabilities into work settings in the Netherlands. A description of these strategies designed to stimulate employment follows later in this section. The measures that have been collected and analyzed in this study are directed at these three phases.

European Policies That Affect School-to-Work Initiatives in the Netherlands

At an international level, there are three organizations engaged in the (re)integration of persons with disabilities into education and a life in work. These are the European Union, the Council of Europe, and the United Nations.

The European Union

In the 1980s initiatives were developed through the European Union aimed at promoting the social and economic integration of persons with disabilities. These initiatives found expression in the first community action program, aimed at the social integration of persons with disabilities (1983–1987), the Helios I program (1988–1991), and the Helios II program (1993–1996). The Helios I and II action programs have as their aim the provision of support to vocational education and the creation of employment opportunities. These European programs are so-called "transnational programs" that are intended to develop innovative activities, focusing on the integration of persons with disabilities, and to exchange expertise and experiences between projects from all the European Union countries that are participating. Initially, attention was focused particularly on the integration of persons with physical disabilities. Since 1985, increasing attention has also been focused on realizing work opportunities in regular work settings for people with a (slight) mental disabilities. This shift of attention has also led to the study of new methods by which persons with disabilities can acquire jobs. After the third action program, Helios II, preparations for a follow-up program have been initiated.

In the aforementioned European programs, persons with "handicaps" are defined as people with serious disorders, limitations, or handicaps that are the result of physical (including sensory), mental, or psychological disorders, which hamper or prevent the performance of activities or a function that would be considered as normal for able-bodied people. (Note: The term "handicapped" is used commonly in Europe, instead of the term "persons with disabilities." However, "persons with disabilities" will be substituted throughout this document.) Given that the first community action program was only a pilot study, attention in this study is focused on the Helios I and II programs.

Helios I (1988–1991).   Helios I has as its main aim a coherent and comprehensive policy in respect to all the problems of persons with disabilities in the area of educational integration, economic integration, social integration, and an independent life. For each area of action a network of local projects has been set up, spread over all the member states of the EU. In this study, analysis has been limited to projects that are aimed at the areas of educational integration and economic integration and that focus on physical and the mental disabilities.

The European Commission evaluated the Helios I program in 1992. From its report on the implementation of the program, it was concluded that this program has contributed to the realization of the conditions necessary for the integration of persons with disabilities. Against this, however, it was pointed out that the program's general effectiveness and coherence could be improved. An improvement could be achieved by extending the program to include other areas, such as the integration of persons with disabilities into educational systems, support for older clients, and accessibility to work settings.

As regards the progress of the implementation of the policy aimed at the educational integration of young persons with disabilities, the European Commission has ascertained that national legislation relating to integration has improved continuously since 1987. Moreover, this legislation has tended to include more and more innovative elements. The commission has made a number of recommendations for the future:

- It points emphatically to the need for more regulations, for national programs to be relaxed and modified, as well as for evaluations geared to the individual;
- It stresses the necessary evaluation of the attitudes of all those involved and of all instruments for integration into education;
- Finally, it points to the fact that the transition between school and the labor market, as well as future opportunities at the end of compulsory education, must still be studied in depth.

Helios II (1993–1996).   Helios II is intended to promote equal opportunities and the integration of persons with disabilities in the EU. The areas of action are functional rehabilitation; integration into education; vocational education, vocational rehabilitation, and economic integration; social integration; and independent living. The activities that will be carried out within this action program are:

- The continuation of the development of the data bank "handynet";
- The financing of a large number of the activities of organizations for the handicapped (so-called nongovernmental organizations);
- The promotion of a consciousness-raising process among the public at large; and
- The exchange of experiences and experts between the member states.

The final evaluation of Helios II is currently taking place, the results of that study are not available at this time.

The Council of Europe

In April 1992 the Council of Europe passed Resolution (92)6 (Council of Europe, 1992). This resolution provided a coherent policy for the rehabilitation of persons with disabilities. It proposed a model for a rehabilitation and integration program for national governments. This resolution specified 12 chapters of coherent policies that indicate the direction that policy on persons with disabilities should follow in the years ahead. The areas of activity on which this policy focuses are:

- Prevention and health information or education;
- Detection and diagnosis;
- Treatment and therapeutic help;
- Education;
- Vocational orientation and education;
- Employment;
- Social integration and everyday environment;
- Social, economic, and legal protection;
- Training of people who are involved in the rehabilitation process and the integration of the handicapped into society;
- Information; and
- Statistics and research.

The United Nations

The General Assembly of the UN accepted the Standard Rules on the Equalization of Opportunities for Persons with Disabilities in December 1993. This is an international document intended to draw worldwide attention to the need for equal rights and opportunities for persons with disabilities. The Standard Rules are not a list of ambitious objectives, but are practical instruments for governments to improve quality of life and to remove the barriers that deter persons with disabilities from participating in society. The areas covered in this document are:

- Conditions for equal participation: increasing consciousness, medical help, rehabilitation, support services;
- Target areas for equal participation; accessibility, education, work, retention of income and social security, family life and personal integrity, culture, recreation, sport, and religious belief;
- Implementation of instruments: information and research, policymaking and planning, legislation, economic policy, coordination of work, organizations of handicapped persons, personal training, national control and evaluation of programs for persons with disabilities in the Rules, technical and economic cooperation, and international cooperation; and
- Control mechanisms.

Dutch Policy

Over the past five years the Dutch government has continued to reduce its efforts to find solutions in the field of national legislation, as it was becoming increasingly complicated to do so for one sector or group without aggravating the problems for another. Instead, the goal is to increase the guiding, coordinating, and problem-solving capacities of local authorities and regions, educational institutions, health insurance companies, and other intermediary bodies. On the basis of this principle, it formulated the "Long Range Intersectoral Policy for the Handicapped" for the years 1995–1998 (Tweede Kamer der Staten Generaal, 1995). This long-range plan presents a survey of the cabinet's policy principles and policy resolutions. The long-range plan is, of necessity, broad in its scope. Its objectives are:

1. To stimulate the problem-solving capacity of persons with disabilities, through such measures as the introduction of a person-related budget;
2. To promote the integration and involvement of persons with disabilities in all sectors of society (including education and work integration);
3. To gain better insight into the most vulnerable categories of persons with disabilities;
4. To stimulate self-regulation, aimed at such areas as quality improvement, being customer-oriented, and an integrated, objectified medical indication policy.

Integration Into Education and Work

The policy resolutions of the Dutch government in the area of integration into education and work are: pupil-related financing in special education; the creation of opportunities to promote attendance at regular secondary education and improvement of general accessibility to regular secondary vocational education; measures aimed at (re)integration, such as a regulations related to supplemented wages; labor costs subsidy; encouragement for starting up companies; incentives for older employees with a work-related handicap; broadening training opportunities and trial placement while retaining benefit; and extending the use of the personal support allowance for employees with disabilities.

Disability-Related Legislation in the Netherlands

In the Netherlands there is a hodgepodge of rules and laws designed to help persons with disabilities enter and remain in work settings. This large body of laws and regulations has resulted in many people, employees, and employers alike overlooking opportunities. The most frequently applied regulations are found in the Provision of Sheltered Workshops Act (WSW) and the Disabled Workers Employment Act (WAGW). These laws still do not function optimally.

The WSW "provides the opportunity to perform work under modified circumstances to persons who are indeed able to work, but who, as a result of a disability or other 'factors related to the person', can find no regular employment." WSW's aim is to use work as the means to maintain, recover, or promote the ability to work. The WSW needs to obtain adequate funding, so that the sheltered workshops can retain employees who function well. Sheltered workshops have begun seconding employees, but this has not yet been fully developed. The supervision required is not being provided effectively.

The WAGW was designed to promote participation by persons with disabilities and reinforce the positions of employees with disabilities. This law can best be seen as a collection of instruments to encourage disabled or partially disabled employees to continue to participate or to participate again in employment. These instruments are:

1. Rehabilitating resumption of work;
2. Temporary revision of the disability benefit;
3. On-the-job provisions;
4. Training-wages dispensation;
5. A helping hand [community support services when needed].

Many persons responsible for enforcing these laws find the WAGW too complicated. Problems include: a limited number of possible adaptations required to meet individual abilities, low subsidies, doubts that sanctions will be implemented, a lack of agreement on the desirability of a quota ruling, and possible disruptions of employer-employee relations as well as those between employer and the enforcing authority. These problems are believed to be the result of too many authorities being involved in implementation, unclear demarcation between the WAGW and the Arbowet (Working Conditions Act), and confusion about the definition of term "handicapped employee."

Secondment represents an approach sometimes used for members of target groups with a relatively good chance of success. The results are, in spite of everything, very mixed. It is proving to be particularly difficult to turn a secondment placement into a permanent job. The word "secondment" is a British term, meaning "to temporarily transfer a person or employee to another organization." While normal temporary employment efforts typically are brokered by commercial temporary employment agencies, secondment involves situations in which temporary employees have labor agreements directly with the organizations for whom they are working (instead of employment agreements with temporary employment agencies). In addition, secondments allow contracted employees to work longer than six months or 1000 hours for the same employer, time constraints that typically apply to temporary employment placement agencies).

In the local projects that were researched, the targeted population's medical service providers concluded that "help in finding employment" seemed to represent the strategy with the best chance of succeeding. Personal contacts and an efficient network of service providers seemed to represent the key factors that enhanced the success of local projects.

Supported employment is a method aimed at a particularly difficult target group, people with severe mental disabilities, and is often the only method that offers a real likelihood of community reintegration for this group. Supported employment is a method where the participants follow selected outlined procedures and also receive on-the-job supervision. The supported job employment method has the following phases: assessment, job finding, job analysis, job matching, and job coaching. The results of the supported job employment are mixed: great number of projects' clients show some progress toward work, but the risk of dropping out remains high.

Individual counseling is aimed at different groups. The determining factor for success is whether the parties are able to create good working relationships with the organizations that provide those parts of their route.

Many positive and negative points appear to apply, in varying degrees, to all approaches discussed above. The most significant negative aspects are: obstructions caused by laws and regulations at the time of the enforcement of these activities, the negative image that laws and regulations have, as well as unfamiliarity with those laws and regulations, inflexible attitudes among enforcing authorities, and the proliferation of projects. Moreover, the projects' lack of insight into the targeted populations with disabilities, their numbers, and their objectives is problematical. Unfamiliarity with the details of laws and regulations, inaccurate assessment of work productivity, and the risk of persons with disabilities dropping out all make job placement difficult. One favorable remark regularly heard is that enforcing authorities' employees have positive attitudes and are willing to analyze these problems and to become more involved in finding solutions. Finally, an important positive influence is a good working relationship between the various parties, enforcing authorities, and employers.

Local Projects

Local projects use various methods to achieve work integration. These methods include reorientation training, work rehabilitation, work experience, training projects, secondment, and help in finding work (Ernste, Wijnands, Schooten, & Van Baas, 1995). Reorientation training is aimed particularly at people who have no idea of the vocational opportunities open to them and who are motivated to end their disability-related unemployment. Local projects' training courses aim to give their participants an understanding of skills deemed necessary for entering or returning to employment.

Work rehabilitation is designed particularly for people who are far removed from the labor market, especially those with mental disabilities. Rehabilitation trainees can experience work rhythms, learn to keep appointments, and to deal with functional relationships during work rehabilitation projects. Despite the remoteness of these participants from the labor market, some progress to paid work is apparent here.

Work experience is aimed at people who are close to the labor market. In general, progress toward achieving paid employment seems to be greater here than in the case of work rehabilitation.

Training projects are available for all target groups. Retraining and refresher courses are deployed here as in those in search of employment. Training projects are organized very frequently and can differ greatly in length of training, direction of training, level of training, the form of the practical component, and the deployment of various instruments, such as job application training, supervision on the job, and so on. Progress to paid work is greater than for work rehabilitation.

THE WORK FORCE AS AN EMERGING FACTOR WITHIN SOCIETY

Reich (1990) noted that the press, politicians, and trend mongers have recently been getting much attention with a continuing series of warnings about the dreadful state of the American workforce. These warnings have claimed that: one out of five 18-year-olds is functionally illiterate (a higher percentage than in any other industrialized nation); and the workforce is becoming far more diverse (only 15% of the net additions will be white male, three out of five will be women and 25% will be minorities; by 2020, two-thirds of America's will be female or minority, groups that historically have tended to have less education and training). These data seldom include any discussions of the increasing proportion of our society with disabilities or of the expanding legal protections for their civil rights and of their access to meaningful career opportunities.

Reich (1990) felt that American businesses should recognize the enormous potential of the American workforce, which needs to be nurtured and developed. Rather than abandon American workers who lack minimal skills and competence, Reich suggested that businesses should pay more than lip service to improving public education and worker training programs. To do so will draw increased attention to the feasibility of hiring persons with disabilities who have often been overlooked as viable members of the American workforce. For example, Goldstein (1988) reported that some estimates indicate that America now assumes the 1.5 million people with unusable skills are enemployable each year, most of whom will require assistance to reenter the workforce. Those companies that do find successful solutions to the complex challenges will be rewarded with stable, productive employees. Geber (1990b) noted that people with disabilities represent a large group from which future employees could be drawn. For example, of the 13.3 million people in America with disabilities that affect their ability to work, 33.6% are in the workforce and 15.6% are unemployed, a rate twice as large as the rate for the nondisabled population.

Diversity Among Individuals With Disabilities

A wide array of diverse individuals representing populations with unique traits, often including special learning needs, continue to be underemployed and unemployed group in the United States. Yet there are many persons with special learning needs who are successfully employed and who are successfully integrated into to their communities. However, it is important that society also recognize that special learning needs affect people without regard to backgrounds, gender, age (before and birth), and ability level. For example, persons with disabilities in the 1991 U.S. workforce, depicted in Table 11.1, were spread across a wide range of demographic categories (as cited in Carnavale & Stone, 1995, p. 385).

Why Have Disability-Related Accommodations in School-to-Work Programs?

Why should we seek to increase the health and productivity of an increasingly diverse workforce? Given the demographic projections that point out approaching changes in the American workforce, representatives of industry, labor, individual workers, and educators are realizing that it is imperative to collaborate in partnerships designed to enhance the health and productivity of a workforce that is more competitive internationally, as well as at the local and national levels (Akabas, Gates, & Galvin, 1992). The following factors substantiate the importance of efforts effectively address the unique needs of our country' increasingly diverse work force:

   1. *The United States is Experiencing Global Competition and Increasing the Importance of Having a Highly Productive Workforce.*   The quality and commitment

TABLE 11.1
Work Force Status of United States Civilians With Disabilities In 1991,
Ages 16 to 64, by Gender, Race, and Hispanic Origin

		With a Work Disability		No Work Disability	
	Total	Number	Percent in work force	Number	Percent in work force
Total	160,123	14,648	34.4	144,506	79.9
Female	81,511	7,380	29.3	74,052	71.1
Male	78,612	7,268	39.5	70,454	89.1
White	135,033	11,553	37.5	122,711	80.7
African American	19,130	2,661	21.5	16,305	76.5
Hispanic*	13,597	1,188	26.1	12,349	73.5
Veteran	19,543	2,828	43.8	16,715	90.7
Vietnam	7,612	974	60.7	6,639	96.5
Korean Conflict	3,965	787	28.9	3,178	82.3
World War I	11,340	383	18.9	957	55.3
Other Service	6,626	685	51.0	5,941	94.3
Nonvet.	140,580	11,819	32.1	127,791	78.5

*Persons of Hispanic origin may be of any race.
Source: Compiled by Janice Hamilton Outtz from U.S. Bureau of the Census, Current Population Survey (unpublished estimates).

of America's workforce is a powerful component of efforts to be competitive in the global economy. A demanding, unsupportive environment will not accommodate the changing needs of our country's workforce, thus limiting its productivity.

2. Work, and Other Aspects of Life as Well, is Increasingly Stressful for Most People. The levels of competition and rates at which change is occurring are increasing geometrically, and the ensuing illnesses, accidents, and long-term disabilities have resulted in a whole new class of claims for stress-induced problems that have proved ambiguous in their cost and remediation and difficult to treat in customary ways (Akabas, Gates, & Galvin, 1992, pp. 6–7).

3. Written Philosophy and Values Can Have a Positive Impact on an Organization and its Environment. The philosophy and values appropriate to special needs learners are no different from those that have been identified consistently as encouraging the development of a productive workforce. They are results-oriented and are tied to the following:

- Recognition that employees are the organization's most valuable asset.
- Commitment to the growth, development, and protection of that employees as assets by enabling employees to make their own voluntary selections from available options.

- Creation of safe and healthy work settings and climates that empower worker participation.
- Expectation that attention to these issues will improve morale and, therefore, productivity.
- Understanding that the workforce and management are in a partnership arrangement to achieve these conditions, and that mutual rights and responsibilities result.
- Effective policy statements help create a culture based on positive attitudes. They enlist everyone in the management mission. They promote the maximum yield from an organization's workforce. Although management often gives lip service to these principles, special learning needs management hinges on action, not just words. It is essential, therefore, to act according to these principles if disability management is to have any significant impact. It is necessary to:
    - Show that management cares by initiating contact with persons experiencing special learning needs.
    - Offer growth experiences by training and promoting employees regardless of special learning needs.
    - Mitigate the conditions that seem to result in accidents and illnesses that cause special learning needs.
    - Share, with workers and/or the union, decision-making power concerning special learning needs-related issues.
    - Provide work place responsiveness through accommodation to persons' special learning needs (Akabas, Gates, & Galvin, 1992, pp. 105–108).

4. Organizational Objectives. Workplace accommodations are desirable when they satisfy both humane and cost-containment objectives. Such efforts enhance each organization's human assets by focusing on rehabilitation as well as prevention. Thus, reduced costs and increased morale, commitment, and well-being within work settings are important evidence of the success of organizations' efforts to accommodate individuals with special learning needs (Akabas, Gates, & Galvin, 1992, pp. 104–107).

5. Types of Barriers. There are a wide variety of obvious barriers to the complete integration of individuals with disabilities, as well as other special learning needs, into the workforce. However, the following represent some of the school-to-work implementation barriers that Tracey (1995) concluded will require attention by advocates, practitioners, and policymakers:

1. Low expectations.
2. Lack of work experience.
3. Public attitudes.

4. Management attitudes.

5. Co-worker insensitivity.

6. Inadequate social skills.

7. Inaccessible facilities.

8. Meager instructor know-how.

9. Communication problems.

10. Learning problems.

11. Lack of accommodations and training opportunities.

12. Cost of accommodations.

13. Performance evaluation (pp. 97–101).

The following additional categories of barriers were specified by Charner (1996b) as issues that he concluded should be addressed by all school-to-work-related system reform initiatives:

Legal and Regulatory Barriers. Implementers of school-to-work reform efforts often encounter some of the following legal and regulatory barriers when seeking to create workplace learning opportunities:

1. Full-time equivalents (FTE), seat time, occupational safety issues, regulations for grants disbursement, and child labor laws.

2. Postsecondary admission requirements: for example, when postsecondary institutions arbitrarily decide which high school courses will be considered for credit, with strong distinctions between the acceptability of academic and vocational course work. It will be important for state postsecondary institutions to cooperate with state school-to-work and K–12 systems to ensure that these artificial barriers are eliminated. A key issue will be the stance that postsecondary systems take on alternate assessment, such as portfolios (Charner, 1996b, p. 1).

Preservice and Inservice Teacher Training Program Barriers. Effective school-to-work programs require pedagogical and curricular approaches that are not usually accorded much consideration in teacher training programs.

1. Both preservice and inservice teacher training will require reform in order to prepare instructors for the contextual, interactive, more flexible approaches demanded by school-to-work programs.

2. Teacher training programs need to incorporate school-to-work into instruction concerning curriculum, pedagogy, and assessment.

3. Teacher training programs seldom offer internships and other opportunities for teachers and prospective teachers to explore firsthand a variety of workplaces (Charner, 1996b, pp. 1–2).

Business Partners' Barriers.   Policymakers and practitioners cannot expect that businesses will participate in school-to-work out of altruism. Incentives will be needed to help businesses assist in the educational system.

1. Businesses are not adequately aware of the range of benefits that can accrue to them through school-to-work participation (Charner, 1996b, p. 2).

Parent Partners' Barriers.   Charner's (1996b) study found one key group of partners was typically absent from school-to-work initiatives focused on parents.

1. It is crucial for policy makers and practitioners to engage parents in school-to-work.
2. Parents that school-to-work programs often have not been integrated into effective strategies for students who go directly to work after high school, as well as for those who go on to two- and four-year colleges.
3. More and better publicity about school-to-work is needed locally, nationally, and at the state level to help parents, teachers, and employers better understand school-to-work, how it could benefit themselves and their children, students, and prospective employees.
4. Too few policymakers appreciate how regulatory or financing systems create arbitrary and unnecessary barriers.
5. Inadequate reform strategies for practitioners and policymakers to simultaneously assemble new school-to-work systems and disassemble old barriers (Charner, 1996b, p. 2).

BEST PRACTICES ASSOCIATED WITH EFFECTIVE SCHOOL-TO-WORK SYSTEM REFORM EFFORTS

The U.S. Department of Education's Office of Educational Research and Improvement recently funded a four-year study by the Academy for Educational Development's National Institute for Work and Learning (Charner, 1996a). This study focused on the planning, design, implementation, and impact of effective school-to-work transition system reform initiatives. By documenting the design and integrity of exemplary programs and by assessing program experiences and impacts, this study identified critical issues and practices related to adapting or adopting programs that effectively link schools with the business community to improve the transition from school-to-work. Through individual case studies, best practices were identified and documented from which others could learn. Twelve "critical elements or building blocks of school-to-work system reform" (p. 2) were identified by the researchers' cross-case analyses. Thus, the final component of this chapter presents those 12 system reform suggestions drawn from

Charner's project report. Readers (wherever they reside internationally) are encouraged to closely examine the following quotes from Charner's report and apply them to their school-to-work-related efforts for persons with disabilities:

Leadership from executives—Where school-to-work finds an advocate at the executive level, the reform is more likely to take root throughout the educational system. Where that advocacy is absent, school-to-work is likely to remain a tenuous and fragmented activity, however strong the support from other sectors. Successful transition systems require executives who are able to develop a shared vision, clear goals, and a comprehensive strategy, enlisting the support and involvement of all stakeholders. Beyond vision and advocacy, these executives typically operate with a keen sense of politics, both in understanding the process and knowing the players. They are also willing to take risks and recognize that change demands time, mistakes, and a tolerance of failure.

Leadership from program deliverers—The category of program deliverers covers a variety of roles, including those of instructor, counselor, transition specialist, school-to-work coordinator, and others. Some delivery roles typically belong to certain positions—instructors usually provide classroom training, for example—but other roles, such as communication with business partners, may be delegated or shared in various ways. As managers, program deliverers must possess excellent organizational and communication skills. As reformers, they must have substantial knowledge of pedagogy, curriculum, the industry, and the student population. Whether their training is academic or experiential, effective program deliverers also understand youth development and learning theory, including the variety of learning styles and the stages of adolescent development. Effective program deliverers also have some understanding, usually earned through actual experience in the industry, of the occupational area within which the school-to-work program provides training.

Professional development for teachers and staff—For any reform effort to take root successfully in a school system, practice in classrooms, counseling sessions, and administration must change. Professional development is one route that school-to-work initiatives adopt in order to engage school staff in the reform, ensuring that at least some will change their professional practice sufficiently to support the vision and strategies of the reform. The executive of the educational system must make professional development a priority for that school, district, or regional entity. Like so many aspects of school-to-work, professional development conflicts with standard school schedules and logistics, which can block the effort unless an administrator in a position of some authority clears the way.

Cross-sector collaboration—A school-to-work transition system is by definition dependent on effective collaboration among all of the stakeholders. The first step in developing a representative system is taking stock of the range of partners in a community. It is important to engage partners early in the process in order to foster a sense of empowerment and ability to influence the shape of the system. Effective long-term collaboration requires not only broad and inclusive recruitment, but also continuous nurturing of partnerships, so that all the partners recognize the rewards, risks, and long-term outcomes they can expect for themselves and, more importantly, for the students. Different partners are going to require different types of support or reassurances that the system will work for them. The goal of such extensive and carefully nurtured partnerships is an atmosphere of shared vision, beliefs, and, ultimately, resources.

Student self-determination—In order to help students prepare for a lifetime of learning, fulfilling work, and productive adult lives, school-to-work transition systems must support the development of self-determination in all students. Students should be encouraged to take responsibility for their learning, to understand and manage their career options, and to develop social skills and a maturity level that will help them interact positively with adults and peers. This is especially true for at-risk students, as the school system may be the only vehicle for them to learn how to cope with the complexities of adult life.

School-based curriculum and instruction—At the heart of school-to-work reform is a transformation of curriculum and instructional practice so that learning is 'contextual,' that is, learning that occurs in a real life context, or a close simulation of a real life context. Curriculum and instruction in transition systems must provide multiple points of connection between the experiences of work and learning. The successful school-to-work curriculum in some manner integrates demanding academic study with up-to-date vocational instruction and work-readiness preparation. Whatever the classroom curriculum, it must connect in a rational and supportive way to the workplace learning experience, and in schools that have instituted articulation agreements, with that postsecondary curriculum as well. The measurement of learning that occurs in settings so unlike the traditional classroom requires assessment practices which are correspondingly different. Many school-to-work programs have drawn up comprehensive sets of competencies, often in consultation with business partners, which students in that program are expected to acquire, at certain minimum levels. Others have established comprehensive standards toward which all the programs within a school or district are expected to strive. Others have experimented with portfolio assessment as the most accurate way to document a student's education.

Work-based learning strategies—Successful transition systems offer a variety of work-based learning experiences, building on local labor market conditions and allowing for differences in student interest, aptitude, and developmental stage. Transition systems can include a menu of options such as business-based experiences, school-based enterprises, entrepreneurial programs, youth apprenticeships, mentorships, cooperative education, and service-learning. Programs also use a range of strategies—paid or unpaid work experiences, for five or fifty students, during the school day or after school, based in the school classroom or in a 'community classroom'—with programs customized to fit the needs of youth, schools, business, and the local community. Regardless of which particular options or strategies a system utilizes, it must provide appropriate support services to students, staff, and business partners.

Integrated career information and guidance system—Another critical component for effective transition systems is the integration of career counseling into the system. In addition to career information, assessment, and guidance, many programs provide mentoring and personal counseling activities. These services are not appendages, but essential components of the system. Services must be ongoing, and each student should have an individual educational and career plan that is regularly updated. As part of the system, career counseling must link back into earlier grades: age-appropriate activities should start in elementary school. There must be multiple points at which counseling can occur, and it must be ongoing and consistently available to students. Equally important, the school's counseling system must tie into reliable, up-to-date labor market and job information sources.

Progressive system starting before grade 11—Programs that do not start until eleventh grade will miss the chance to make a difference for many students. It is crucial to reach younger students before they become discouraged, disengaged, or drop out. Common sense and research both support the concept that a student who understands the connection between school and work—between lifelong learning and a successful life—will be much more motivated to succeed in school. Programs must take a progressive, sequential approach that includes preparatory, age-appropriate "feeder" programs starting as early as elementary or middle school.

Postsecondary articulation—Just as an effective school-to-work system begins before eleventh grade, it also extends beyond high school graduation. Programs must provide multiple connections to postsecondary institutions, beginning when the student is still in high school and extending to provide post–high school education and training options. Articulation with postsecondary institutions while the student is in high school may take the form of dual/concurrent enrollment, college credit for high school courses, the acceptance by postsecondary institutions of alternative forms of assessment such as portfolios or certificates of mastery, or an agreement that the postsecondary institution will grant credit for alternative instruction such as work-based learning experiences. These arrangements at once greatly expand the training immediately available to high school students, and offer them a ladder of opportunity toward progressively more advanced training and advantageous employment after high school.

Creative financing—Obtaining seed money for reform in its early stages is almost always a critical element of school-to-work initiatives. Many initiatives have drawn on federal funding, including Perkins Act and other vocational and special populations grants. Where the state government has supported tech prep and related reforms, state funds have made a significant difference. In some states, funds for educational reform, including specific set-asides for school-to-work transition, have helped schools initiate school-to-work reforms. Business has provided funds, in- kind contributions, and human resources that have not only underwritten specific programs, but offered evidence of corporate support that often helps leverage additional support. Interagency agreements that allow education programs to draw on other governmental funds, particularly those set aside for employment and training or for special populations, have greatly benefited school-to-work transition systems in several states.

Application of research—A number of the sites studied by the Academy for Educational Development consciously drew upon existing research, conducted their own research, or commissioned new research in order to plan, assess, or strengthen their school-to-work system. They made use of the research to provide a foundation for a program model; to assess the local labor market and economy; and to measure the impact of the program on students, specifically how their graduates fared in the worlds of work and postsecondary education. Using research in these ways also brought a number of secondary benefits, as the findings helped justify the school-to-work system, affirm to the staff the importance of their work, leverage additional resources for its support, and provide feedback that could be used to improve and refine different aspects of the reform initiative.

An educational reform that engages as many players and as many levels of the educational system as does school-to-work transition reform has the potential to achieve significant outcomes for many people and institutions. The National Institute for Work and Learning's study documented evidence of such outcomes for students, business partners, schools (from elementary grades through college), and other partners to the school-to-work collaboration (Charner, 1996, pp. 2–4).

REFERENCES

Akabas, A., Gates, L., & Galvin, D. (1992). *Disability management: A complete system to reduce costs, increase productivity, meet employee needs, and ensure legal compliance.* New York: AMACOM.

Carnevale, A., & Stone, S. (1995). *The American mosaic: An in-depth report on the future of diversity at work.* New York: McGraw-Hill.

Charner, I. (1996a). *Study of school-to-work initiatives: Studies of educational reform (Executive summary).* Washington, DC: Office of Educational Research and Improvement, U.S. Department of Education.

Charner, I. (1996b). *Study of school-to-work initiatives: Studies of educational reform (Implications for policy and practice).* Washington, DC: Office of Educational Research and Improvement, U.S. Department of Education.

Commissie Dualisering (1993). *Beroepsvorming langs vele wegen* [Many roads lead to occupational training]. Zoetermeer: Ministry of Education and Science.

Copeland, L. (1988a). Learning to manage a multicultural workforce. *Training, 25* (5), pp. 52–56.

Copeland, L. (1988b). Valuing diversity, part 1: Making the most of cultural differences at the workplace. *Personnel* (June), pp. 52–60.

Copeland, L. (1988c). Valuing diversity, part 2: Pioneers and champions of change. *Personnel* (July), pp. 44–49.

Cox, T. H., Jr., & Nkomo, S. (1990). Invisible men and women: A status report on race as a variable in organizational behavior research. *Journal of Organizational Behavior, 11,* 419–431.

Department of Work, Community, and Family Education. (1996). *Proposal for a School-to-Work Certificate.* Unpublished manuscript, Department of Work, Community, and Family Education, College of Education and Human Development, University of Minnesota, St. Paul.

Dreyfuss, J. (1990, April 23). Get ready for the new work force. *Fortune*, 165–181.

Erneste, D. E., Wijnands, Y., Schooten, P., & Van Bass, L. M. (1995). Reinterpretation projects for people receiving a disability benefit. The Hague: Ministry of Social Welfare and Employment.

European Commission. (1997). Helios II, guide to good policy: Toward equal opportunities for all persons with disabilities. Luxembourg: Bureau for Official Publications of the European Community.

Geber, B. (1990a). Managing diversity. *Training, 27*(7), 23–35.

Geber, B. (1990b). The disabled: Ready, willing, and able. *Training* (December), 29–36.

Goldstein, M. (1988, August 15). Tomorrow's workforce today. *Industry Week*, 41–43.

Harris, P., & Moran, R. (1987). *Managing cultural differences.* Houston: Gulf Publishing.

Hasan, A. (1994). Ontwikkelingen op de arbeidsmarkt en onderwijs-en opleidingsbeleid [Labor market developments and education and training policy]. *Europees Tijdschrift Beroepsopleiding* [*European Journal Vocational Training*], *2*, 14–22.

Institute for Applied Social Sciences: Ministry of Education and Science. (1988). *The Dutch education system.* Zoetermeer: Ministry of Education and Science.

Jamieson, D., & O'Mara, J. (1991). *Managing workforce 2000: Gaining the diversity advantage.* San Francisco: Jossey-Bass.

Johnston, W. B., & Packer, A. E. (1987). *Work and workers for the 21st century.* Indianapolis, IN: Hudson Institute.

Loden, M., & Rosener, J. (1991). *Workforce 2000: Managing employee diversity as a vital resource.* Homewood, IL: Business One Irwin.

Ministry of Education and Science. (1993). The changing role of vocational and technical education and training. In OECD (1994), *Vocational training in the Netherlands: Reform and innovation.* Paris: OECD.

National Transition Network. (1994). *Policy update: Youth with disabilities and the School-to-Work Opportunities Act of 1994.* Washington, DC: Office of Special Education and Rehabilitation Services. U.S. Department of Labor.

Nijhof, W. J., & Streumer, J. N. (Eds.). (1994). *Flexibility in training and vocational education.* Utrecht: Lemma.

NRC/Handelsblad. (1996, September). *Leerlingwezen na daling nu stabiel* [Number of Apprentices is stable now]. (Research report).

Reich, R. (1990, November). Metamorphosis of the American worker. *Business Month*, 58–66.

Sailor, W. (1989). *Transition in the U.S. and Western European nations.* Office of Special Education and Rehabilitative Services. ED 365047.

School-to-Work Opportunity Act of 1994 (STWOA), Pub. L. No. 103–239 (1994), 20 U.S.C.A. § 6101 *et seq. U.S Statutes At Large.*

Sekaran, U., & Leong, F. T. L. (1992). *Womanpower: Managing in times of demographic turbulence.* Newbury Park, CA: Sage.

Stern, D., Bailey, T., & Merritt, D. (1996). *School-To-Work policy insights from recent international developments* (Research report). National Center for Research in Vocational Education.

Streumer, J. N., & Feteris, A. (1994). CNC machining and flexible production automation. In *Vocational training in the Netherlands: Reform and innovation.* Paris: OECD.

Thomas, R. R., Jr. (1990). From affirmative action to affirming diversity. *Harvard Business Review, 68*(2), 107–117.

Thomas, R. R., Jr. (1991). Beyond race and gender: Unleashing the power of your total workforce by managing diversity. New York: Amacom.

Tomervik, K. (1994). *Work force diversity in Fortune 500 corporations headquartered in Minnesota: Concepts and practices.* Unpublished doctoral dissertation, University of Minnesota, St. Paul-Minneapolis.

Townley, P. (1991, April). *Managing diversity: Demographics are destiny.* Presentation to United Way of Eastern Fairfield County, Bridgeport, CT.

Tracey, W. R. (1995). Training employees with disabilities: Strategies to enhance learning and development for an expanding part of your workforce. New York: American Management Association.

Tweede Kamer der Staten Generaal [Lower House of the Dutch Parliament]. (1995). De perken te buiten [Exceeding the limits]. The Hague: SDU Publishers.

CHAPTER 12

Vocational Preparation and Employment Options for Adults with Disabilities: An International Perspective

JAY W. ROJEWSKI
The University of Georgia

Throughout the world, nations and private organizations provide a vast and complex array of vocationally related services to adults with physical, mental, behavioral, or emotional disabilities. Many of these services are surprisingly similar in different countries, especially those found in the more industrialized countries of North America, Western Europe, and Japan. Other services remain uniquely associated with a certain country or culture, particularly in some less-developed countries found in Central America, Africa, or Asia. Without question, the types of vocational services offered to adults with disabilities reflect a country's unique combination of culture, tradition or history, the availability of employment, and degree of industrialization.

This chapter provides an international perspective of prominent vocationally related services provided to adults with disabilities in the United States and select countries throughout the world. While not an exhaustive review, important and relevant issues related to the vocational preparation and employment of adults with disabilities are addressed including guiding legislation and mandates; types of vocational services available to adults with disabilities; major employment preparation and placement models; and the types of hiring incentives, services, and benefits used by countries to increase opportunities for employing adults with disabilities. A description of vocational service delivery in the United States will serve as a basis for describing and understanding the types of programs and services offered elsewhere in the world. International agencies and organizations that provide support for the vocational preparation and employment of adults with disabilities will also be briefly identified.

GUIDING PHILOSOPHIES, LEGISLATION, AND MANDATES

The past several decades have been unprecedented in the amount and scope of progressive legislation focused on disability issues in countries around the world. Throughout Europe, North and South America, Asia, and Africa laws reflecting the rights of persons with disabilities to equality of treatment and access to opportunity have been adopted (Groce, 1992). In addition, clear and positive trends are emerging in many countries that reflect a comprehensive approach to vocational service delivery for adults with disabilities that is increasingly deinstitutionalized and more community-based (Satapati, 1989).

Lunt and Thornton (1994) described two dominant approaches to the development of national legislation on disability employment issues. National policy in the U.S., Canada, and Australia tends to be more comprehensive in scope and usually focuses on issues of human rights and antidiscrimination, of which employment is just one aspect. Legislative schemes typically employed by Western European countries have had a compartmentalized approach to disability policy where legislation is connected with distinct issues (e.g., employment, physical access) or specific government agencies or departments.

Comprehensive Approach to Disability Employment Legislation

In the United States, federal legislation and policies covering the training and employment of adults with disabilities has undergone extensive changes in recent years. The rapidly emerging disability consumer movement of the 1970s, as well as international legislative efforts, exerted considerable influence on federal legislation resulting in an increased emphasis on environmental accessibility, consumer self-advocacy and empowerment, and the provision of independent living services (Groce, 1992; Rubin & Roessler, 1995). Since then, a myriad of specific measures (e.g., Rehabilitation Act Amendments of 1992, Individuals with Disabilities Education Act [IDEA] of 1990, the Americans with Disabilities Act of 1990; Social Security Work Incentives, Pub. L. No. 99-463) have generally endorsed the principles of access, empowerment, and inclusion for citizens with disabilities (McGaughey, Kiernan, McNally, Gilmore, & Keith, 1995; Whitehead, Davis, & Fisher, 1989).

Federal rehabilitation and disability-related legislation in the United States (e.g., the Developmental Disabilities Act of 1984 and the Rehabilitation Act Amendments of 1992) clearly establishes individuals with disabilities as consumers who are empowered to make choices about their rehabilitation program rather than passive recipients of services (Goldberg, 1989; Wehman & Kregel, 1995). Another important change in rehabilitation services has been a shift from employability to employment-based outcomes (Arkansas Research and Training Center in Vocational Rehabilitation, 1993). Federal mandates also call for a renewed commitment to track and serve individuals with severe disabilities, develop and maintain interagency collaboration and service coordination, plan for and provide services to young adults with disabilities preparing to transition from school to adult life, expand services for individuals with developmental disabilities, and advance the civil rights of persons with disabilities (Gilbride, Stensrud, & Johnson, 1994; Rubin & Roessler, 1995).

The Americans with Disabilities Act (ADA) of 1990 further advances the civil rights of individuals with disabilities. The ADA, which prohibits discrimination on the basis of disability, has been referred to as the most comprehensive and advanced legislation on disability in the world (Groce, 1992; Rubin & Roessler, 1995). The ADA is a broad civil rights statute guaranteeing equal access for people with disabilities in virtually every aspect of life including employment, and the services and benefits of state and local governments such as public education and transportation (Brown & Johnson, 1994).

Compartmentalized Approach to Disability Employment Legislation

Some countries, particularly those in Western Europe, have adopted a more focused or specialized approach to disability and employment issues. Yet, despite a segmented or compartmentalized approach to legislation and public policy, vocational service delivery in these countries tends to be comprehensive and well-coordinated.

The basic legislation governing vocational services in Germany was enacted in the mid-1970s (e.g., Employment Promotion Act, Order of the Governing Body of the Federal Institute of Employment on Industrial and Vocational Rehabilitation of People with Disabilities) and has been amended several times (Goldberg, 1989). As a whole, these laws provide a comprehensive, multidisciplinary system of interlocking institutions that provide for the educational, medical, social, and vocational needs of German adults with disabilities (Council of Europe, 1993).

In the United Kingdom, vocational services to adults with disabilities are provided under the auspices of the Employment Service, which was originally designated by the Employment and Training Act of 1973 as amended in 1988 and 1989. This law established two agencies responsible for the delivery of services to citizens with disabilities throughout Great Britain, the Employment Service and the Training Agency. These agencies provide a wide range of rehabilitative and supportive services including vocational assessment, vocational training and placement, communication, and adaptive aids and services. In an effort to provide comprehensive vocational service delivery, the Disabled Persons (Services, Consultation, and Representation) Act of 1986 fostered closer cooperation between agencies providing medical, educational, social, and vocational services. Other long-standing UK legislation (e.g., the Disabled Persons [Employment] Acts of 1944 and 1958, and the 1986 amendments) requires all workers with disabilities to register at local Employment Service offices, requires vocational assessment toward the end of an individual's school involvement, and allows the Secretary of State for Employment to designate certain occupations, such as car park attendant or passenger electric lift attendant, as especially suitable for people with disabilities and restrict entry to those persons (Council of Europe, 1993; Fish, 1990).

Other European countries such as Belgium, Spain, France, Denmark, Italy, Sweden, and Luxembourg also have extensive legislation and policies governing vocational services including occupational counseling, educational and occupational training, sheltered employment, and material or social assistance. Legislative mandates in these countries tend to reflect a philosophy of employment for all. In an effort to attain this ideal, a variety of measures have been enacted including social security (e.g., disability insurance, special allowances for citizens with disabilities, and unemployment benefits), compensation, vocational rehabilitation, and intervention schemes (Council of Europe, 1993; Sailor, 1989).

One typical response from many European governments has involved establishing legal requirements to change employers' behavior regarding the training and hiring of potential workers with disabilities. Since the end of World War I, the most commonly adopted legislative strategy has involved the use of quota systems and reserved employment (Lunt & Thornton, 1994). The basic feature of quota systems, or affirmative action measures, is a requirement that businesses must hire workers with disabilities at legally established standards (Konig & Schalock, 1991; Rubin & Roessler, 1995). While many nations rely on quota systems, Bordieri (1986) observed that specific hiring mandates vary widely across countries. Quotas may range from approximately 2% for Japanese employers to 15% or more for businesses with more than 35 employees in Italy. Other examples are found in Spain and the Netherlands (2%), England and Ireland (3%), Israel and Egypt (5%), Germany (6%), and France (7%). Quite recently, China has begun to test the efficacy of a quota system for hiring citizens with disabilities on a trial basis in nine Chinese cities (Yun, Piao, & Gargiulo, 1995).

Although not part of the European community, legislative mandates and service options found in Japan are quite comparable to those found in Europe. The Physically Handicapped Persons Employment Promotion Law was enacted in 1960 as the first major employment law for individuals with disabilities in Japan. The importance of this legislation was several-fold. Perhaps most importantly was a change in philosophy from social welfare to employment opportunity for persons with disabilities. The employment of persons with physical disabilities was promoted through an employment quota system, on-the-job adjustment training program, and assistance grant system. In addition, vocational guidance and placement services were developed and made available at local Public Employment Security Offices (PESOs) throughout Japan (Matsui, 1994).

Recent changes to Japan's fundamental legislation on employment and disability reflect the changing needs of its citizens and the culmination of an international effort during the 1980s, sponsored by the United Nations, to highlight the needs of persons with disabilities. One of these changes occurred in 1987 with the Law for the Employment Promotion, and so forth of the Disabled, which reflected a theme of full participation and equality. More recently, amendments have strengthened the measures for Japanese citizens with intellectual, behavioral, and emotional disabilities. Recent passage of related legislation (e.g., Employment Measures Law, Employment Insurance Law) has reflected an intent of the Japanese government to offer vocational training and employment services to persons with disabilities in an integrated and systematic fashion (Japan Association for Employment of the Disabled, 1992; Matsui, 1994).

Approaches to Disability Employment Legislation in Developing Countries

While the use of quota systems appears to be positive for many industrialized nations, quota systems may not be appropriate for many developing nations (Mintaredja, 1978). As a whole, less industrialized countries have not been as responsive to the social or vocational needs of their citizens with disabilities. For example, legislative efforts aimed at providing vocational services to adults with disabilities in India are practically nonexistent. As a result of limited legislative support and a lack of formalized services, the delivery of vocational services are usually developed and provided by family members or relatives (Scorzelli, 1995).

Even though a need exists to develop stronger and more comprehensive vocational legislation and services for adults with disabilities in developing countries, considerable advancements have been made in recent years (Armstrong, 1993). Couch (1993) reported that legislative efforts currently underway in many Central American countries may eventually pave the way to awareness of disability and employment issues and the development of formalized vocational service structures like those found in industrialized nations.

VOCATIONAL REHABILITATION AND OTHER VOCATIONAL TRAINING OPTIONS

United States

An estimated 20 million Americans have work-related disabilities (Gilbride et al., 1994). The general system of vocational services available to these adults has been characterized as a collection of many independent rehabilitation services that use many different approaches, innovations, and models (Goldberg, 1989). One positive aspect to this arrangement is that services are often creative in design and implementation. Even so, services tend to be uncoordinated, fragmented, and guided by different agencies and philosophies (Sailor, 1989). Fragmentation of services in the U.S. may result in inadequate service provision for some adults with disabilities.

In the U.S., adults with disabilities are often eligible for vocational rehabilitation services offered through state offices of the Department of Vocational Rehabilitation (Brown & Johnson, 1994). Vocational rehabilitation services were created shortly after the end of World War I. These government services were designed to support persons with industrial accidents, physical disabilities, and primarily ambulatory impairments in reaching their fullest potential in work and independent living (Gilbride et al., 1994; Goldberg, 1989). Since its inception, vocational rehabilitation professionals in the U.S. have stressed employment as the primary outcome of service provision (Sailor, 1989).

While the goal of employment has remained relatively intact over the years, a fuller and more comprehensive approach to rehabilitation has recently emerged. From a singular focus on employment, multiple service priorities have developed including a commitment to facilitate independent living services and strengthening client involvement in the entire rehabilitation process. In addition, the types of disabilities considered eligible for services has expanded over the years to be more inclusive of a wide range of disabling conditions. Eligibility for vocational rehabilitation services is now typically based on the presence of a disability that presents a significant barrier to employment and the assumption that the person with a disability could benefit from rehabilitation services (Rubin & Roessler, 1995).

According to the 1992 Amendments to the Rehabilitation Act, the purpose of vocational rehabilitation in the United States is

> to provide comprehensive employment opportunities for individuals with disabilities; to maximize employability, independence, and integration; to direct the provision of rehabilitation services to recognition of career choice of persons with disabilities, and to establish systems of service and support for their career advancement; and to lead states and service providers to promote meaningful, gainful employment and independent living. (Arkansas Research and Training Center in Vocational Rehabilitation, 1993, p. 14)

Vocational rehabilitation represents a state-federal collaboration. The federal government (Rehabilitation Services Administration, RSA) provides the bulk of funding, technical assistance in program implementation, and leadership to state programs. RSA also provides a broad framework for program structure and operations. However, states are responsible for the day-to-day administration of rehabilitation programs such as establishing state-wide eligibility criteria (Brown & Johnson, 1994; Clearinghouse on Disability Information, 1993).

Rehabilitation counselors have an impressive list of services at their disposal including medical, psychological, and vocational assessments to determine functional strengths and limitations; counseling and guidance, referral and placement in necessary services; work adjustment and vocational training; job-seeking skills and employment placement; interpreter services; rehabilitation technology services; and postemployment services deemed necessary to maintain or regain suitable employment (American Share Foundation, 1996; Office of Special Education and Rehabilitative Services, 1996). The Arkansas Research and Training Center in Vocational Rehabilitation observed that "vocational rehabilitation is undergoing a transformation in employment services to respond to redefined priorities, diverse populations, changing labor markets, state-of-the art technologies, legislative mandate, and economic factors" (1993, p. 1).

The services that participants receive depend on each person's unique set of circumstances and identified needs. Identified needs form the basis for an individualized written rehabilitation plan, jointly developed between participant and rehabilitation counselor, which guides service provision (Clearinghouse on Disability Information, 1993). Rubin and Roessler noted that the job role of rehabilitation counselors is a demanding one that "calls for broad-based knowledge and skills related to affective counseling, vocational assessment, vocational counseling, case management, job development, and placement counseling" (1995, p. 215).

Bordieri (1986) observed that the U.S. emphasized competitive employment for adults with disabilities but has few national policies that promote the hiring of adults with disabilities. While not as broad or extensive as many European countries, the U.S. government does provide a variety of incentives and benefits to employers in an effort to encourage hiring workers with disabilities. Current incentives include tax credits, employer reimbursement for training periods, and indirect supports provided by job coaches (Whitehead et al., 1989). Examples of specific skills training programs and incentives for hiring adults with disabilities include (Pozner & Hammond, 1993; Simmons & Flexer, 1992):

- The Jobs Training Partnership Act (JTPA), which was created in 1981 "to prepare youth and unskilled adults for entry into the labor force and to afford job training to economically disadvantaged individuals and others facing serious barriers to employment who are in special needs of training to obtain productive employment" (Office of Special Education and Rehabilitative Services, 1993, p. 19).
- The Targeted Jobs Tax Credit (TJTC), which allows businesses tax credits of up to $2,400 for hiring workers with disabilities.
- Tax deductions of up to $35,000 are available for expenditures related to the modification or adaptation of business facilities. A little-known incentive, the Second Injury provision of the Workmen's Compensation Fund, provides protection for a business if an injury occurs to a worker as a direct result of the employee's disability.
- The Department of Labor provides waivers that allow employers to pay workers with disabilities less than the prevailing industry wage to allow time for training and establishing competitive work pace.

- One often overlooked benefit is the availability of employment specialists who provide placement, training, and follow-along support services to workers with disabilities. Funding is also available to defray excess costs associated with training and accommodations of employing persons with disabilities from Vocational Rehabilitation, the United States Employment Services, and Private Industry Councils.

Several Social Security benefits programs (Supplemental Security Income and Social Security Disability Income) provide monthly income and Medicare benefits to adults with disabilities and their families. These programs have been criticized by some who maintain that the benefits actually serve as a disincentive for obtaining employment. However, recent attempts have begun to include work incentives such as a nine-month trial work period, during which an individual may work and earn any amount of money without losing any benefits, reimbursement of disability-related work expenses, an extended period of program eligibility (up to 36 months after the trial work period), and a continuation of Medicare coverage for persons with disabilities who work (Office of Special Education and Rehabilitative Services, 1993; Rubin & Roessler, 1995; Shrey, Bangs, Mark, Hursh, & Kues, 1991).

Industrialized Nations

Western Europe. Despite differences in bureaucratic arrangements and service provision structures, Western European nations provide a wide range of vocational services to adults with disabilities. Like the United States, these countries offer vocational assessment, guidance and counseling, vocational training, sheltered or supported employment, and job placement assistance. Most nations also have elaborate systems of assistance that include financial support for travel, purchase of specialized equipment or workplace modifications, and employer benefits or incentives to hire workers with disabilities (Council of Europe, 1993). Holland, for example, has a long tradition of providing comprehensive protective, welfare-based services to its citizens with disabilities (Sailor, 1989). In many European countries (e.g., the United Kingdom, Denmark, and Italy), several important initiatives have emerged in recent years that reflect a philosophy of empowering individuals with disabilities to be involved in the decision-making process and a shift toward integration in school-based programs and community-based employment (Fish, 1990; Thomson, Ward, & Wishart, 1995).

The German system of vocational services for adults with disabilities is characterized by its comprehensive and coordinated nature. Goldberg (1989) noted that while the German system does offer extensive social, recreational, and work opportunities for citizens with disabilities, they are more likely to be provided in segregated environments or institutions than in other European or North American countries. This may be due to a combination of several factors including the philosophical objections of German educators and vocational service providers, as well as cultural beliefs and traditions that uphold discipline, order, and a respect and deference to authority. Vocational training is provided in one of several dozen occupational training centers (*Berufsbildungswerke*) throughout Germany, where young adults with disabilities choose and complete a course of training. Involvement in this training program includes room and board. Despite the criticism of segregated service delivery, Goldberg praises the German vocational rehabilitation system as ingenious, creative, coordinated, and well-funded.

Luxembourg has developed four distinct levels of rehabilitation services with defined target groups including a general school level, prevocational training level, public and private vocational training levels, and rehabilitation facilities for adults. General school services are provided to adolescents with disabilities (ages 15–22 years) to support the successful completion of a lower secondary, technical/vocational, or domestic science school curriculum. Prevocational training is available to young adults with intellectual or other severe disabilities and provided in designated special schools located throughout the country. Vocational training is provided in both the public and private sector. Public sector training usually results in a vocational or technical training certificate in manual skills. In the private sector, employers are charged with training a job applicant but receive support from the Placement and Vocational Rehabilitation Office for Handicapped Workers (a government agency). Rehabilitation facilities are also available and provide long-term, sheltered work opportunities for adults with disabilities (Council of Europe, 1993).

A variety of government policies, initiatives, and legal requirements such as quota systems, government grants and tax credits to employers, wage subsidies, and reserved employment are evidenced in many Western European countries to encourage businesses to hire adults with disabilities (Bordieri, 1986; Lunt & Thornton, 1994). The central element of quota systems, also known as employment equity or affirmative action programs, is the call for specially designed proactive measures to increase workforce participation, usually through reserving a certain number of jobs for persons with disabilities.

Noncompliance with established quotas typically result in fines being assessed against the offending business. Fines are usually placed in a public fund that is then spent on providing vocational services, employment opportunities, salary subsidies, and workplace accommodations to adults with disabilities (Konig & Schalock, 1991; Raskin, 1994). For example, revenues received from English and German businesses have been used to cover expenses associated with job site accommodations and transportation to the workplace (Bordieri, 1986; Lunt & Thornton, 1994).

Several other types of incentives are used by European governments to encourage hiring workers with disabilities. Wages subsidies are used to compensate for lost productivity. In Great Britain, the Job Introduction Scheme is a national

program that offers financial grants to employers to subsidize the salary of a
worker with disabilities for up to 13 weeks of trial employment, as well as to
modify existing worksites to ensure retention of these workers. One drawback to
a wage subsidy policy is the attention drawn to the limitations of workers with
disabilities rather than their work-related abilities (Lunt & Thornton, 1994).
Other available incentives provide rewards/bonuses or grant tax credits to those
businesses who employ individuals with a disability (Bordieri, 1986; Goldberg,
1989; Thomson et al., 1995).

Eastern Europe. Russia, with a disabled population estimated at 10 million,
faces a number of formidable challenges in the provision of vocational services and employment. First, unlike its Western European and North American
neighbors, Russia does not have a legislative history of establishing the rights
of its citizens with disabilities. As a result, issues like physical accessibility or
employment are addressed on a case by case basis with differing degrees of success. Negative attitudes, pervasive discrimination toward persons with disability,
a lack of government resources, and a weak economic base have created additional problems. Russians with disabilities are typically classified into one of
three categories making them eligible for government pensions and services. Unfortunately, once categorized, adults with disabilities are often actively discouraged from pursuing advanced education or employment opportunities (Impact,
1995/1996).

Recent developments in Russia hold promise for improvements. The All-
Russian Society of the Disabled is a private organization that has a leadership
role in protecting and expanding the rights of Russians with disabilities. The
potential of this group to make substantive changes in Russia is evident in its
membership of over 2.2 million persons with disabilities and large bureaucratic
network of regional, district, and local offices spread across the country. The organization currently owns and manages over 1,350 businesses employing approximately 19,000 people with disabilities (Impact, 1995/1996).

Asia. A number of vocational rehabilitation efforts have also been observed
in Asian countries like China, Japan, and Hong Kong. The National Institute on
Disability and Rehabilitation Research (1993) noted that the unique sociocultural
values and beliefs of citizens in these countries tends to influence the treatment
of individuals with disabilities. Examples of these beliefs include the social stigma
attached to persons with disabilities, the influence of Confucianism, and a pre-
occupation with social order and the collective. One general outcome of cultural
beliefs is the reluctance of persons with disabilities to seek assistance from professionals outside the immediate family. This results in a substantial delay before
professional help is sought and attained.

The vocational rehabilitation system in Hong Kong is modeled on both the

U.S. and British delivery systems and has aggressively undergone substantial revisions the past several years. Whether or not these changes will be retained and enacted given the recent return of Hong Kong to Chinese control remains to be seen. Regardless, recent legislative efforts such as the Disability Discrimination Ordinance of 1995 and the White Paper on Rehabilitation, have resulted in a comprehensive policy to guide vocational policy and services for persons with disabilities for the next decade. Currently, vocational rehabilitation policy is detailed in the Rehabilitation Program Plan that describes the role of government departments, statutory bodies, and over 70 nongovernment organizations that provide vocational services to adults with disabilities. The country's Vocational Training Council operates five skills training centers for adults with disabilities. In addition to specific skills training, the Vocational Assessment Center and the Technical Aids and Resource Center provide vocational assessment, guidance and counseling services, develop job accommodations, adaptations, and technical aids needed to obtain or maintain employment, and job placement assistance (Hong Kong Rehabilitation Services, 1996; National Institute on Disability and Rehabilitation Research, 1993).

China, with over 52 million citizens with disabilities, faces enormous obstacles to the development and delivery of vocational services to adults with disabilities, including the largest disabled population in the world, the social stigma and discrimination associated with disability, availability of limited resources, and a lack of qualified rehabilitation and education professionals. In addition, China does not have a long history of providing specialized vocational services to adolescents or adults with disabilities. Despite the obstacles, China has focused considerable attention and effort on improving special education and vocational rehabilitation services within the past 15 years. Emerging vocational policies in China reflect a philosophy of community integration and self-reliance (Yun et al., 1995).

China's Disabled Persons' Federation has been at the forefront of recent government efforts to reduce discrimination and increase resources to enhance employment opportunities for adults with disabilities. Vocational training goals were detailed in the Work Program for Disabled Persons during the Period of the 8th Five-Year National Development Plan (1991–1995). This plan established specific career paths for persons with disabilities who are trained in one of 30 segregated vocational training schools. Customary vocational paths for individuals with visual impairment include massage training and piano tuning, while persons with hearing impairments are often directed toward carpentry and tailoring occupations. Citizens with intellectual disabilities are usually employed by special government factories (Yun et al., 1995).

In contrast with China's struggling vocational rehabilitation efforts, Japan maintains a highly complex and interconnected system of vocational services for adults with disabilities. A number of government agencies are directly or indirectly involved in providing vocational programs and services. Public Employment Security Offices (PESOs), established according to provisions found in the

Employment Security Law, play a central role in providing vocational assessment, guidance and counseling, training and employment referrals, and job placement services. While PESOs provide vocational assistance to all Japanese citizens, a top priority is to promote the hiring of persons with disabilities. Local vocational centers for persons with disabilities bear the primary responsibility for vocational training and support and are located in each of the 47 prefectures in Japan. A variety of vocational training programs are available to participants including sheltered employment and facility-based or on-the-job training (Japan Association for Employment of the Disabled, 1992; Matsui, 1994).

In Japan, the Law for Employment Promotion, etc., for the Disabled established a two-pronged system of allocating employment for adults with disabilities: "an employment quota system which obligates employers to hire a certain minimum ratio of disabled persons, and a levy and grant system to compensate the financial burdens involved" (Japan Association for Employment of the Disabled, 1992, p. 42). As with European counterparts, the fines and levies collected from Japanese businesses are redistributed to businesses in compliance with the quota requirements to subsidize wages and modify existing work sites.

Developing Nations

A large portion of the world's disabled population is located in developing nations. These individuals are among the poorest and least powerful members of society (Osuala, 1993). Understanding the incidence of and meanings attached to disability in developing nations is often complex and intricately tied to the social and cultural conditions found in a particular country. The problems faced by persons with disabilities in developing countries are often not limited to the complications associated with disability but include a myriad of other problems that affect daily living including large-scale unemployment, poverty, and overpopulation. These conditions make finding suitable vocational opportunities extremely difficult (Satapati, 1989).

Given the challenging situations encountered in many developing countries, it is not surprising that most government-sponsored vocational services are uneven in the nature and scope of services provided. Bordieri (1986) observed that both time-limited services or long-term vocational support to persons with disabilities is usually not a high human service priority for developing nations. When services do exist, "less industrialized nations seem to pattern their rehabilitation efforts on techniques used in the United States. [However,] they are generally not as comprehensive given their more pressing social and health concerns" (p. 5).

Satapati (1989) explained that while governments in developing countries often have a limited or ineffective role in vocational service provision, nongovernmental organizations do provide some assistance. When available, four basic approaches to providing vocational services to adults with disabilities can be identified, including institutional, center-based, extension, and special opportunity approaches. Institutional approaches often draw participants from a relatively large area and provide vocational training and assistance at one location, typically an institution. This approach has been criticized for being cost-intensive and isolating persons with disabilities from their communities. Centers usually provide in-house, short-term training opportunities, while extension staff go to homes and communities to deliver vocational services. Special opportunities are vocational training opportunities often sponsored by institutions but based in the community. Despite the rather bleak picture regarding the availability of vocational services for adults with disabilities in developing countries, vocational service provision in some developing countries have seen marked improvements in recent years (Armstrong, 1993).

Central America. Individuals with disabilities in Central America encounter a number of serious barriers to adequate vocational preparation and employment. First, these countries are collectively among the most underdeveloped and poorest in the world. Second, individuals with disabilities face pervasive unemployment, ranging from 9% to 45% over the past decade. To further complicate matters, a general prevailing attitude exists that maintains people with disabilities cannot be expected to hold jobs. These factors have almost eliminated opportunities for persons with disabilities to enter normal labor markets (Couch, 1993).

Couch (1993, 1994) conducted an extensive study on the condition of vocational services in seven Central American countries. He observed that, like developed countries, the official positions and approaches taken by various Central American governments concerning individuals with disabilities followed logical and predictable patterns: that is, first providing medical care and maintenance, next establishing special education and vocational training opportunities, and finally offering vocational rehabilitation. Although most Central American countries are moving in this direction, few opportunities currently exist to obtain vocational services and the few that do exist are limited to urban areas.

Despite limited service availability, Couch (1993, 1994) reports a number of innovative measures being implemented across Central America in rehabilitation programming, job development, and job placement alternatives for individuals with disabilities. Efforts to tie secondary and postsecondary vocational services initiated in Belize and Panama are now being adopted by the ministries of education in other countries of the region. Costa Rica, Guatemala, Panama, El Salvador, and Honduras have recently established national offices for the employment of persons with disabilities. Their ministries of labor offices are small but have made impressive efforts in job placement and could eventually evolve into national vocational rehabilitation systems. Guatemala, the most heavily industrialized and populated country in Central America, recently established a cooperative venture with private business called the Institute for Vocational

Training. This venture provides employers and their workers with disabilities a combination of formal vocational training held at a local training center and on-the-job training conducted at the regular work site. The least-developed country, Honduras, provides approximately 1,600 of its citizens with disabilities (4% of the total disabled population) some type of educational, vocational, or rehabilitative services in one of seven major education/rehabilitation facilities in the country. Although some government-sponsored programs exist, a majority of services are provided through the private sector.

India. Most vocational services provided to adults with disabilities in India are initiated by the private sector, often a family member or nongovernmental organization (Satapati, 1989). This arrangement may be due in part to a paternalistic attitude that maintains individuals with disabilities are incapable of providing for themselves or of functioning independently. The caste system, which defines traditional social categories and roles in India, also contributes to the limited role assumed by the Indian government. Although limited, recent developments in some parts of India have begun to address the lack of vocational services. The adult center provides prevocational training for adolescents with disabilities who are close to completing their education and postgraduate training leading to job placement for adults. The job placement center in Calcutta provides vocational training in food service, printing and packaging, leather works, and computer programming (Scorzelli, 1995).

JOB PLACEMENT SYSTEMS AND ALTERNATIVES

Most job development and employment placement services for adults with disabilities in industrialized countries can be categorized into one of four delivery systems: general rehabilitation counselor, specialized placement professionals, contracted services, and supported employment. The general rehabilitation counselor system is probably the most established approach to placement assistance and continues to dominate the United States state-federal system of vocational service delivery. The specialized professionals model first emerged during the 1970s and is characterized by the use of placement specialists who provide job-seeking skills, job club, employer development, and other technical services. A third delivery method known as contracted services moves placement functions closer to the employer. On-the-job training and Projects with Industry programs are examples of attempts to support employers in the hiring and training of workers with disabilities. Supported employment represents a dramatic departure from the first three systems in that prerequisite employability skills and pre-placements services are de-emphasized. Rather, the focus is on post-placement training, integration, and ongoing services as needed to maintain employment.

Emerging trends designed to assist in placing adults with disabilities into employment include marketing individual and organizational needs through environmental assessment and strategic planning, team networking and mentoring, and demand-side job placement that prepares and supports employers in hiring workers with disabilities (Fish, 1990; Gilbride et al., 1994; McGaughey et al., 1995; Satapati, 1994).

Vocational outcomes related to the use of these four options span a continuum defined by the level of supports needed to be successful and encompass potential work settings that are fully or partially integrated (e.g., full competitive employment, individual supported employment, and group supported employment), as well as environments that are sheltered or nonvocational (e.g,. facility-based work and nonwork programs). Primary distinctions are made for adults with disabilities in integrated settings based on the need for time-limited or long-term/ongoing support (Bordieri, 1986). While the trend in U. S. vocational service delivery is for integration in normal work environments (Sailor, 1989), facility-based work and nonwork environments continue to be options for many adults with disabilities. Facility-based programming is distinguished primarily on whether or not the major function is work. Nonwork programs focus on therapy and prevocational skills development rather than paid work (McGaughey et al., 1995).

INTEGRATED WORK ALTERNATIVES FOR ADULTS WITH DISABILITIES

United States

Of all integrated or semi-integrated employment models available in the U.S., the supported employment model has, by far, received the greatest attention over the past decade (Wehman & Kregel, 1995). The emergence of supported employment as a viable employment option has been preceded by several important developments. Demonstrations that persons with severe disabilities are capable of work, as well as major trends that stress individualization, community-based services, consumer empowerment, and the perceived inadequacy of traditional rehabilitation services have resulted in a growing realization that adults with disabilities can be productive and integrated members of their community if they receive necessary training and support (Konig & Schalock, 1991; Office of Special Education and Rehabilitative Services, 1993; Whitehead et al., 1989).

Federal legislation has established the parameters of supported employment and describe necessary program components. The Rehabilitation Act of 1986 defined supported employment as

> Competitive employment in integrated settings (a) for individuals with severe handicaps for whom competitive employment has not traditionally occurred, or (b) for individuals whom competitive employment has been interrupted or inter-

mittent as a result of a severe disability and who, because of their handicap, need ongoing support services to perform such work. (Federal Register, May 12, 1988)

Wehman and Kregel (1995) argued that long-term support and follow-along services have proven to be necessary components in the successful vocational placement of many adults with severe disabilities.

Supported employment programs are typically operated using public funds and administered by government and nongovernment organizations or university-affiliated programs. Currently, five separate U.S. government agencies (Department of Education, Administration of Developmental Disabilities, Social Security Administration, Department of Labor, and the Office of Planning and Evaluation in the Department of Health and Human Services) provide supported employment funding and employment opportunities to adults with disabilities (McGaughey et al., 1995).

Several different models of supported employment have been developed to address the diverse employment and support needs of persons with disabilities including individualized placement, enclaves, and mobile work crews (Konig & Schalock, 1991; McGaughey et al., 1995). Mobile work crews and enclaves involve small groups of workers with disabilities being actually situated or contracted by a host business to perform work tasks in a competitive work environment and are primarily entrepreneurial in nature (Pozner & Hammond, 1993; Simmons & Flexer, 1991). Whitehead et al. (1989) noted a relative balance throughout the U.S. in the prevalence of these three major external supported employment models.

These primary supported employment models use a variety of innovative, community-based approaches—unsubsidized employment, transitional employment schemes that help adults with disabilities try work in competitive employment for up to six months while being subsidized and supported by a job coach, and long-term supported employment with ongoing support provided by a job coach—to provide individualized assistance deemed necessary to be successful (Goldberg, 1989). Although various approaches and combinations of approaches exist, all supported employment models emphasize a place-train approach to competitive job placement, provide the normal benefits of working to participants, and accommodate all disabilities, especially the most severe (Bordieri, 1986; Simmons & Flexer, 1992).

A number of benefits have been cited for supported employment models. Wehman and Kregel observed that supported employment offers many adults with disabilities "their first choice between a lifetime of performing meaningless tasks for inconsequential wages in segregated workshop settings and the opportunities and challenges of a real job in their local communities" (1995, p. 286). Other major benefits include a raise in wage earnings (up to 150% in some cases), integration and interaction with the nondisabled community, and an enhanced sense of worth and independence (Whitehead et al., 1989). Supported employment can also result in a significant return on the investments needed for training and support over the long-term. However, initial start-up costs are often quite high (Konig & Schalock, 1991). Despite the benefits associated with supported employment models, Wehman and Kregel suggest that the early momentum of the supported employment movement appears to have slowed. While program advocates envisioned a vocational employment system without sheltered employment options, most service providers "still maintain policies that refer to supported employment as merely one of an array of appropriate vocational options for individuals with disabilities" (p. 289).

Industrialized Nations

The concept of supported employment originated in the United States but has been adopted by many industrialized nations (Pozner & Hammond, 1993). The development of supported employment in the United Kingdom is fairly representative of the process followed in other European countries. Until recently, citizens with disabilities in the United Kingdom basically had two employment options: employment in a competitive industry or sheltered workshop (Bordieri, 1986; Thomson et al., 1995). Although supported employment has offered another job placement alternative, it has developed on a more modest scale than found in the United States. Pozner and Hammond characterized the growth of supported employment programs in the United Kingdom as slow and sporadic. They noted that "funding is piecemeal and fragile with little long-term funding available to agencies" (p. 22).

Supported employment agencies in the United Kingdom have gradually begun to place increasing numbers of adults with disabilities into competitive and supported employment. The national charity, the Royal Society for Mentally Handicapped Children and Adults, has pioneered employment services for adults with disabilities for several decades and operates a network of local service agencies through its Pathway Employment Service model. As part of the Pathway Employment model, employers who hire workers with disabilities are reimbursed for expenses for a trial period of up to 12 weeks before they must commit themselves. A foster worker, appointed from within the business, is responsible to support the new employee and help with the adjustment to competitive employment. A number of back-up support services are also available for employers, employees, and others (Pozner & Hammond, 1993). Current emphasis in the United Kingdom is on assisting sheltered employment workers into competitive employment, although long-term goals include expansion of services to include adolescents with disabilities preparing to transition from school to adult life (Bordieri, 1986; Pozner & Hammond).

Examples of supported employment programs can also be found in Italy, France, Australia, and Japan. Konig and Schalock (1991) reported on an employment project in Genoa, Italy designed to integrate adults with disabilities into competitive employment. Genoa project participants are matched with appropriate jobs and signed to a one-year contract with the host business. The project reimburses employers for the worker's wages, while the employer agrees to subsidize job training and support activities. The Genoa project boasts a high degree of success; over 90% of participants have achieved continuous, fully compensated, and integrated employment. In France, a not-for-profit organization (the Groupments Interprofessionels Regionauz pour la Promotion de L'Emplo, des Personnes Handiapees [GIRPEH]) has promoted the employment of workers with disabilities in integrated and semi-integrated environments since 1977. GIRPEH promotes the hiring and full integration of workers with disabilities, provides support for businesses in managing workers with disabilities, and develops ties between business and organizations that offer sheltered work areas for adults with disabilities (Bordieri, 1986).

Although not a supported employment setting in the strictest sense, Centre Industries of Australia provides an excellent example of an affirmative industry. An affirmative industries model offers fully integrated and meaningful employment to workers with and without disabilities working together on challenging tasks. Originally developed in 1961 as a sheltered workshop, Centre Industries now offers fully integrated employment to approximately 300 workers with disabilities and 400 workers without disabilities. No preferences are given to workers with disabilities; everyone uses the same equipment and earns the same piece rate. The affirmative industry model of Centre Industries was adopted by the Japanese government in the late 1970s as the model factory program. Model factory programs provide employment opportunities to adults with (and without) disabilities in light manufacturing industries. Workplaces sanctioned as model factory businesses are provided some government support in the form of low-interest loans (Bordieri, 1986).

Developing Nations

Community-Based Approaches.   Despite the advances made in supported employment models for adults with disabilities in industrialized nations, modern innovations and programs are often far too expensive to be readily available to a vast majority of people in developing countries (Groce, 1992). In response, the international community (e.g, International Labor Organization, Rehabilitation International) has increasingly focused on establishing decentralized, community-based training and employment programs in countries such as the Philippines, Indonesia, Malawi, Ethiopia, and Zimbabwe (Konig, 1990). Community-based rehabilitation (CBR) is a grassroots effort designed to provide vocational services to adults with disabilities by people in the local community. Vocational services provided by rehabilitation professionals are de-emphasized. Instead, community responsibility is emphasized and existing community resources (including volunteers, friends, and family members without full professional training) are used to provide the vocational services necessary for adults with disabilities to become successfully employed (Groce, 1992; International Labor Organization, 1994; Scorzelli, 1995). The CBR approach attempts to offer local solutions to vocational training and employment problems (Brouilette & Margia, 1993). Types of services typically offered through the CBR approach include

> identifying and opening training and employment opportunities in the community, identifying the needs and potential of disabled people, arranging for the training in agricultural and rural occupations, helping them find jobs, supporting the establishment of cottage industries, facilitating access to credit, assisting disabled people to join cooperatives, and with promotional activities and the like. (Momm & Konig, 1989, p. 506)

CBR can include a range of possible outcomes including domestic, subsistence, or salaried forms of employment. "In agrarian economies, work for barter or in-kind payment can be more appropriate than work for pay. In places were regular integrated employment is competitive, cooperative and revolving loan schemes are ways to establish employment alternatives" (Brouilette & Margia, 1993, p. 28).

Satapati (1989) reported that the concept of community-based rehabilitation has become fairly widespread, resulting in numerous programs being implemented in developing countries. Yet, despite the success and appeal of CBR at the local level, many developing countries are reluctant, from a political standpoint, to adopt the advice of international aid agencies that may have hidden or unknown cost implications. In their critique, Momm and Konig (1989) concluded that "government agencies, local communities, and the disabled themselves view CBR as something that has yet to prove its value" (p. 505).

Entrepreneurial Efforts. Couch (1993) speculated that individual and group placement approaches to supported employment would not be successful in most Central American countries due to economic and attitudinal barriers prevalent throughout the region. He noted, however, that entrepreneurial ventures appeared to be successful in some developing nations. And, in fact, self-employment is increasingly recognized as a viable way for adults with disabilities to participate in the labor force (Konig, 1990).

Central American countries have successful introduced cooperatives and microbusinesses as two means of self-employment. Examples of successful cooperatives include a mattress factory in El Salvador that employs workers with visual impairments and an agricultural cooperative sponsored by the Guatemalan Social Security Rehabilitation Center that hires workers with visual or intellectual disabilities. Costa Rica also has a number of agricultural-based cooperatives. A common type of microbusiness in many Central American countries is the cottage industry. In a cottage industry sponsored by the Guatemalan Center for Education and Vocational Rehabilitation, yarn is shipped to rural workers that have received training in weaving native textiles. When the handicrafts are completed, they are returned to the Center for sale (Couch, 1993, 1994).

Successful entrepreneurial ventures like self-employment, cooperatives, and microbusinesses are also evident in other developing countries. In Malaysia, the Society of Orthopedically Handicapped—Malaysia (POCAM), a self-help and advocacy organization, encourages self-employment for persons with physical disabilities because it is amenable to both rural and urban settings (Armstrong, 1993). A business run by Nepal's Association for the Welfare of Mentally Retarded Persons operates a business that provides employment for adults with intellectual disabilities. Workers with disabilities manufacture natural peanut butter from peanuts grown in Southern Nepal. A third example of entrepreneurship in developing countries can be found in the African nation of Mauritius. Here, adult workers with intellectual disabilities grow flowers, which are then exported to Europe (Brouilette & Margia, 1993).

SEGREGATED WORK ALTERNATIVES FOR ADULTS WITH DISABILITIES

United States

Sheltered Employment.   Simmons and Flexer (1992) observed that traditional vocational service systems for adults with disabilities have relied heavily on sheltered employment and various near-work and nonwork options provided by public and private rehabilitation facilities. Sheltered employment usually involves segregated work settings for individuals with disabilities who perform prevocational or subcontracted work tasks. Historically, sheltered employment has been viewed as an appropriate alternative for persons with intellectual or severe disability. However, in recent years, sheltered workshop placements have been criticized for warehousing adults with disabilities rather than providing vocational skill development and placement in competitive employment opportunities (Whitehead et al., 1989). As a result, a shift has been occurring in the U.S. and other industrialized countries from providing sheltered to supported employment opportunities (Lunt & Thornton, 1994).

The provision of sheltered employment services has generated a large and complex service provider network throughout the U.S., composed primarily of private not-for-profit organizations. And in spite of calls for replacing segregated systems with integrated employment opportunities, the current system of activity centers and sheltered workshops remains largely intact, leading McGaughey et al. (1995) to exclaim that a dual service system providing both sheltered and supported employment exists in the United States. Proponents of supported employment for adults with disabilities continually call for the conversion of reha-bilitation facility-based day programs and sheltered employment to integrated and meaningful employment outcomes (Wehman & Kregel, 1995). However, it is doubtful that a complete transformation like this will occur anytime soon (Whitehead et al., 1989).

Rehabilitation Facilities. Private, not-for-profit, and for-profit rehabilitation facilities also provide a variety of internal and external vocational services to adults with disabilities. Examples of services available from rehabilitation facili-ties include both time-limited and long-term sheltered employment, as well as various ancillary services like case management, assessment, vocational training, job placement, job coaching, and follow-along support services. Facilities may also provide or coordinate other types of services such as job redesign, employer consultation, transportation, housing, and financial assistance (Gilbride et al., 1994; Rubin & Roessler, 1995; Whitehead et al., 1989).

Industrialized Nations

Western Europe. In recent years, many European countries have embraced the underlying philosophy of providing integrated work settings for adults with disabilities. Even so, limited progress has been made toward developing inte-grated work alternatives (Pozner & Hammond, 1993). A variety of reasons exist for slower movement toward adopting and implementing philosophies of inte-gration and program options like supported employment. In Great Britain, for example, high rates of unemployment, chronic labor problems, and poor eco-nomic conditions have shaped government policies to favor sheltered placement. Switerland's heavy reliance on high competitive work production standards pro-vides little or no incentive to offer integrated work opportunities to adults with disabilities. Finally, the social insurance systems in countries such as Great Brit-ain, Switzerland, and France are also cause for limited integrated work opportu-nities. In these countries, many adults with disabilities choose employment in a sheltered work setting to avoid the risk of losing governmental benefits (Sailor, 1989).

Bordieri explained that "when compared to the sheltered employment in the United States, however, the workshops of Sweden, Denmark, Hungary, The Netherlands, Great Britain, Poland, and The Federal Republic of Germany are operated differently. . . . workshops in these countries are run like businesses" (1986, p. 28). Most European sheltered workshops stress an industrial orientation rather than rehabilitation and training. Holland, for example, has equipped its sheltered workshops with state-of-the-art equipment and technology, allowing them to successfully compete with private business and industry. As a result of this investment, the Dutch government "is unlikely to easily embrace a plan that rapidly replaces these programs with more integrated alternatives" (Sailor, 1989,

p. 44). Denmark operates a two-tiered system of sheltered employment based on level of productivity. High-production workshops are time-limited and have a high rate of job placement in integrated employment settings, while low-production workshops provide segregated work experiences and day care programs for adults with severe disabilities.

Sheltered workshops in many parts of Europe tend to be viewed as self-contained programs rather than automatic extensions of the vocational service delivery system. Vocational services in many European countries are provided by separate rehabilitation facilities not directly affiliated with sheltered workshops. While in other countries, like France, community rehabilitation facilities often provide comprehensive services to adults with disabilities (Sailor, 1989).

Bordieri provided a brief comparison of the major differences between sheltered workshops found in Europe and those in the United States.

> Sheltered workshops in Europe tend to be larger than workshops in the USA, utilize more modern technology in their operations, pay workers competitive or near competitive wages, provide workers with typical fringe benefits found in industry, tend to be more integrated with disabled and nondisabled employees working together, and emphasize long-term rather than transitional employment. (1986, p. 28)

Despite Bordieri's positive review, Lunt and Thornton (1994) paint a different picture. They argued that sheltered employment in Europe is associated with low wages, reliance on social security benefits, and underemployment.

Asia.   In China, adults with disabilities are classified into two groups: those who have working ability and those without an ability to work. Sheltered employment and self-employment are two primary employment options available for individuals capable of working. Sheltered employment is provided in one of approximately 50,000 government-subsidized (welfare) factories located throughout China. Each factory is provided exemptions for all or part of its tax liability for hiring workers with disabilities (Yun et al., 1995).

The number of sheltered workshops for adults with disabilities has been steadily rising in Japan as competitive employment opportunities for these individuals have steadily decreased (Japan Association for Employment of the Disabled, 1994). Matsui (1994) reported that approximately 4,000 public and private sheltered workshops (e.g., rehabilitation and welfare) currently exist in Japan. Although the goal of sheltered workshops is to assist their clientele in obtaining competitive employment, annual placement rates for individuals with disabilities in competitive employment has remained at or below 2% annually.

Developing Nations

Brouilette and Margia (1993) noted that sheltered employment opportunities are limited in many developing countries. While a less attractive alternative than community-based, integrated work opportunities, they suggested that when available sheltered employment can be a viable option for vocational training and income and can even support CBR initiatives in developing countries. "Employees training in sheltered environments will have a greater opportunity for assimilation into regular employment" (p. 28).

Funding is an issue for most sheltered workshops and rehabilitation facilities, regardless of the country. However, the problem is often greater in developing countries due to the limited economic and material resources at government disposal. Couch (1993) described innovative methods for raising funds in several Central American countries. Examples of funding methods include using proceeds from national lotteries or special raffles, sponsoring an annual telethon devoted to raising funds for vocational training and employment facilities, or concentrating the efforts of the sheltered workshop on prime manufacturing that earns profits for the facility. Local churches and missionaries are often supportive of the work of sheltered workshops and rehabilitation facilities.

INTERNATIONAL AGENCIES AND ORGANIZATIONS

There has been a consistent and substantial effort put forth by the world community to enhance the quantity and quality of vocational services for adults in developing countries with disabilities. Examples of these types of activities include programs and agencies initiated by the United Nations (e.g., the International Labor Organization) and other agencies like Rehabilitation International, the World Rehabilitation Fund, Disabled Peoples' International, and the World Institute on Disability.

United Nations' Efforts to Improve Vocational Services to Adults with Disabilities

International Decade of Disabled Persons. The United Nations and several UN-affiliated agencies have been at the forefront of efforts to "ensure the fullest possible integration of and equal participation by people with disabilities in all aspects of the life of their communities" (Satapati, 1989, p. 5). The UN's commitment to the international disabled community was firmly established by two proclamations made in the early 1980s. First, 1981 was declared the International Year of Disabled Persons. This was followed with an announcement of the International Decade of the Disabled (1983–1992). These two declarations were "the logical culmination of a series of initiatives, directives, and proclamations that had built up over the preceding decade" (Groce, 1992, p. 105).

Programmatically, international efforts have focused on shifting vocational service efforts to the community level, fostering community integration, and eliminating barriers to services (Satapati, 1989). Campbell (1990) explained that this focus is embedded in a larger UN agenda adopted in 1982 that supports the prevention of disability, develops education and rehabilitation services, and attempts to equalize opportunities for all individuals with disability. Despite high expectations, few of the proposed national plans for improvements have been implemented (Groce, 1992). A lack of recognition by organizations from industrialized countries of the need for vocational service delivery has contributed to this situation (Satapati, 1989).

The UN sponsors a number of agencies that provide advice, technical assistance, and direct services to countries, as well as to people with disabilities. One of these organizations, the International Labor Organization, emphasizes vocational service delivery and employment issues (Campbell, 1990).

International Labor Organization (ILO).   The ILO, based in Geneva, Switzerland, is the UN's specialized agency that promotes international labor rights and standards. The ILO's responsibility is broad in scope and includes technical assistance and establishment of minimum standards for the international community on an entire spectrum of work-related topics (ILO Mandate, 1996; Konig & Schalock, 1991). The ILO's primary role with individuals with disabilities is to ensure that they have equal access to vocational training and integrated employment opportunities in the productive sector of their society (Konig, 1990; Momm & Konig, 1989).

One ILO initiative, the Global Applied Disability Research Network for Employment and Training (GLADNET), deserves particular mention. GLADNET is a global research network that focuses on sharing and discussing concrete ways to achieve equality in training and employment for persons with disabilities. The network was launched in 1995 with the cooperation of over 50 social policy research institutions from around the world. Interestingly, the Internet is used as the primary means of communication among researchers, policymakers, and service providers. The rationale for developing such a system is the relatively small body of knowledge available from different countries about effective vocational programs and services. GLADNET hopes that access to information about cost-effective and successful vocational preparation and placement systems will help countries develop appropriate legislation, workplace policies, and equitable vocational training and employment models for their citizens with disabilities. This type of network holds promise for advancing our knowledge of vocational services to adults with disabilities (Fact Sheet: Gladnet, 1996; Gladnet Background, 1996; Gladnet Home Page, 1996).

Other Agencies Dedicated to the Improvement of International Vocational Service Provision

A variety of international organizations provide vocationally-related technical support and services including Disabled Peoples' International, the World Rehabilitation Fund, Rehabilitation International, and the World Institute on Disability. Each of these organizations serves an advocacy role for individuals with disabilities and emphasize a comprehensive range of educational, vocational, social, and legislative issues. For example, the central role of Rehabilitation International is to serve as a clearinghouse for all types of disability-related materials, information, and networking. Although broad in scope, this agency does collect and disseminate information on vocational rehabilitation and employment issues. Several agencies sponsor idea and expertise exchange programs; for example, the International Exchange of Experts in Information in Rehabilitation Project and the International Disability Exchanges and Studies Project, which have advanced the delivery of vocational services in many countries (Groce, 1992; National Institute on Disability and Rehabilitation Research, 1994; Rehabilitation International, 1996).

SUMMARY

This review was not intended to represent an exhaustive or definitive treatment on vocational services for adults with disabilities from an international perspective. Rather, an attempt has been made to describe and synthesize widely scattered, and sometimes sketchy, information about the vocational services available to adults with disabilities in a number of industrialized and developing countries. Available information reveals major differences between industrialized and nonindustrialized countries on legislation, service availability and delivery, and employment options and job placement efforts for adults with disabilities. Developing countries face entirely different challenges when considering vocational services for their citizens with disabilities. High general unemployment, limited governmental resources, and a lack of qualified professionals often limit the effectiveness of programs that are often successful in more industrialized countries. The introduction of community-based rehabilitation is one promising approach for providing vocational services in developing countries.

A need exists to continue our development of an international perspective of the vocational services available to adults with disabilities from countries around the world. The globalization of national economies and growing international competition is placing increasing pressure on industrialized and developing countries alike to critically exam the effectiveness of their vocational service delivery systems. Hopefully, knowledge of successful and cost-effective programs and services can help countries develop informed national employment and disability policy, design and implement equity-oriented vocational training and employment models for adults with disabilities, and formulate new strategies to integrate disability issues into mainstream social, economic, and labor markets (Gladnet Background, 1996).

REFERENCES

American Share Foundation. (1996). *Rehabilitation in process* [on-line]. Available on the World Wide Web: http://www.asf.org/mktplace/asf/dfg/rehab.html.

Arkansas Research and Training Center in Vocational Rehabilitation. (1993). *The name of the game: Employment.* Hot Springs, AR: National Institute on Disability and Rehabilitation Research, Author. (ERIC Document Reproduction Service No. ED 378 744)

Armstrong, M. J. (1993). Disability self-help organizations in the developing world: A case study from Malaysia. *International Journal of Rehabilitation, 16,* 185–194.

Bordieri, J. E. (1986). *Employment alternatives for workers with disabilities: An international perspective.* Menomonie: University of Wisconsin-Stout, Stout Vocational Rehabilitation Institute.

Brouilette, R., & Margia, L. (1993). *Community-based approaches for individuals with mental handicap: An African experience.* Brussels: International League of Societies for Persons with Mental Handicaps.

Brown, S. E., & Johnson, K. L. (1994). Recent Federal legislation and the role of vocational rehabilitation in the transition from school to community. *Rehabilitation Education, 8,* 67–78.

Campbell, L. F. (1990). An international disability network. *Journal of Visual Impairment and Blindness, 84,* 333–336.

Clearinghouse on Disability Information. (1993). *Pocket guide to Federal help for individuals with disabilities.* Washington, DC: U.S. Department of Education, Office of Special Education and Rehabilitative Services.

Couch, R. H. (1993). Rehabilitation innovations in Central America. *International Journal of Rehabilitation Research, 16,* 13–22.

Couch, R. H. (1994). Living with disability in Central America. *Vocational Evaluation and Work Adjustment Bulletin, 27,* 82–87.

Council of Europe. (1993). *Legislation on the rehabilitation of people with disabilities in sixteen member states of the Council of Europe* (5th ed.). Strasbourg, Germany: Council of Europe Press.

Fact Sheet: Gladnet. (1996). *Fact sheet: GLADNET* [on-line]. Available on World Wide Web: http://infoweb.magi.com/craskin/netfact.html.

Federal Register. (1988, May 12). *Rehabilitation Act Amendments of 1986: The state of supported employment service program; final regulations (34 CFR Part 363), 53*(92), 16981-16986. Washington, DC: Department of Education.

Fish, J. (1990). *Transition to adult life for people with disabilities* [Bulletin No. 3]. London: Center for Educational Research and Innovation, Further Education Unit. (ERIC Document Reproduction Service No. ED 320 001)

Gilbride, D. D., Stensrud, R., & Johnson, M. (1994). Current models of job placement and employer development: Research, competencies and educational considerations. *Rehabilitation Education, 7,* 215–239.

Gladnet Background. (1996). *International Labour Office, Geneva: Global Applied Disability Research Network for Employment and Training (GLADNET)* [on-line]. Available on World Wide Web: http://www.infoweb.magi.com/craskin/gladbk.html.

Gladnet Home Page. (1996). *GLADNET: Global Applied Disability Research Network for Employment and Training* [on-line]. Available on World Wide Web: http://www.infoweb.magi.com/craskin/index.html.

Goldberg, R. T. (1989). Comparison of the German and American systems of rehabilitation. *Journal of Rehabilitation, 55*(1), 59–62.

Groce, N. E. (1991). A history of international rehabilitation: An American perspective. *OSERS News in Print, 4*(2), 5–8. (ERIC Document Reproduction Service No. ED 343 372)

Groce, N. (1992). *The U.S. role in international disability activities: A history and a look towards the future.* Washington, DC: National Institute on Disability and Rehabilitation Research, International Disability Exchanges and Studies Project. (ERIC Document Reproduction Service No. ED 375 581)

Hong Kong Rehabilitation Services. (1996). *Topical information from A to Z: Rehabilitation* [on-line]. Available on World Wide Web: http://www.info.gov.hk/info/frehab.html.

ILO Mandate. (1996). *International Labour Organization: ILO mandate* [on-line]. Available on the World Wide Web: http://www.unicc.org/ilo/mandate/mandate.html.

Impact. (1995/1996, Fall & Winter). *Russians take home ideas and inspiration* [Semi-annual report, 3(1), 6–7]. Oakland, CA: World Institute on Disability, Author.

International Labor Organization. (1994). *Community-based rehabilitation for and with people with disabilities.* Geneva, Switzerland: Author. (ERIC Document Reproduction Service No. ED 375 552)

Japan Association for Employment of the Disabled. (1992). *Vocational rehabilitation in Japan.* Tokyo: National Institute of Vocational Rehabilitation.

Konig, A. (1990). Toward participation and equality: The UN's International Labour Organization. *Journal of Visual Impairment and Blindness, 84,* 332–333.

Konig, A., & Schalock, R. L. (1991). Supported employment: Equal opportunities for severely disabled men and women. *International Labour Review, 130*(1), 21–37.

Lunt, N., & Thornton, P. (1994). Disability and employment: Toward an understanding of discourse and policy. *Disability & Society, 9,* 223–238.

Matsui, R. (1994). Employment measures for persons with disabilities in Japan: Recent developments. *International Journal of Rehabilitation Research, 17,* 368–372.

McGaughey, M. J., Kiernan, W. E., McNally, L. C., Gilmore, D. S., & Keith, G. R. (1995). Beyond the workshop: National trends in integrated and segregated day and employment services. *Journal of the Association for Persons with Severe Handicaps, 20,* 270–285.

Mintaredja, H. (1978). *Problems concerning a quotum systems for the disabled in the local market in developing countries.* Paper presented at the Second International Conference on Legislation Concerning the Disabled, Manila, Philippines.

Momm, W., & Konig, A. (1989). Community integration for disabled people: A new approach to their vocational training and employment. *International Labour Review, 128,* 497–509.

National Institute on Disability and Rehabilitation Research. (1993). *Developing awareness of disability in the world: Looking at issues relevant to disability in Asia, the Pacific, and Africa through the eyes of the U.S Fellows* (Monograph 54). Durham: University of New Hampshire, Author. (ERIC Document Reproduction Service No. ED 375 582)

National Institute on Disability and Rehabilitation Research. (1994). *An international resource directory of disability-related organizations.* Durham: University of New Hampshire, Institute on Disability, International Exchange of Experts and Information in Rehabilitation. (ERIC Document Reproduction Service No. ED 375 578)

Office of Special Education and Rehabilitative Services. (1996). *Special education and rehabilitative services programs* [on-line]. Available on World Wide Web: http://www.ed.gov/pubs/TeachersGuide/pt12.html.

Osuala, J. D. C. (1993). Employment problems of the adult disabled in Nigeria. *International Journal of Rehabilitation Research, 16,* 343–345.

Pozner, A., & Hammond, J. (1993). *An evaluation of supported employment initiatives for disabled people.* London: Employment Department Group, OUSET Consultancy Services.

Raskin, C. (1994). Employment equity for the disabled in Canada. *International Labour Review, 139,* 75–88.

Rehabilitation International. (1996). *Rehabilitation International* [on-line]. Available on World Wide Web: http://www.who.ch/programmes/ina/ngo/ngo147.html.

Rubin, S. E., & Roessler, R. T. (1995). *Foundations of the vocational rehabilitation process* (4th ed.). Austin, TX: PRO-ED.

Sailor, W. (1989). *Transition in the U.S. and Western European nations.* San Francisco: San Francisco

State University, California Research Institute. (ERIC Document Reproduction Service No. ED 365 047)

Satapati, P. R. (1989). *Rehabilitation of the disabled in developing countries.* Frankfurt, Germany: AFRA-Verlag.

Scorzelli, J. F. (1995). The development of educational and rehabilitation services for people with cerebral palsy in India. *Journal of Rehabilitation, 61*(2), 68–71.

Shrey, D. E., Bangs, S. A., Mark, L. S., Hursh, N. C., & Kues, J. R. (1991). Returning Social Security beneficiaries to the work force: A proactive disability management model. *Rehabilitation Counseling Bulletin, 24,* 257–273.

Simmons, T., & Flexer, R. (1992). Business and rehabilitation factors in the development of supported employment programs for adults with developmental disabilities. *Journal of Rehabilitation, 58*(1), 35–42.

Thomson, G. O. B., Ward, K. M., & Wishart, J. G. (1995). The transition to adulthood for children with Down syndrome. *Disability and Society, 10,* 325–340.

Wehman, P., & Kregel, J. (1995). At the crossroads: Supported employment a decade later. *Journal of the Association for Persons with Severe Handicaps, 20,* 286–299.

Whitehead, C., Davis, P. K., & Fisher, M. (1989). The current and future role of rehabilitation facilities in external employment. *Journal of Applied Rehabilitation Counseling, 20*(3), 58–64.

Yun, X., Piao, Y., Gargiulo, R. M. (1995). *Special education in the People's Republic of China: Characteristics and practices.* Paper presented at the annual convention of the Council for Exceptional Children, Indianapolis, IN. (ERIC Document Reproduction Service No. 384 185)

PART IV

Cross-Cultural Future

CHAPTER 13

Transfer of Beliefs, Knowledge, and Experiences Between Countries

DAVID MITCHELL
University of Waikato
Hamilton, New Zealand

In recent years, beliefs, principles, knowledge, and practices relating to special education and rehabilitation increasingly have been transferred between countries, with the result that there is a remarkable degree of convergence, both in ideology and in practices, across all types of nations. This chapter will examine the following questions:

- Who transfers beliefs, knowledge, and experiences?
- What beliefs, knowledge, and experiences are transferred?
- What are the issues involved in transferring beliefs, knowledge, and experiences?

WHO TRANSFERS BELIEFS, KNOWLEDGE AND EXPERIENCES?

Knowledge and experiences relating to people with disabilities are transferred between countries in varied ways by a range of organizations and individuals. These sources fall into seven categories:

1. International governmental and intergovernmental organizations.
2. Regional governmental and intergovernmental organizations.
3. International and regional nongovernmental organizations.
4. Bilateral arrangements between countries.
5. Influential legislation and policies from specific countries.

6. Associations and individuals involved in rehabilitation.
7. The Internet.

International Governmental and Intergovernmental Organizations

International agencies have been actively promoting a consistent set of philosophies regarding persons with disabilities. These have been expressed in several key documents that have been promulgated by the United Nations and associated agencies (e.g., UNESCO, UNICEF, UNDP, WHO, ILO) over the past half century. The most important of these are as follows:

- The Universal Declaration of Human Rights, adopted by the UN General Assembly (1948).
- The Declaration on the Rights of Mentally Retarded Persons, adopted by the UN General Assembly (1971).
- Declaration of the Rights of Disabled Persons, adopted by the UN General Assembly (1975).
- The International Covenant on Economic, Social and Cultural Rights adopted by the UN General Assembly in 1966, and entered into force in 1975.
- The International Year of Disabled Persons (1981).
- The UN Decade of Disabled Persons (1983–1992), and the associated UN World Programme of Action Concerning Disabled Persons (1983).
- The International Labour Organization Convention concerning Vocational Rehabilitation and Employment of Disabled Persons (1983).
- The Convention on the Rights of the Child adopted by the UN General Assembly in 1989, and entered into force in 1990.
- The World Declaration on Education for All (1990).
- The Standard Rules for the Equalization of Opportunities for Persons with Disabilities, adopted by the UN General Assembly (1993).
- The Salamanca Statement and Framework of Action on Special Needs Education, adopted by UNESCO (1994).

Several of the aforementioned documents warrant special mention. The International Year of Disabled Persons, and the follow-up Decade of Disabled Persons with its 201-paragraph World Programme of Action Concerning Disabled Persons, both had major impacts on the development of policies around the world. Several countries—Senegal, Pakistan, India, Japan, and the Republic of Korea, to name a few, created legislation that can be directly attributed to the policies promoted during this period (Kim, 1993; Lynch, 1994; Mazurek & Winzer, 1994). For example, in India, it led to a National Plan of Action that included the following objectives: (a) to evolve a national policy for full social integration and legal protection for disabled persons, (b) to initiate a few practical programs that would carry immediate benefit for the integration of disabled persons, and (c) to initiate public campaigns to create greater awareness among the people regarding the causes, prevention, and effects of disability and the potentials of disabled persons (Agrawal, 1994). According to O'Hanlon (1995), the International Year of Disabled Persons also formed a basis for the European Union's response to the social and economic needs of people with disabilities, and led directly to the establishment of the first action program, the Social Integration of Disabled People—a Framework for Community Action. This document contained the recommendation that member states should promote measures to prepare handicapped people for an active life, in particular by integrating them in normal education and training whenever possible. This first action program led directly to the second action program, Handicapped People in the European Community Living Independently in an Open Society (HELIOS), which ran from 1988 to 1991. A third program, known as HELIOS II (1993–1996), focused on the exchange of information, experiences, and good practices in the fields of functional rehabilitation, education, employment, and independent living. For the first time, older disabled people have been identified as a separate priority group within the European Union program (Merceron, 1996).

The 1983 World Programme of Action was further clarified by the UN Secretary-General in 1984, when he emphasized nine priorities for member states: continuing and extending national disability committees established during the International Year, reviewing national legislation, collecting basic data, preventing disability, establishing regulations to ensure accessibility, providing technical aids, equalising opportunities in education, informing the public, and— at the international level—establishing effective services for the exchange of information.

In turn, the World Programme of Action led to the development of *The Standard Rules for the Equalization of Opportunities for Disabled Persons*, which were adopted by the UN General Assembly in 1993 (United Nations, 1994). This document is of special significance because it represents a contemporary and authoritative distillation of all preceding UN documents on disability. It was drafted by representatives of 74 governments who took part in three different conferences from 1991 to 1992. The *Standard Rules* comprises 22 general rules, with a total of 132 more detailed guidelines. As Rowland (1996) points out, one of the attractive features of the *Standard Rules* is that while they are specific, they are not overly detailed and are thus adaptable to different legal systems and cultures. In countries that are in transition, they provide a basis for formulating disability policy and legislation as witnessed, for example, in South Africa and Namibia (Rowland, 1996). The UN was not satisfied with merely promulgating the *Standard Rules*, but instead set up a mechanism for monitoring and furthering their implementation, with three responsible agents, the Permanent Commission of the UN, the Commission for Social Development, and a Special Rapporteur assisted by a 10-member panel of experts. Initially, the Rapporteur and panel of experts have focused on surveying and promoting six of the rules: education, employment, legislation, accessibility, the position of organizations of disabled people, and the distribution of government responsibilities.

Almost contemporaneous with the development of the *Standard Rules* was the development of the *Salamanca Statement and Framework of Action on Special Needs Education*. The latter document had its specific origins in the World Declaration on Education for All (1990), which resulted from the World Conference on Education for All held in Jomtien, Thailand in 1990 and convened by UNESCO, UNICEF, UNDP, and the World Bank (Inter-Agency Commission, 1990). This conference brought together government representatives from 155 countries and over 150 organizations. One of the major outcomes of this conference was the convening by UNESCO of a series of high-level regional seminars on policy, planning, and organization of education for children and young people with special needs, with an emphasis on inclusive education. These seminars culminated in a meeting in 1994 of representatives of 92 governments and 25 international organizations who drew up the document known as the *Salamanca Statement* (UNESCO, 1994). Included in this document were statements of beliefs and an appeal to governments to give priority to developing and implementing policies on special education, with particular attention to inclusive education. It provides a "Framework for Action" that contains 85 specific recommendations to do with policy and organization, school factors, recruitment and training of educational personnel, external support services, priority areas, community perspectives, resource requirements, and guidelines for action at the regional and international levels.

Many examples can be found of the direct role played by the UN and its agencies in transferring policies and practices to countries around the world. A few will suffice here. Firstly, Diaconescu, Ionescu, Chis, and Daunt (1995) outline how, in 1991, with the sponsorship of UNESCO and UNICEF, the Romanian authorities organized a conference to review the system of special education. While there were some reservations, considerable interest was shown in the concepts of integration and normalization. The three foreign consultants attending the conference under UNESCO's auspices prepared a draft proposal for the setting up of pilot projects to promote the educational and social integration of children and young people with disabilities of whatever kind or severity. In 1993, the government accepted the proposal and two projects were launched, with UNESCO continuing to provide technical support and UNICEF some funding.

One of the major determinants of international convergence of policies and practices in social areas is undoubtedly the World Bank. While it has not been particularly active in defining policies related to people with disabilities, the World Bank, as noted by Torres (1995–96), is already a major player in the transnationalization of knowledge, influencing the discourse of education and educational reforms, not only in developing countries, but worldwide. The underlying ideology thus projected, according to Torres, is that of neoliberalism. The World Bank made its first loan for education in 1963 and is now the largest single source of external financing for education in developing countries, accounting for about a quarter of all such aid (World Bank, 1995). In developing countries, it has the ultimate influence to bring about change: money. In its own words, "Bank financing will generally be designed to leverage spending and policy change by national authorities" (World Bank, 1995, pp. 14–15). Its priorities for reform therefore bear close study in the broader context of forces underlying the transfer of ideology and knowledge. In a recent publication, these were summarized as being in six key areas: (a) giving higher priority to education, (b) setting priorities with reference to outcomes, (c) emphasizing basic education, (d) attending to equity, (e) involving households in the governance of schools, and (f) granting schools the autonomy to use instructional inputs according to local school and community conditions, with accountability to parents and communities. The bank's principal policy instrument for reducing the high incidence of physical and learning disabilities in developing countries is through the improvement of child nutrition and health. It notes, too, that the "unit costs" for special education can be reduced by using community-based approaches, referring in this context to the existence of community-based rehabilitation programs (see next section) in many countries, including India, Indonesia, Jamaica, Kenya, Malaysia, Nepal, the Philippines, and Zimbabwe.

In the light of its relevance to the theme of this book, it is appropriate to look more closely at the World Bank's view on equity, which it defines as having two principal aspects:

> (a) everyone's right to a basic education—the basic knowledge and skills necessary to function effectively in society—and (b) the government's obligation to ensure that qualified potential students are not denied education because they are poor or female, are from disadvantaged ethnic minorities or geographically remote regions, or have special educational needs. (World Bank, 1995, pp. 10–11)

It will be noted that the reference to "qualified potential students" raises doubts as to whether this statement's coverage extends to all learners with special needs.

Regional Governmental and Intergovernmental Organizations

Regional-level governmental and intergovernmental organizations have adopted and promoted policies on persons with disabilities. Examples drawn from Europe, Asia, and Latin America will suffice to illustrate this point.

Europe. In Europe, as O'Hanlon (1993, 1995) points out, the movement towards integration has been heavily influenced by the Community's (and now the Union's) belief in human rights. Observance of human rights was originally embedded in the Convention for the Protection of Human Rights and Fundamental

Freedoms within the Council for Europe, which was signed by member states in 1950. Since that time, the preservation of basic human rights has formed the foundation of all measures adopted by the Council for Europe. However, while the European Union (EU) has wide powers to formulate and implement policy, it does not have harmonization of educational systems as an overt aim and individual countries can opt out of certain policy instruments such as the Social Charter (which the UK has done). O'Hanlon notes that although there is no specific EU legislation for inclusive education, there is evidence of the development of similar policies within member states in relation to this matter. The Council of Ministers, for example, has been considering the possibility of developing more prescriptive general guidelines for the inclusion of pupils with special educational needs in education, with the intent that member states will bear these in mind when passing their own legislation. Such a development would be consistent with the *Resolution of the Council and the Ministers of Education of 31 May 1990* concerning the integration of children and young persons with disabilities into ordinary systems of education (O'Hanlon, 1995). Also, as noted by Merceron (1996), the treaties are currently being revised and discussions on Social Europe are high on the agenda.

As well as legislative moves, there are other mechanisms in place in Europe that play an important role in transferring knowledge and practices among countries, both within the EU and between it and countries in the former Communist bloc. At the governmental and intergovernmental level, the most important of these would be the ERASMUS and TEMPUS programs of the EU (Mittler & Daunt, 1995). The European Community Action Scheme for the Mobility of University Students (ERASMUS) aims at increasing the number of EU students undertaking a period of study in another member state, promoting cooperation among higher education institutions, and promoting the mobility of teaching staff. One such program was concerned with the integration of children with disabilities and involved universities in Bologna (Italy), Cologne (Germany), Malaga (Spain), and Manchester, Birmingham, and London (UK). TEMPUS is the acronym for Trans European Mobility Programme for University Staff, a program in which several universities collaborate on joint projects involving, especially, countries in Central and Eastern Europe. One such project is that between Manchester Metropolitan University, the Institut Universitaire de la Formation des Maîtres, Grenoble, and the Siauliai Pedagogical Institute in Lithuania, which is concerned with good practice in inclusive education and the teacher training structures that underlie it. As described by Johnson, this project aims "to empower the teachers by encouraging them to have confidence in their personal expertise and not to look constantly for the advice of 'experts'" (1995, p. 83). A second TEMPUS project deals with special educational needs in the mainstream and involves a partnership between the Bárczi Gusztáv College for Special Education in Hungary, which acts as both coordinator and contractor, along with the Budapest Teacher Training College, Manchester and Cambridge Universities in

England, the Heidelberg Pädagogische Hochschule in Germany and the Instituut voor Doven (a school for the deaf) in the Netherlands (Csanyi, 1995).

Asia. During the last decade or so, several conferences and seminars relevant to special education have been held in the Asia Pacific Region and have yielded a wide range of policy recommendations in the field of special education (Mitchell & Chen, 1996). Preeminent among these is the series of regional seminars on special education, which have been held annually since 1981 under the auspices of UNESCO's Asia Pacific Programme of Educational Innovation for Development. These seminars have been hosted by Japan's National Institute of Special Education and largely funded by the Japanese National Commission for UNESCO. Participants have usually included representatives from Australia, Bangladesh, China, India, Indonesia, Japan, Malaysia, Nepal, New Zealand, Pakistan, the Philippines, the Republic of Korea, and Sri Lanka. As an example of the these seminars, the one held in 1996 focused on the transition from schooling to postcompulsory education.

Another important regional initiative in Asia is the Asia Pacific Decade of the Disabled (1993–2002), with an agenda that includes national coordination, legislation, information dissemination, public awareness, training and employment, education, rehabilitation services, and regional cooperation.

Latin America. In 1993, the *Declaration of Managua* was signed by representatives of 36 Latin American countries who had come together to develop policies concerning the human rights of people with intellectual disabilities. The impact of this declaration is shown, for example, in the Dominican Republic where in 1995 the Catholic Church issued a public statement at every mass supporting its principles. As well, the church is gradually moving towards inclusive education in its schools and is recognizing the needs of children with disabilities in its policy on strengthening the Dominican family (Inclusion International, 1996).

Other regional or multinational organizations that are having or have the potential to impact on policies and practices of their member states include OECD, APEC, the Organization of American States, the Organization of African Unity, and the Arab League.

International and Regional Nongovernmental Organizations

Nongovernmental organizations (NGOs) play a very important role in developing and promoting policies on people with disabilities. As pointed out by Mitchell & Chen (1996), although NGOs are not in a position to take on nationwide responsibility, they can join forces with the national authorities, assisting in areas like community-based programs and working on small-scale innovative projects to demonstrate new approaches. In this respect, they act as catalysts for change. Thus, it is very important that NGOs be involved in planning and coordinating their work with the public sector provision.

Of particular relevance here is the impact of worldwide organizations such as Rehabilitation International and Inclusion International (formerly known as the International League of Societies for Persons with Mental Handicap), Disabled People's International, the World Blind Union, the World Federation for the Deaf, the Islamic World Council on Disability and Rehabilitation, and the World Federation of Psychiatric Users (Helander, 1993).

A second group of NGOs comprises those that have their origins in a single country, but are involved in one or more other countries. For example, the German NGO Blindenmissen operates in several countries, Diakonia from Sweden operates in areas such as the West Bank and the Gaza Strip (Mazurek & Winzer, 1994, p. 62), and the Swedish voluntary organization, Radda Barnen, is introducing community rehabilitation centers in the Republic of Yemen (Qirbi, 1993). As well, the Japanese Society for the Rehabilitation of Disabled Persons is developing cooperation with Thailand, Vietnam, and the Philippines, is assisting in the establishment of a printing and computer training workshop in Thailand and is marketing products made in Vietnamese workshops in Japan (Niwa, 1996). A useful case study of the role of NGOs is afforded by Romania, where, since 1990, many new developments have been initiated by NGOs. As noted by Diaconescu et al. (1995), the Romanian NGOs that promoted these activities began to be important elements in the implementation of reform, "able to transmit messages to and from the citizens and the authorities, and even more importantly, able to establish international contacts and cooperation" (p. 68). Of particular interest is the contact generated by the Danish Red Barnet (Save the Children) between three Romanian NGOs in County Dolj and a number of different Danish counties.

Lynch (1994) also draws attention to the role played by NGOs in developing services with national counterparts. For example, Helen Keller International has established an Asia Pacific regional office in Bangkok where it conducts regional training workshops; it has also set up field offices in nearly all developing Asian nations. A similar range of programs has been established by the UK Save the Children Fund. Yet another example is the work of the Cheshire Foundation, which has established projects for disabled children and adults in over 50 countries throughout the world (McConkey, 1996).

At times, the range of NGOs operating can create problems in coordination —a point developed in more detail in the next section. Lynch (1994) cites the case of Nepal in 1988, when there were no fewer than 32 international agencies assisting in the development of services:

> Helen Keller International, the German Blindenmission, Norwegian, British and American Save the Children, Action Aid, SEVA, United Missions to Nepal, Norwegian Association for the Mentally Retarded, Mary Knoll Fathers, the World Union of the Blind, Perkins School for the Blind, Special Olympics, Sight Savers, and Jaycees, among others. (p .12)

The role of NGOs is also apparent in Indonesia, where private voluntary agencies provide 55% of the resources for special education (World Bank, 1995).

Private organizations and NGOs also play a significant role in the provision of special education in the Philippines. Of the 4,470 special education facilities, one-third are operated by NGOs or private corporations/foundations; this is especially the case with special and residential schools. (Mitchell & Chen, 1996). While not all of the NGOs in Indonesia and the Philippines are from outside the country, these figures serve to illustrate the critical role that NGOs play in some countries' provisions for individuals with disabilities.

While, strictly speaking, they are not classifiable as NGOs, it is worth mentioning here the important role that church groups and missionaries have played in the evolution of special education in several developing countries. Some such influences are noted in the above description. Another example is afforded by the Republic of Korea, where Kim (1993) acknowledges the work of an American missionary, Rosetta S. Hall, who set up education programs for the blind and the deaf in the late 19th and early 20th centuries, and another American missionary, Edward Adams, who initiated education for physically disabled children in 1959. In Jordan, the first school for children with disabilities was set up in 1964 by Father Andeweg, a Dutch Anglican priest (Moulton, Andrews, & Smith, 1996).

Bilateral Arrangements Between Countries

Several countries are active in providing bilateral aid to developing countries in the field of disability and rehabilitation. As noted by Lynch (1994), the Scandinavian countries in particular have made significant contributions to Asian national efforts to train personnel and provide initial services in provisions for people with disabilities. For example, the Swedish International Development Agency supported the Sri Lankan Ministry of Education in the area of staff training, development of sign language, the establishment of a resource and teacher training center for special education, and the maintenance of a Braille press; the Norwegian Agency for Developmental Cooperation helped to provide teacher training facilities in Bangladesh and services development in Nepal; the Australian International Development Assistance Bureau funded a Childhood Disabilities Project in some of the island states of the South Pacific; the Canadian International Development Agency funded the development of a disability diploma in the Gaza Strip (Brown, Abu Ghazaleh, and Neufeldt, 1996); and the United States Agency for International Development provided funding for programs for disabled people in the Gaza Strip. The Japanese Government–funded National Institute for Special Education is another example of bilateral aid that has had a pronounced influence on regional development.

Influential Legislation and Policies From Specific Countries

In the field of disability, there are perhaps three landmark reports or sets of legislation, with associated research, which have had effects well beyond the countries that generated them. The first of these is undoubtedly the Scandinavian legislation and practices that gave rise to the notion of "normalization" (e.g., Nirje, 1969, 1985) These have been acknowledged by several writers as having had a major impact on their countries' approaches to special education and rehabilitation: for example, Australia (Swan, 1994), New Zealand (Mitchell and Mitchell, 1987), and Japan (Misawa, 1994).

The second influential event is the U.S. Public Law 94-142 and its successor, the Individuals with Disabilities Education Act (IDEA) 1990. Their significance has been acknowledged in countries as diverse as Australia (Brown, 1997; Swan, 1994), Brazil (Kerns & Cavalcante, 1997), Canada (Winzer, 1994), Japan (Misawa, 1994), New Zealand (Mitchell & O'Brien, 1994), Nigeria (Abang, 1994), and Taiwan (Chen & Lu, 1994).

The Warnock Report in the UK (Warnock, 1978) is the third landmark event to have had an impact, with countries such as Japan (Misawa, 1994), Hong Kong (Crawford & Bray, 1994), Australia (Brown, 1997; Swan, 1994), and New Zealand (Mitchell and O'Brien, 1994) all being influenced by its principles.

Associations and Individuals Involved in Rehabilitation

The final major way in which knowledge and experiences are transferred between countries is via various associations and individuals with interests in disabilities. In the field of mental retardation, the pre-eminent bodies in this regard are probably the International Association for Scientific Studies on Intellectual Disability and the American Association for Mental Deficiency, with the Asia Federation for the Mentally Retarded playing a very important regional role. Networks of organizations in the field of disability and rehabilitation also facilitate the dissemination and implementation of knowledge. An example of such a network is given by Hekking (1996), who describes the European Platform of Vocational Rehabilitation, a transnational network of European rehabilitation institutions, established in 1993. This was set up in part because of the growing political integration of the EU and the likelihood of a growing integration of the European labor market. It has four main strategies: (1) the development of a common European understanding of vocational rehabilitation, (2) the promotion of research and innovation in vocational rehabilitation, (3) developing the skills of professionals, and (4) improving service quality by such means as establishing common guidelines for European quality standards.

The Internet

Including all of the above, but extending beyond them, is the Internet, with its enormous and growing array of information on disability, special education, and rehabilitation. As noted by Mitchell (1996), the Internet, with its access to E-mail and the World Wide Web, is the prime current exemplar of how technology facilitates one's capacity to independently reach out and find information. The introduction of E-mail has dramatically changed the character and speed of communication, with participants able to simultaneously exchange information with a large number of people in a way that uniquely combines ease, speed, immediacy, and (increasingly) cheapness.

In recent years there has been a burgeoning network of sites on disability, special education, and rehabilitation. For example, GLADNET (Global Applied Disability Research and Information Network on Employment and Training) has been developed by the ILO to promote policies, programs, and projects to further equal opportunities for people with disabilities. This network is based in Geneva with a mirror home page in Ottawa and hyperlinks with over 50 disability sites. As of mid-1996, it comprised 160 members. Similarly, in 1995 ILO published a network of 53 organizations on the Web with information to do with disability. A third network of relevance is the one on inclusive education (inclusive-education@mailbase.ac.uk). One of its originators, David Skidmore of the University of Reading, UK, has also compiled a list of World Wide Web sites about inclusive education, disabilities, and other related subjects. The list (updated frequently) comprises a mix of U.S., Canadian, and U.K. sites. It may be accessed at http://www.mailbase.ac.uk/lists/inclusive-education/files/inclusion_sites.txt.

WHAT BELIEFS, KNOWLEDGE, AND EXPERIENCES ARE TRANSFERRED?

Taking the foregoing organizations together, the philosophies expressed by them cohere around principles such as the following:

- disability should be seen in a societal, rather than an individualized context;
- persons with disabilities should be treated as being self-responsible, rather than dependent;
- persons with disabilities have the right to access physical environments, information, education, health care services, rehabilitation services, communication, employment, and recreation; and to make choices, develop individuality, and participate fully in citizenship;
- multisectorial approaches to dealing with disability should be implemented at national levels, with coordinated, complementary, and collaborative approaches among different agencies and ministries;
- the public should be educated and informed about the rights of disabled persons to participate in and contribute to various aspects of economic, social, and political life;
- persons with disabilities should be helped in their physical and psychological adjustment to society;

- every child has a fundamental right to education and must be given the opportunity to achieve and maintain an acceptable level of learning;
- those with special educational needs must have access to regular schools that should accommodate them within a child-centered pedagogy capable of meeting these needs;
- regular schools with an inclusive orientation are the most effective means of combating discriminatory attitudes, creating welcoming communities, building an inclusive society, and achieving an education for all; moreover, they provide an effective education to the majority of children and improve the efficiency and ultimately the cost-effectiveness of the entire education system;
- greater effort should be invested in early identification and intervention strategies;
- transition programs should be seen as an integral part of a continuous process of development ranging from early childhood and school to postschool programs; these programs need to include greater employment opportunities and other appropriate activities;
- emphasis should be placed on the provision of programs that include the development of vocational skills.

In terms of vocational inclusion, the *Standard Rules for the Equalization of Opportunities for Persons with Disabilities* (United Nations, 1994) contains a clear indication of what is being asserted as internationally acceptable principles pertaining to persons with disabilities. Rule 7, which deals with employment, asserts that states should recognize the principle that persons with disabilities must be empowered to exercise their human rights, particularly in the field of employment. It goes on to note that in both rural and urban areas, they must have equal opportunities for productive and gainful employment in the labor market and that laws and regulations in the employment field must not discriminate against them and must not raise obstacles to their employment. Further, states should actively support the integration of persons with disabilities into open employment, through such measures as vocational training, incentive-oriented quota schemes, reserved or designated employment, loans or grants for small business, exclusive contracts or priority production rights, tax concessions, and contract compliance or other technical or financial assistance to enterprises employing workers with disabilities. States' action programs should include measures (a) to design and adapt workplaces and work premises in such a way that they become accessible to persons with different disabilities; (b) to support the use of new technologies and the development and production of assistive devices, tools, and equipment for persons with disabilities to enable them to gain and maintain employment; (c) to provide appropriate training, placement, and ongoing support for workers with disabilities; (d) to initiate and support public awareness-raising campaigns designed to overcome negative attitudes and prejudices concerning workers with disabilities; and (e) to create training and employment opportunities through such means as flexible hours, part-time work, job-sharing, self-employment, and attendant care for persons with disabilities. Over all, the aim should always be for persons with disabilities to obtain employment in the open labor market. For persons with disabilities whose needs cannot be met in open employment, small units of sheltered or supported employment may be an alternative, with the caveat that the quality of such programs should be assessed in terms of the extent to which they provide opportunities for persons with disabilities to gain employment in the open labor market.

In recent years, one of the major philosophies to have taken root in developing countries is Community-Based Rehabilitation (CBR), defined by ILO, UNESCO, and WHO (1994) in a joint position paper, as

> a strategy within community development for the rehabilitation, equalization of opportunities and social integration of all people with disabilities. CBR is implemented through the combined efforts of disabled people themselves, their families and communities, and the appropriate health, education vocational and social services.

The aim of CBR is to allow people with disabilities to live in their communities and to fully participate in all types of activities, including employment (Murray, 1996). It is a comprehensive approach that should involve the community in the planning, implementation, and evaluation of the program and, as such, is part of the process of community development whereby the community seeks to improve itself (O'Toole, 1991). As noted by Tjandrakusuma (1996), an underlying assumption of CBR is that problems faced by people with disabilities result not only from their individual impairments, but from the attitudes and beliefs of their communities. It therefore aims at enabling community members to increase their understanding about disability issues, to become involved in the disability prevention activities and to "provide a positive environment . . . to improve the quality of life of persons with disabilities" (p. 2).

As well as promulgating broad principles, international and regional bodies have been increasingly involved in attempting to ensure the implementation of policies at a very practical level. Two examples will suffice. Firstly, as alluded to above, major steps have been taken in several developing countries to implement CBR (Narayan, 1996; O'Toole, 1991; Thorburn, 1996; Tjandrakusuma, 1996). Secondly, in the field of education the impact of UNESCO's *Teacher Education Resource Pack* (Ainscow, 1994) must be noted. This is aimed at encouraging member states to develop strategies for responding to children's special needs in ordinary schools and was developed through regional and national workshops sponsored largely by UNESCO. It contains four modules: (1) introduction to special needs in the classroom, (2) special needs: definitions and responses, (3) towards effective schools for all, and (4) help and support. Each module contains several units with instruction sheets discussion materials and videos. Developments such as those reflected in the *Resource Pack* are very timely as countries strive to upgrade the quality of teaching. Referring to special education in the Asian region, Lynch (1994) noted that "much of the useless theory, often deriving from models current in western teacher education in the 1960s and 1970s" (p. 14), is being replaced by curriculum-led developments, with an increasing emphasis on group work, multigrade teaching, continuous pupil assessment, and ways to motivate a diversity of children to learn.

WHAT ISSUES ARE INVOLVED IN TRANSFERRING BELIEFS, KNOWLEDGE, AND EXPERIENCES?

The transfer of beliefs, knowledge, and experiences between countries is a complex matter that raises both technical and moral issues. In this section, five such issues will be discussed: coordination of international assistance, the universal design of technology, differential access to the Internet, convergence or diversity among cultures, and guidelines for introducing innovations.

Coordination

In most countries where rehabilitation provisions exist, they come under the auspices of a diverse range of governmental, NGO, and private service providers, a diversity that is often compounded by the involvement of several governmental ministries or departments—social welfare, health, employment, and education. Even in the most developed countries, the issue of service coordination is one that has constantly to be addressed, notwithstanding the arguments of advocates of the market economy that there are merits in having some duplication of services, as this introduces an element of contestability and competition that will lead to improved service efficiency and quality, provided consumers have genuine choice.

In developing countries, where there are often negligible resources available for the rehabilitation sector, the notion of contestability may seem to be an esoteric, if not luxurious, Western economic model, even if it is promoted by the World Bank. Perhaps a higher priority in such countries is the need to attend to international coordination. This has received attention from the UNDP, where Helander (1993) talks about his personal frustrations in bringing this about. He cites difficulties arising from (a) the choice of representatives attending meetings (too many administrators without technical knowledge of disability, too many professionals from industrialized countries with limited experience in developing countries, and too few national rehabilitation managers); (b) the choice of subject matter (too much on industrialized countries, too much focus on information exchange, and too little on cooperative planning); (c) the expected outcomes (mainly confined to annual repetitions of rituals of producing documents that do not bring forth much in terms of services to persons with disabilities); and (d) the policymaking mechanisms of international organizations (insufficient concern for innovation, inward-looking structures). Helander concludes his critical review by stating that "the present forum for international co-ordination is not effective as an instrument of change" and that "a thorough review is needed of the entire effort of international co-ordination" (p. 196). He suggests the following steps: (a) creating a new coordination mechanism in particular countries (or in a region), involving all potential partners—UN agencies, governmental international development organizations, and NGOs; (b) commissioning a group of experienced national program managers and field experts to propose a new set of policies for the coordinating agency; (c) formulating detailed guidelines within each developing country regarding the approaches to be applied; (d) reaching an agreement between donor/development agencies on how work can be divided up so as to avoid the present concentration on a few countries; (e) joint planning by all those who work in a specific country under the leadership of the government; and (f) creating a joint mechanism for follow-up and evaluation.

Universal Design

As rehabilitation services expand, particularly in the area of assistive technology, there will be an increasing need for some degree of international standardization. In a recent international conference on rehabilitation, the importance of developing universal and adaptable designs—a "design for all"—was emphasized by Seelman (1996). This principle draws attention to the importance of developing standardized approaches to the design of various assistive devices, ranging from the wheelchairs to computer software. Seelman noted that international cooperation between people and nations in assistive technology is at a formative stage, with dialogue about assistive technology and cooperation among nations currently taking place, for example, between the United States and Europe and between the United States and Japan. As well, the European Union has established a program called TIDE (Technology for the Integration of the Disabled and Elderly People) aimed at increasing the availability in technology in Europe. Currently, the European Commission is arguing for the adoption of technical rules and standards before assistive technology devices can be put on the European market.

Differential Access to the Internet

Several features of the Web make up its special character. Firstly, like no other form of information sharing, the Web is fundamentally egalitarian in that it gives all people with access to it a forum for expressing their views and for seeking and sharing information (Burbules, 1995; UNESCO, 1996). Interactive media will soon make it possible not only to send and receive information, but to engage in dialogue and to transmit information and knowledge unconstrained by distance or operating time. Secondly, because every node in the Web is linkable to any other node, the structure is decentered and nonhierarchical; or, as described by Burbules (1995) it is "hypertextual and rhizomatic." Thirdly, the Web has multimedia capability (i.e., it is able to integrate multiple sources and forms of information). Networked multimedia systems will provide general, efficient, enduring, and multimodal (as distinct from a hitherto predominantly verbal) access to cultural works of nearly every form conceivable (McClintock, 1995, p. 262).

The Internet is often described as being "anarchic," in the sense that it is not under the control of any authority, nor is it susceptible to such control. This view is somewhat glib, however, for there are various levels of control that can be and currently are being exercised over the medium. While it is true that anyone can put on or pull down information from the Internet, it is not equally accessible. Firstly—and most obviously—not everyone has physical access to it, either because they cannot afford it, or their country lacks the infrastructure of telephones or electricity to support it, or they lack the individual skills to enter into it. Secondly, the Internet has created a new class of what Burbules and Callister call "knowledge producers and knowledge organizers" (1996, p. 44)—those who act as interpreters and makers of knowledge, deciding on the inclusion and exclusion of materials in hypertexts and the links between them and who create the filters that help users sort through the enormous volume of information available. Burbules and Callister feel that these people will control access to information in ways that are potentially much less democratic and more restrictive than is now possible with simpler informational systems. In a similar vein, the International Commission on Education for the Twenty-first Century (UNESCO, 1996) notes with concern the differences that will arise between societies that will be capable of producing the content and those that will merely receive the information without taking a real part in the exchanges.

Finally, we must be aware that the opportunities afforded by information technology and its increasing role in all aspects of life will not be equally accessible to all members of a society, let alone to all societies. This means that there could well be growing disparities in knowledge and basic skills "between those who have access to the wonderworld of opportunities afforded by computers and those who have not, between those who can pay for the service and those who cannot" (Roll, 1995, p. xii).

Convergence or Diversity

Perhaps the key issue underlying the transfer between countries of beliefs, principles, knowledge, and practices relating to special education and rehabilitation is the one to do with cultural propriety. Is it appropriate for the ideas generated in one society with a particular culture and world view to be transferred to another? Who should decide? What safeguards should be put in place if cultural imperialism is to be avoided? Is this a real issue, or are the forces of globalization inexorably leading to cultural convergence?

As noted by Mitchell (1996), globalization is a trend that is well under way and will gather pace as we move into the what Kennedy (1993) refers to as the "transnational world" of the 21st century. In this world, we will experience "the intensification of worldwide social relations which link distant localities in such a way that local happenings are shaped by events occurring many miles away and vice versa" (Giddens, 1990, p. 9). In a transnational world, the sovereignty of nation-states will increasingly be challenged by forces that lie well outside their borders (Kennedy, 1993), a process which Torres (1995–96, p. 312) refers to as "denationalization." As nations become more interdependent, there will be more frequent and broad-ranging exchanges of goods and services across national boundaries (Wilson, 1988). This trend towards globalization is the product of such factors as the emergence of a global economy, the development of intergovernmental and quasi-supranational institutions, the establishment of regional political federations and alliances, and the expansion of transnational economic and cultural links (Held, 1991). To these economic and geopolitical factors, we must add the impact of increasing communications interconnectivity (Negroponte, 1995), which will lead to many of the values of the nation-state giving way to those of both larger and smaller electronic communities, with their own cultures (Rheingold, 1993). Increasingly, we will socialize in digital neighborhoods and engage in electronic commerce on a global scale (Butler, 1996). Societies will increasingly depend on telecommunications to move information to where it is needed, physical space will be irrelevant and time will play a different role (Negroponte, 1995; Tiffin & Rajasingham, 1995). In his controversial book, *The End of History and the Last Man*, Fukuyama (1992), goes so far as to suggest that as countries modernize they must increasingly resemble one another, "regardless of their historical origins or cultural inheritances" (p. xiv). This homogenization reflects the "universal economic nexus of modern consumerism, . . . centering around technologically-driven economic growth and the capitalist social relations necessary to produce and sustain it" (p. 126). It must be noted, however, that contrasting positions are taken on this issue. There are those who, like Fukuyama, perceive a convergence of cultures, but there are others who see the post–Cold War world leading to cultural identities shaping the patterns of cohesion, disintegration, and conflict. Such a view is espoused by Huntington (1996) in his recent book, *The Clash of Civilizations and the Remaking of World Order*. A third position is that there is truth in both views, in that there is both convergence and divergence, depending on the activity. Whatever the mix of values that emerges in different countries, these will have profound implications for education and rehabilitation.

In terms of education, recent years have seen what McNeely and Cha (1994) refer to as "a remarkable degree of convergence in both educational ideology and educational structure across all types of nation states," a situation that reflects the trend towards nation-states becoming increasingly subject to world-level ideological prescriptions and practices, as mediated by such agencies as the UN and the OECD. Such agencies exercise considerable authority, according to McNeely and Cha, influencing national systems through a number of normative and rule-creating activities, four in particular. Firstly, international organizations act as a major forum for the transnational exchange of ideas and information via their publications, through the provision of consultants, and by sponsoring various types of conferences, meetings, and workshops. Secondly, in order to become members of these international organizations, countries have to sign up to their charters and constitutions, which typically contain professions of adherence to global principles, norms, and procedures. A third and related means of bringing about international convergence can be found in standard-setting instruments such as declarations and recommendations. Although these may not be legally binding, "they may be both inspirational and educational." As noted in a previous section of this chapter, international bodies have already had a major impact on special education and rehabilitation. This is likely to continue, if not accelerate, in the future as the *Salamanca Statement and Framework for Action on Special Needs Education* (UNESCO, 1994) and *The Standard Rules on the Equalization of Opportunities for Persons with Disabilities* (United Nations, 1994) exert their influences. Finally, and in some circumstance perhaps most importantly, international organizations exert their influence through direct financial assistance or through the provision of development experts, both of which are usually linked to the adoption of certain ideas and policies.

Despite the evidence of convergence, the emergence of a transnational world with shared social values will not be achieved easily. Disputes are bound to occur. For example, in a recent publication, UNESCO's International Commission on Education for the Twenty-first Century identify six main tensions that will be central to the problems of the next century (UNESCO, 1996):

- *global and local:* people will need to become world citizens without losing their roots and continuing to participate in their nation and community;

- *universal and individual:* people will need to adapt to a globalized culture without submerging their unique individual character;

- *tradition and modernity:* people will need to adapt to the new information age without turning their backs on the past;

- *long-term and short-term:* this tension is sustained by the prevalence of the ephemeral and instantaneous in a world when an over-abundance of information and fleeting emotion keeps the spotlight on immediate problems;

- *competition and equality of opportunity:* the pressure of competition has driven many authorities to lose sight of their mission to give every human being the means to take advantage of every opportunity; three forces must be reconciled: competition (which provides incentives), cooperation (which gives strength), and solidarity (which unites);

- *spiritual and material:* education should stimulate everyone to reach out to the universal and to a measure of self transcendence. (pp. 16–18)

Some writers have expressed their disquiet regarding the way in which Western principles and practices are often imported into countries in ways that undermine the indigenous culture. In an analysis of the impact of Western practices on Indonesia, Kugelmass (1995) studied a group of parents of 14 mentally handicapped children. She found that all had consulted *dukuns* (spirit doctors) regarding the care and treatment of their child and believed in magic that held out the promise that some day their child would be cured. Notwithstanding this, Indonesian parents have begun to question the value of traditional approaches to caring for one another as they look towards technological and institutional solutions to provide a "cure" for their children: "The physician is replacing the dukun and medical knowledge is becoming his or her magic" (p. 45). Kugelmass notes that while some professionals recognized *dukuns* as an important component of Indonesian health care who, at the very least, provide emotional support for families, most had not incorporated them into their treatments, and were not recognizing the value of the community-based systems that have sustained Indonesian families for centuries. Instead, they were relying solely on Western approaches and were imitating Western practices and styles (e.g., the use of IQ tests). Kugelmass expresses concern at this importation of technologies into a culture based on very different assumptions, values, and patterns of thinking than the culture from which they originated. She cites Fitch and Webb's (1989) summary of the set of values underlying Indonesian belief systems, inviting a comparison with Western values. The former comprise the notions that wisdom always comes from experience; change is always possible, but one cannot change one's destiny; duties of office are predetermined and one must accept them and act accordingly; everything has its place in the universe according to one's status and morality and one must do what is appropriate and avoid what is not; and people should know their place and task. She concludes that in order for the artifacts of one culture to be adopted appropriately by another, the subjective and objective aspects of both must be fully understood and respected.

In a similar vein, Kerns and Cavalcante (1997) note that the model of inclusion developed in the United States cannot be applied directly to Brazilian schools. They argue that Brazilian educators and parents need to create their own model of inclusion, taking into consideration their social, economic, political, and cultural singularities. They cite DaMatta (1987) as describing the spectrum of social life in Brazil and in the United States of America following "radically different logics":

> The historical-cultural process of Brazil (and Latin America) is one of having to open a social and political space for local and individual manifestations since everything is rigidly overseen and dominated by an enormous political, religious and legal centralism. The historical North American experience is one of generat-

ing laws which can invent or save totalities greater than local systems. In Brazil, individualism is created with effort, as something negative and *against* the laws which emanate from the state and define totality. In the United States, individualism is positive, and the thrust has been to create a *union*, a totality. (p. 314)

The explicit or implicit cultural imperialism that has accompanied much of the transfer of beliefs, knowledge, and experiences in the past is particularly pernicious in the case of countries that have gone though extended periods of colonialism. Ajuwon (1996), for example, is very critical of the ways in which "the forces of urbanisation and the dependency pattern of development, coupled with missionary activities" (p. 192) in Africa have led to the collapse of kinship systems and community-based learning experiences for children.

A further example of the need for senstivity on transferring beliefs and practices across cultures is provided by New Zealand, where the indigenous people, the Maori, embrace a model of well-being referred to as *Whare Tapa Wha*. This model translates literally as "the four walls of the house," with each being necessary to ensure strength and balance (Durie, 1994). These walls comprise *taha wairua* (the spiritual side), *taha hinengaro* (thoughts and feelings), *taha tinana* (the physical side), and *taha whanau* (the extended family). Many cultures have a similar holistic perception of well-being and it behooves those engaged in the cross-cultural transfer of knowledge to work within such models if they wish to have their ideas accepted.

In his review of disability in the context of Eastern religions, Miles (1995) provides a salutary reminder for Westerners of the fact that "at least 70% of global disability is experienced in countries and contexts upon which western ethics and philosophy impinge only peripherally" (p. 50). Furthermore, he asserts, current formulations of the rights of the disabled "rest upon a largely western liberal consensus of views" (p. 61) and as such constitute "unintended cultural colonialism" that largely ignores "the history and anthropology of disability outside the dominant culture of the western educated classes" (p. 62). Miles concludes that as global efforts are made to improve the lot of disabled people, beliefs and attitudes present in the world's major non-Christian religions (Islam, Hinduism, and Buddhism) must be taken more fully into account.

Various projects have taken steps to guard against imposing outside solutions in the process of transferring beliefs, knowledge, and practices. For example, Johnson (1995) outlines how, in the Lithuania project described earlier in this chapter, the philosophy of the project was based on the principle that all those potentially affected by changes should have a voice and, if possible, an involvement in the events leading to such changes: "Application of this principle enhances the likelihood that any resulting structures and processes will be Lithuanian in character because they have been derived by Lithuanians" (p. 79). A second example of an attempt to redress potential power imbalances that are inherent between aid donors and recipients is afforded by UNESCO's Parent Education Project implemented in Malawi, Sri Lanka and Uganda (McConkey, 1993). This project utilizes indigenously produced video programs as a medium for educating families and local communities about childhood disabilities. In a similar vein, a Training for Work video course has been developed by the Chesire Foundation International using video programs recorded on location throughout the Asia Pacific Region (McConkey, 1996).

Introducing Innovations

A useful analysis of how educational innovations should be introduced is provided by Baine (1996). He identifies three phases: initiation, implementation, and institutionalization. The initiation phase involves a needs assessment; deciding whether to undertake innovation; mobilizing resources; and developing initial commitment. Planning plays a most important role during this phase. Strategic planning involves selecting and prioritizing objectives and selecting broad implementation strategies. Here a balance has to be struck between narrowing the focus to those objectives that can reasonably be achieved with existing or easily obtainable resources and bringing about sufficient change to improve quality (Rondinelli, Middleton, & Verspoor, 1990). Operational planning involves translating broad program objectives into specific policy actions, implementation schedules, and procedures that will allow the achievement of the strategy objectives. The implementation phase involves putting an innovation into practice, with attention to ongoing personnel training, consultation, project coordination, commitment, maintenance, materials dissemination, conducting pilot studies, program evaluation, innovation revision, and diffusion. Institutionalization involves removing the novelty of the innovation and making it part of the normal, continuing administrative and professional practice. Derham (1988) describes this phase in terms of sustainable systems development, with local responsibility playing the critical role.

A complementary perspective to the foregoing is provided by the Norwegian Agency for Development Cooperation, which has put forward a set of principles it requires NGOs to meet to be eligible for financial support. These coalesce around three basic values: justice (e.g., development assistance should benefit poor and marginalized population groups), participation (e.g., development assistance should promote democratization), and sustainability and self-reliance (e.g., development assistance should promote self-reliance at individual, community and national levels).

PROSPECTS FOR THE FUTURE

As we approach the 21st century, it is timely to consider ways in which the transfer of beliefs, knowledge, and experiences relating to special education and rehabilitation should take place in the future. Such projections need to take account of a range of contextual factors—many of which have negative connotations for people with disabilities—which have been identified by writers such as Merceron (1996), Mitchell (1996), Murray (1996), and Rehabilitation International (1996). These include: (a) the acceleration of globalization processes, which are facilitating both integration and fragmentation; (b) the increasing disparities of living standards, both within and between countries; (c) a rethinking of the concept of social protection, arising from concerns at the growing costs of the welfare state and an increased emphasis on economic efficiency at the expense of social justice; (d) longer average life expectancies, resulting in the trend for young people with disabilities to survive to adulthood and to outlive their parents' ability to care for them; (e) the expansion of automation, resulting in the elimination of less sophisticated tasks, especially in industries with a low-skilled, labor-intensive content—the sector frequently occupied by disabled people; (f) the increasing sophistication of assistive devices, but a corresponding diminution of access by many people with disabilities, especially in developing countries; and (g) the wide variation among countries with respect to issues such as human rights, quality of life, and personal choice.

If the negative effects of these social and economic trends for people with disabilities are to be ameliorated, and if greater equality is to be achieved both within and between countries, it is clear that there will have to be improvements in the ways in which beliefs, knowledge, and experiences—and, of course, capital—are transferred. As explained in this chapter, international instruments such as *The Standard Rules for the Equalization of Opportunities for Persons with Disabilities* and the *Salamanca Statement* provide a sound basis for future developments and are already exerting considerable influence on many countries' policies. The challenge remains, however, of finding ways to convert these good intentions into actual practices across the world in all its diversity: the rural areas of Malawi, the isolated mountain villages of Nepal, the subarctic communities of Siberia, the nomadic tribes of Jordan, the slums of Calcutta, the former communist countries of Eastern Europe, the strife-torn societies of Rwanda and Albania, the island states of the South Pacific. As pointed out in this chapter, there already exist complex networks of international, national, and regional agencies working in the field of rehabilitation. In developing countries, some of these networks are coordinated, but more often they are uncoordinated; some work within sustainable parameters, while others create over-dependence on external assistance; some are sensitive to indigenous cultures, whereas others import inappropriate technologies; some can independently access the most recent developments in the field through such means as the Internet, whereas others are dependent on external consultants or "knowledge brokers."

The challenge to both exporters and importers of philosophies and practices is to determine how far should indigenous philosophies, ideologies, and practices be encouraged, respected, challenged, overthrown, or blended with those from "outside." There are ultimately three approaches to this dilemma (Mazurek

& Winzer, 1994). One is to adopt a position of social relativism, which asserts that because social enterprises reflect their cultural milieu, it would be inappropriate and culturally imperialistic to seek to radically change their policies or practices, even if authorities in the importing country would seem to encourage such new ideas. A second approach is to have recourse to "human and cultural universals that provide the touchstones against which ideas and practices may be measured and evaluated" (Mazurek & Winzer, 1994, p. xxiii), as expressed, for example, in the recent UN-sponsored *Standard Rules*. The third perspective represents a midpoint of the foregoing and would see change arising from a process of reflection upon existing policies and practices (Ainscow & Hart, 1992), with countries taking ownership of the process (Brown, Baine, & Neufeldt, 1996) and being supported in the development of their own models. An essential element of this approach is that of capacity building, in which institutional and human resources are developed to enhance the countries' abilities to solve their problems in a sustainable manner. In this context, the role of the external consultant is one of facilitating rather than directing change (Brown, Abu Ghazaleh, & Neufeldt, 1996; Davies & Johnson, 1996; Silverman, 1996).

A final word needs to be added. As outlined in this chapter, much of what has taken place in the transfer of beliefs, knowledge, and experiences between countries has been characterized by one-way traffic—from richer to poorer countries, from high-technology to low-technology countries, from Western to non-Western countries. It is to be hoped—and expected—that the future will see sincere steps taken to redress this assymetrical transfer (King, 1991) and that there will not only be an increase in collaborative projects (Barcham & Upton, 1993), but also greater appreciation among developed countries of what can be learned from the experiences and perceptions of those from developing nations (Brown, Baine, & Neufeldt, 1996). Ultimately, wherever one lives, it will be the judicious blending of outside ideas and existing cultural practices that will bring about sustainable changes that are likely to improve the quality of life of people with disabilities.

REFERENCES

Abang, T. B. (1994). Nigeria. In K. Mazurek & M. A. Winzer (Eds.), *Comparative studies in special education* (pp. 71–87). Washington, DC: Gallaudet Press.

Agrawal, R. (1994). India. In K. Mazurek & M. A. Winzer (Eds.), *Comparative studies in special education* (pp. 179–203). Washington, DC: Gallaudet Press.

Ainscow, M. (1994). *Special needs in the classroom: A teacher education guide.* Paris: UNESCO; London: Jessica Kingsley Publishers.

Ainscow, M., & Hart, S. (1992). Moving practice forward. *Support for Learning, 7*(3), 115–120.

Ajuwon, P. M. (1996). Educational and rehabilitation aspects of visual impairments in developing countries. In R. Brown, A. Neufeldt & D. Baine (Eds.), *Beyond basic care: Special education and community rehabilitation in low income countries* (pp. 183–199). North York, ON: Captus Press.

Baine, D. (1996). Introducing changes to educational and rehabilitation programmes in developing countries. In R. Brown, A. Neufeldt, & D. Baine (Eds.), *Beyond basic care: Special education and community rehabilitation in low income countries* (pp. 307–319). North York, ON: Captus Press.

Barcham, L., & Upton, G. (1993). Towards the comparative study of special education. In R. J. Michael & G. Upton (Eds.), *The Viewfinder, Volume 2: Expanding boundaries and perspectives in special education* (pp. 50–52). Reston, VA: Division of International Special Education and Services, The Council for Exceptional Children.

Brown, R., Baine, D., & Neufeldt, A. H. (1996). Introduction. In R. Brown, A. Neufeldt, & D. Baine (Eds.), *Beyond basic care: Special education and community rehabilitation in low income countries* (pp. 1–7). North York, ON: Captus Press.

Brown, R. I. (1997). Legislation in Australian special education intent and effect: The impact on child, family and teacher. In D. Mitchell & J. Kugelmass (Eds.), *The Viewfinder: Volume 4, New Models for Re-forming Special Education.* Reston, VA: Division of International Special Education and Services, The Council for Exceptional Children.

Brown, R. I., Abu Ghazaleh, H., & Neufeldt, A. (1996). Challenges to rehabilitation—A case example. In R. Brown, A. Neufeldt, & D. Baine (Eds.), *Beyond basic care: Special education and community rehabilitation in low income countries* (pp. 280–306). North York, ON: Captus Press.

Burbules, N. C. (1995). Technology and changing educational communities. Paper presented to AESA, Fall 1995. Available online at: http://www.ed.uiuc.edu/coe/eps/NickB.html.

Burbules, N. C., & Callister, T. A. (1996). Knowledge at the crossroads: Some alternative features of hypertext learning environments. *Educational Theory, 46*(1), 23–50.

Butler, G. (1996). *Impact 2000: How information technology will change New Zealand.* Wellington: Information Technology Advisory Group and Information Technology Association of New Zealand.

Chen, Y-H., & Lu, T-H. (1994). Taiwan. In K. Mazurek & M. A. Winzer (Eds.), *Comparative studies in special education* (pp. 238–259). Washington, DC: Gallaudet Press.

Crawford, N., & Bray, M. (1994). Hong Kong. In K. Mazurek & M. A. Winzer (Eds.), *Comparative studies in special education* (pp. 286–304). Washington, DC: Gallaudet Press.

Csanyi, Y. (1995). Special education and teacher training in Hungary. In P. Mittler & P. Daunt (Eds.), *Teacher education for special needs in Europe* (pp. 138–144). London: Cassell.

DaMatta, R. (1987). The quest for citizenship in a relational universe. In J. Wirth, E. Nunes, & T. Bogenschild (Eds.), *State and society in Brazil: Continuity and change* (pp. 307–335). Boulder, CO: Westview Press.

Davies, R., & Johnson, P. R. (1996). Consulting in the Middle East—A personal perspective. In R. Brown, A. Neufeldt, & D. Baine (Eds.), *Beyond basic care: Special education and community rehabilitation in low income countries* (pp. 261–279). North York, ON: Captus Press.

Derham, M. (1988). The right kind of development. *TEAR Times, 39,* 4–6. [Cited by Ager, A. (1990). Planning sustainable services: Principles for the effective targeting of resources in developed and developing nations. In W. I. Fraser (Ed.), *Key issues in mental retardation research* (pp. 385–394). London: Routledge.]

Diaconescu, R., Ionescu, M., Chis, V., & Daunt, P. (1995). Teacher training and the integration of children with special needs: Romanian initiatives. In P. Mittler & P. Daunt (Eds.), *Teacher education for special needs in Europe* (pp. 64–74). London: Cassell.

Durie, M. H. (1994). *Whaiora: Maori health development.* Wellington, New Zealand: Oxford University Press.

Fitch, R. M., & Webb, S. A. (1989). Cultural immersion in Indonesia through Pancasila: State ideology. *Journal of Educational Thought, 23*(1), 44–51.

Fukuyama, F. (1992). *The end of history and the last man.* London: Hamish Hamilton.

Giddens, A. (1991). *Modernity and self-identity: Self and society in the late modern age.* Cambridge: Polity Press.

Hekking, K. (1996). Participant in Joint Seminar of Vocational Commission on Organisation and

Administration—Organisation and Administration of Employment Initiatives Through Systems Change. In *Proceedings of 18th World Congress of Rehabilitation International* (pp. 194–200). Auckland, New Zealand, 15–20 September 1996,

Helander, E. (1993). *Prejudice and dignity: An introduction to community-based rehabilitation*. New York: UNDP.

Held, D. (1991). Democracy, the nation-state and the global system. In D. Held (Ed.), *Political theory today*. Cambridge: Polity Press.

Huntington, S. P. (1996). *The clash of civilizations and the remaking of world order*. New York: Simon & Schuster.

ILO, UNESCO, & WHO (1994). *Community-based rehabilitation for and with people with disabilities: A joint position paper*. Unpublished manuscript.

Inclusion International (1996, October). Inclusive education in the Dominican Republic. *Inclusion International*, No. 4.

Inter-Agency Commission (UNDP, UNESCO, UNICEF, World Bank) (1990). *World Declaration on Education for All*. New York: UNICEF House.

Johnson, M. (1995). East-West cooperation for pupils with SEN: A report on a TEMPUS project. In P. Mittler & P. Daunt (Eds.), *Teacher education for special needs in Europe* (pp. 75–86). London: Cassell.

Kennedy, P. (1993). *Preparing for the twenty-first century*. New York: Random House.

Kerns, G. M., & Cavalcante, F. S. (1997). Brazilian special needs education: Conceptual framework and policy for the 1990s. In D. Mitchell & J. Kugelmass (Eds.), *The viewfinder, Volume 4: New models for re-forming special education*. Reston, VA: Division of International Special Education and Services, The Council for Exceptional Children.

Kim, S-K. (1993). Development of special education in the Republic of Korea. In R. J. Michael & G. Upton (Eds.), *The viewfinder, Volume 2: Expanding boundaries & perspectives in special education* (pp. 26–28). Reston, VA: Division of International Special Education and Services, The Council for Exceptional Children.

King, K. (1991). *Aid and education in the developing world: The role of donor agencies in educational analysis*. Harlow, England: Longman.

Kugelmass, J. (1995). The Indonesian system of caring: Beyond technology solutions to human problems. In D. L. Edyburn, R. A. Henderson, & L. Sandals (Eds.), *The viewfinder, Volume 3: International perspectives on special education technology* (pp. 37–48). Reston, VA: Division of International Special Education and Services, The Council for Exceptional Children.

Lynch, J. (1994). *Provision for children with special educational needs in the Asia region*. Washington, DC: World Bank.

Mazurek, K., & Winzer, M. A. (1994). Introduction. In K. Mazurek & M. A. Winzer (Eds.), *Comparative studies in special education* (pp. xvii–xxxix). Washington, DC: Gallaudet Press.

McClintock, R. (1995). *Power and pedagogy: transforming education through information technology*. Available online at: http://www.ilt.columbia.edu/academic/texts/mcclintock/pp/title.html.

McConkey, R. (1993). Video training packages for parent education. In R. J. Michael & G. Upton (Eds.), *The Viewfinder, Volume 2: Expanding boundaries and perspectives in special education* (pp. 34–37). Reston, VA: Division of International Special Education and Services, The Council for Exceptional Children.

McConkey, R. (1996). A valued life in the community. In R. Brown, A. Neufeldt, & D. Baine (Eds.), *Beyond basic care: Special education and community rehabilitation in low income countries* (pp. 151–167). North York, ON: Captus Press.

McNeely, C. L., & Cha, Y.-K. (1994). Worldwide educational convergence through international organizations: Avenues for research. *Educational Policy Analysis Archives*, 2(14).

Merceron, A. (1996). Does technology enhance the quality of life for elderly people? In *Proceedings of 18th World Congress of Rehabilitation International* (pp. 374–385). Auckland, New Zealand, 15–20 September 1996.

Miles, M. (1995). Disability in an Eastern religious context: Historical perspectives. *Disability & Society, 10*(1), 49–69.

Misawa, G. (1994). Japan. In K. Mazurek & M. A. Winzer (Eds.), *Comparative studies in special education* (pp. 221–237). Washington, DC: Gallaudet Press.

Mitchell, D., & Chen, Y-Y. (1996). Special education in East and South East Asia. In R. Brown, A. Neufeldt, & D. Baine (Eds.), *Beyond basic care: Special education and community rehabilitation in low income countries* (pp. 8–42). North York, ON: Captus Press.

Mitchell, D., & O'Brien, P. (1994). New Zealand. In K. Mazurek & M. A. Winzer (Eds.), *Comparative studies in special education* (pp. 420–451). Washington, DC: Gallaudet Press.

Mitchell, D. (1996). What will special education look like in 2021? Paper presented at 18th World Congress of Rehabilitation International, Auckland, New Zealand, 15–20 September 1996.

Mitchell, J., & Mitchell, D. (1987). Integration/mainstreaming. In D. R. Mitchell & N. N. Singh (Eds.), *Exceptional children in New Zealand* (pp. 107–117). Palmerston North, New Zealand: Dunmore Press.

Mittler, P., & Daunt, P. (Eds.) (1995). *Teacher education for special needs in Europe.* London: Cassell.

Moulton, R., Andrews, J. F., & Smith, M. (1996). The deaf world. In R. Brown, A. Neufeldt, & D. Baine (Eds.), *Beyond basic care: Special education and community rehabilitation in low income countries* (pp. 168–182). North York, ON: Captus Press.

Murray, B. (1996). Participant in Joint Seminar of Vocational Commission on Organisation and Administration—Organisation and Administration of Employment Initiatives Through Systems Change. In *Proceedings of 18th World Congress of Rehabilitation International* (pp. 178–189). Auckland, New Zealand, 15–20 September 1996.

Narayan, J. (1996). Special education in India. In R. Brown, A. Neufeldt, & D. Baine (Eds.), *Beyond basic care: Special education and community rehabilitation in low income countries* (pp. 43–62). North York, ON: Captus Press.

Negroponte, N. (1995). *Being digital.* London: Coronet Books, Hodder and Stoughton.

Nirje, B. (1969). The normalization principle and its human management implications. In R. Krugel & W. Wolfensberger (Eds.), *Changing patterns in residential services for the mentally retarded.* Washington, DC: President's Committee on Mental Retardation.

Nirje, B. (1985). The basis and logic of the normalisation principle. *Australia and New Zealand Journal of Developmental Disabilities, 11*(2), 65–68.

Niwa, S. (1996). Developments in creating an Asia/Pacific Network of Centers for Disabled Persons. Paper presented at 18th World Congress of Rehabilitation International, Auckland, New Zealand, 15–20 September 1996.

Norwegian Agency for Development Cooperation, *Guide to planning and evaluating NGO projects* [five parts]. Oslo: Norwegian Agency for Development Cooperation, Division for Non-Governmental Organizations.

O'Hanlon, C. (1993). Inclusion and integration in Europe: A human rights issue. In R. J. Michael & G. Upton (Eds.), *The viewfinder, Volume 2: Expanding boundaries & perspectives in special education* (pp. 47–49). Reston, VA: Division of International Special Education and Services, The Council for Exceptional Children.

O'Hanlon, C. (1995). A comparison of educational provision for pupils with special educational needs in Europe. In P. Mittler & P. Daunt (Eds.), *Teacher education for special needs in Europe* (pp. 1–16). London: Cassell.

O'Toole, B. J. (1991). *Guide to community-based rehabilitation services.* Paris: UNESCO.

Qirbi, A. (1993). Poverty and handicap in the Republic of Yemen. In R. J. Michael & G. Upton (Eds.), *The viewfinder, Volume 2: Expanding boundaries & perspectives in special education* (pp. 12–17). Reston, VA: Division of International Special Education and Services, The Council for Exceptional Children.

Rehabilitation International. (1996). Summary of Congress outcomes. In *Proceedings of 18th World Congress of Rehabilitation International* (pp. 3–9). Auckland, New Zealand, 15–20 September 1996.

Rheingold, H. (1993). *The virtual community.* Reading, MA: Addison-Wesley.

Roll, R. (1995). Foreword. In J. Tiffin & L. Rajasingham, *In search of the virtual class: Education in the information society* (pp. xxi–xvi). London: Routledge.

Rondinelli, D. A., Middleton, J., & Verspoor, A. M. (1990). *Planning educational reforms in developing countries.* Durham, NC: Duke University Press.

Rowland, W. (1996). Participant in the Roundtable Forum on the UN Standard Rules for the Equalisation of Opportunities for Persons with Disabilities. In *Proceedings of 18th World Congress of Rehabilitation International* (pp. 478–479). Auckland, New Zealand, 15–20 September 1996, .

Seelman, K. (1996). Equality through participation. In *Proceedings of 18th World Congress of Rehabilitation International,* Auckland, New Zealand, 15–20 September 1996, pp. 89–99.

Silverman, F. H. (1996). Personal involvement in the development of programmes for persons with disabilities. In R. Brown, A. Neufeldt, & D. Baine (Eds.), *Beyond basic care: Special education and community rehabilitation in low income countries* (pp. 254–260). North York, ON: Captus Press.

Swan, G. (1994). Australia. In K. Mazurek & M. A. Winzer (Eds.), *Comparative studies in special education.* Washington, DC: Gallaudet Press.

Thorburn, M. (1996). Roles and relationships of community-based rehabilitation in Jamaica. In R. Brown, A. Neufeldt, & D. Baine (Eds.), *Beyond basic care: Special education and community rehabilitation in low income countries* (pp. 126–150). North York, ON: Captus Press.

Tiffin, J., & Rajasingham, L. (1995). *In search of the virtual class: Education in the information society.* London: Routledge.

Tjandrakusuma, H. (1996, September). Towards the 21st century: Challenges for community based rehabilitation in the Asian and Pacific Region. Paper presented at 18th World Congress of Rehabilitation International, Auckland, New Zealand.

Torres, C. A. (1995/96). State and education revisited: Why educational researchers should think politically about education. *Review of Research in Education, 21,* 255–331.

UNESCO. (1994). *The Salamanca Statement And Framework For Action On Special Needs Education.* Paris: UNESCO.

UNESCO. (1996). *Report of the International Commission on Education for the Twenty-first Century.* Paris: UNESCO.

United Nations. (1994). *The Standard Rules on the Equalization of Opportunities for Persons with Disabilities.* Paris: United Nations.

Warnock, H. M. (1978). *Report of the Committee into the Education of Handicapped Children and Young People.* London: HMSO.

Wilson, J. (1988). *Politics and leisure.* Boston: Unwin Hyman.

Winzer, M. A. (1994). Canada. In K. Mazurek & M. A. Winzer (Eds.), *Comparative studies in special education* (pp. 370–386). Washington, DC: Gallaudet Press.

World Bank (1995). *Priorities and strategies for education: A World Bank review.* Washington, DC: The World Bank.

CHAPTER 14

Utilizing Technology for the Inclusion of Individuals With Mental Retardation

JANNA SIEGEL
University of Memphis

In today's increasingly technological society, great advances in computers and other mechanical devices have assisted individuals with disabilities to better integrate into society. A multitude of new available devices have given individuals added mobility, increased their communication access, and enabled them to receive instruction through computers. In this current information age, resources, research, and consultations can be obtained through on-line resources. Though these new prospects are exciting and the potential is enormous, the use of technology has not yet significantly improved the lives of most individuals with mental retardation around the world.

The costs of some technology is prohibitive to many individuals, and in many regions access to basic requirements such as electricity may not be found. Much software is only available in developed countries and will only work on state of the art computers, which are not available in many areas. Additionally, software is limited to a few languages, and often not translated into more than one or two languages at best.

On-line resources can be a valuable tool for individuals working with persons with mental retardation. There are on-line journals, research, listservs, newsgroups, chat lines, support groups, and a myriad of services available on the Internet. However, the quality of these services is variable and the time required to sift through much of the information can be daunting. Access to the Internet, though becoming much easier in developed countries, is still quite problematic in many areas of the world. The languages used on the Internet are also limited. Fortunately, many of these concerns are being addressed with the improvement of search engines and the growing use of translation software.

Technology will not be the panacea for individuals with mental retardation. It will not cure their disabilities or even fully compensate for the difficulties they

287

may encounter. Technology can, however, assist individuals in many ways that can improve their ability to integrate themselves into their world. The possibilities of how technology can be used to is just beginning to be explored. As computers get faster, less expensive, and easier to use, the potential benefits of using them will be more accessible and more feasible for individuals with mental retardation worldwide.

CULTURE AND TECHNOLOGY

There are sociocultural aspects to technology to consider, and a need to develop knowledge and skills to cope with the technological environment. Technology is not just computers and machines, but any process or product by which humans have dealt with their environment (Kerka, 1994). People always have lived in a society with new technologies and are continually having to adapt to the changes. But there are concerns that technology can be viewed as either a controlled or a controlling force. People can choose to perceive technology with optimism—that there are technological solutions to every problem; or with suspicion—that technology is going to dehumanize society and possibly destroy civilization (Postman, 1992).

The workforce is currently composed mostly of groups traditionally not targeted by technological advancements. These include females, people with disabilities, culturally diverse individuals, and persons from less developed nations (Selby, 1993). There are also cultural issues to consider, such as respect for the technologies of other cultures, concern for increasing access to technology, and focus technology that is compatible with the values of other cultures (Kerka, 1994).

Society will have to face the following question: "To whom will technology give greater power and freedom? And whose power and freedom will be reduced by it?" (Postman, 1992, p. 11). The answer may impact the future of technology developed for all individuals, including those with mental retardation.

There are several types of current technologies being used to assist individuals with disabilities. These are assistive technology, which includes adaptive and augmented communication devices, and computer-assisted instruction and assessment. Also, there are on-line resources that are available now through the use of new technologies. In this chapter, this author will describe the tools currently being used by individuals with mental retardation and review relevant international research.

ASSISTIVE TECHNOLOGY

Assistive technology is the term used to describe devices that are used by children and adults with mental retardation and other disabilities to compensate for functional limitations and to enhance and increase learning, independence, mobility, communication, environmental control, and choice. It also refers to direct services that assist individuals in selecting, acquiring, or using such devices (The Arc, 1991). Specifically, the user may communicate with others, engage in recreational and social activities, learn, work, control the environment, and increase his or her independence in daily living skills with the assistance of technology (Copel, 1991). For students with physical disabilities, there have been augmented keyboards, touch pads, voice commands, and other assistive devices to help individuals master the physical requirements of computers (Siegel, Good, & Moore, 1996). Computers have been a major component of recent communication devices by nonverbal or limited-verbal individuals (Bigge, 1991).

Assistive technology is used in several ways by individuals with mental retardation. The areas of uses for assistive technology are communication, environmental control, mobility, education, daily living, employment, and recreation. The following is a list of examples adapted from The Arc (1993; formerly Association of Retarded Citizens).

• *Communication:* For individuals with expressive disorders due to physical or cognitive disabilities, there are several communication devices that replace or supplement the voice or hand/motion communication of an individual. Computerized communication devices with vocal output are called augmentative and alternative communication devices.

• *Environmental control devices:* These help individuals to control their environment and are important to people with severe or multiple disabilities or cognitive disabilities, whose ability to move about in the environment and to turn electrical appliances on or off is limited. Assistive technology allows a person to control electrical appliances, audio/video equipment (such as home entertainment systems) or to do something as basic as lock and unlock doors.

• *Mobility.* For a person who does not walk, simple to sophisticated computer-controlled wheelchairs and mobility aids are available. There are also devices available to open doors, and lift people and wheelchairs up stairs, over curbs, and into vehicles. Additional mobility devices are available for personal hygiene such as being lifted/lowered into a bath tub, or into or out of a bed.

• *Education.* For a student with disabilities, the computer becomes a tool for improved literacy, language development, mathematical, organizational, and social skill development. Students with severe and multiple disabilities use technology in all aspects of the classroom learning environment; from academic software to communication. Alternative ways to access computers are available for students who cannot operate a keyboard. Software can be regulated so it runs at a slower pace if a student needs this type of modification for learning.

• *Activities of daily living.* Technology is assisting people with disabilities to successfully complete everyday tasks of self-care. Examples include automated and computerized dining devices that allow an individual who needs assistance at mealtime to eat more independently (Brown, Sauer, Cavalier, Frisch, & Wyatt, 1991).

Devices may be used to assist a person with memory difficulties to retrieve information or complete a task or to follow a certain sequence of steps from start to finish in such activities as making a bed or taking medication. Homes can be designed that use technology to assist a person to become more independent. Various devices can regulate and control many aspects of the living environment. An environment can be computerized to give cues and auditory direction for successfully performing tasks or for navigating. Directional guidance systems with auditory cues can assist a person in traveling from one location to another. Technology can assist a person to shop, write a check, pay the bills, or use the ATM machine.

• *Employment.* With the advent of the Americans with Disabilities Act, employers in the United States are making the workplace more cognitively accessible. For some employees, this requires worksite modifications where the employer adapts the environment, to permit the employee to perform a job. As an example, an audio tape is an accommodation that can be used to prompt a worker to complete each task in a job. Supplying modified keyboards or wheelchair-accommodating office furniture are also examples of employment accessibility support.

• *Sports and recreation.* Computerized games can be adapted for the user with physical limitations. Adaptations can be made to computer games thatallows the game activity to be slowed down for the user who cannot react as quickly to game moves and decision-making. Specially adapted sports equipment is available to compensate for functional limitations and which allow an individual to participate more fully. For example, people with mental retardation can participate in bowling using specially designed ball ramps.

There are several issues concerning the effectiveness of assistive technology for individuals with mental retardation. The first issue is the problem of cost and availability. Although several developed countries have funding available for assistive technology, it is more often allocated for the obvious needs of the physically disabled rather than the less observable needs of individuals with cognitive disabilities. Assistive technology designers and manufacturers often do not consider cognitive limitations when designing their tools. Oftentimes the tools required for cognitive disabilities do not even exist. Although many of the devices designed for augmented communication are adaptable to a variety of cognitive/communication levels, other devices are sometimes complicated and inflexible in design.

Since cognitive difficulties are highly varying, assistive technology needs to be easily modifiable. Many practitioners are not familiar with assistive technology devices; even those who are often are not familiar with the cognitive access designs. This can lead to inadequate instruction for users of the devices (The Arc,

1993). There are a variety of issues that need to be considered when deciding on an assistive technology device. In Figure 14.1, there is an "Assistive Technology Evaluation Checklist" developed to assist families and individuals when making this important decision (The Arc, 1994).

There are other concerns with assistive technology. In an ideal situation, a child would be given assistive tools at a young age and would have them available in every environmental setting. Transitions between tools, settings, and developmental stages would be smooth. Comprehensive assessments of individuals to match them to appropriate tools would be standard. Practitioners would be familiar with the tools and would continually assess their effectiveness. The purpose of promoting independence and inclusion would be checked to insure that devices were not inhibiting skill development. Family members and professionals working with individuals with mental retardation would be familiar with specific devices and support for their maintenance would be available and ongoing. Despite the best intentions of families and professionals, often many of these goals are never achieved for individuals with mental retardation.

A review of the research on the use of assistive technology and individuals with mental retardation shows it to be almost nonexistent. Basically, the only assistive technology regularly used with cognitive disabilities is augmented or adaptive communication, to be discussed and reviewed in the next section. Although other assistive technologies are used with individuals with mental retardation, it is usually only if they have physical limitations as well. Even the research on using adaptive communications is sparse concerning individuals with mental retardation. For years there was a belief that these devices would inhibit development of communication, so they were not utilized for individuals with cognitive disabilities. Most of the older research focuses solely on computer assisted instruction for communication and other cognitive tasks. Only in recent years has this view been modified to include the use of technological devices to assist in communication and other individuals needs.

Augmented and Alternative Communication

Augmented and Alternative Communication (AAC) is a type of assistive technology specifically designed for individuals who require assistance for communication. This is one area of assistive technology where flexibility is essential, because every individual person has their own communication abilities and needs. Unlike most assistive devices, these usually can be adapted for individuals with a range of cognitive / communicative abilities. The following is a brief description of some of the computer assisted AAC devices available.

In AAC, there are two broad methods of inputting information into communication devices. One is random selection of letters, words, symbols, or options, while the other is when access is given to two choices and the individual must choose one. To accomplish this input, communication boards have been devel-

To simplify the decision-making process, The Arc has compiled the following checklist to be used by people with mental retardation and their family members when making decisions about assistive technology. While the checklist cannot provide all the questions you need to address, technology-users and their advocates who address all of the questions on this list will have taken the basic steps needed to evaluate and assess an assistive device. The previous narrative can provide more details about the process covered by each question.

Look at the questions below as you evaluate and select devices. Questions are worded so that the optimal response is always "yes." In some circumstances, the question is not applicable (N/A). However, if, after completing the checklist there are too many "no" responses, you might want to reconsider any decisions about the device, at least until you can fill in your information gaps.

Before you evaluate a device (user questions):

Have you identified your specific need(s) to be addressed by an assistive device?	YES	NO	N/A
Are you familiar with environment where you will use the device?	YES	NO	N/A
Have you written your goals and objectives down and developed a way of tracking your progress?	YES	NO	N/A

Before you evaluate a device (vendor questions):

Does the vendor have a good reputation?	YES	NO	N/A
Does the vendor provide demonstration or trial periods?	YES	NO	N/A
Is deliver available, and if so, is it prompt and reasonably priced?	YES	NO	N/A
Does the vendor provide, or can the vendor direct you to required training for device use?	YES	NO	N/A
Will the vendor assist you in completing papterwork and documentation needed by funding sources?	YES	NO	N/A
Can the vendor modify the device, if necessary, and will the vendor provide ongoing support?	YES	NO	N/A

FIG. 14.1. *(Above and at right)*   The Arc: Assistive Technology Evaluation Checklist.

oped with symbols, pictures, or words to accommodate individual needs. Often current keyboard layouts are not suitable for input due to physical or cognitive limitations. Augmented keyboards include rearranging keys into efficient layouts, reducing keys for less physical demands, and expanding keys for additional message options. There are also encoding alternatives that are available for individuals. The options include ionic encoding (pictures or symbols), semantic compaction (where one symbol may have many possible meaning depending on keys pressed), alphabetic encoding (where one alphabet letter has several meanings), enlarged key keyboards, abbreviation expansion (where a few letters allow the whole word to be spoken), and lexical predication (where a list of likely options is provided after each letter typed). The output is usually provided by computer-

After you identify a device:

Device Performance Evaluation

Have you seen data to backup performance claims?	YES	NO	N/A
Was the device testing conducted by an independent evaluator?	YES	NO	N/A
Was testing conducted under circumstances similar to those in which you will be using the device?	YES	NO	N/A
Are device space, electronics and wiring requirements compatible with your use of the device? With other devices?	YES	NO	N/A

Device Convenience Evaluation

Have you tried out the device and found it to be comfortable and convenient to use?	YES	NO	N/A
Is the device easily or reasonably transported, stored and secured?	YES	NO	N/A
Can you operate all components of the device without training, or, if not, is training available?	YES	NO	N/A
Are installation and assembly requirements reasonable?	YES	NO	N/A
Will the device adapt to changes in your disability?	YES	NO	N/A

Device Reliability and Safety Evaluation

Did performance testing include reliability and durability assessment?	YES	NO	N/A
Are annual and lifetime maintenance and repair costs reasonable?	YES	NO	N/A
Is there a warranty available for the device?	YES	NO	N/A
If there is regular maintenance, is someone available to do this work?	YES	NO	N/A
Does the device meet federal standards for wiring and construction?	YES	NO	N/A
Was safety testing performed in situations similar to those in which you will be using the device?	YES	NO	N/A
Will the device require extensive modification and, if so, have you determined that this will not impact reliability and safety?	YES	NO	N/A

Device Practicality Evaluation

Is the device within your price range?	YES	NO	N/A
Does the device meet requirements identified by your funding source?	YES	NO	N/A
Dopes the device address the needs you identified earlier?	YES	NO	N/A
Is the device available within a reasonable time?	YES	NO	N/A
Is the device consistent with your lifestyle, age, personality and values?	YES	NO	N/A
Do you like the way the device looks, and will you feel comfortable using the device around others?	YES	NO	N/A
Have you compared this device with others performing similar functions?	YES	NO	N/A

ized voices (speech synthesizers), which are now becoming faster, less mechanistic sounding, and more age- and gender-appropriate (Venkatagiri, 1995). Table 14.1 shows a list of companies that provide adaptive keyboards.

The limited research on the use of AAC with individuals with mental retardation has shown some positive results. Two studies with adults found improvement through use of speech synthesizers. In one study, it was demonstrated that synthetic speech improved the efficiency of learning and decreased error rate with three adults with severe mental retardation (Schlosser Belfiore, & Hetzroni, 1995). In the second study (Brown & Cavalier, 1992), the adult with severe mental retardation they examined was able to learn how to use voice commands for environmental devices, differentiate vocalizations for different situations, and experience positive affect. Snyder and colleagues (1994) found that vocabulary acquisition was improved by five primary school students with mental disabilities, even after facilitator prompting was removed.

Unfortunately, not all studies found success using AAC with individuals with disabilities as successful. Koenigsfeld, Beukelman, and Stoefen-Fisher (1993) found, in a study of hearing impaired individuals, that AAC devices provided inconsistent communication success with hearing persons and there was some confusion from a lack of experience with these devices. Morgan, Ames, and Taylor (1995) found that professionals and supported-employment specialists were not sufficiently trained in the uses of assistive technology including AAC.

One interesting finding by Soto, Belfiore, and Schlosser (1993) was that a man with mental retardation who was able to learn two AAC devices had a definite preference for one. This study demonstrates the need for accurate assessment of which tools are the "best fit" for an individual. There are also equal concerns about fitting AAC devices to not only the individual, but to their families and environments (Parrette, 1991, 1994).

TABLE 14.1
Companies That Provide Keyboards Adapted for Persons With Disabilities

Ability Systems Corp., 1422 Arnold Ave., Roslyn, PA 19001

William Bradford Pub., 310 School St., Acton, MA 01720

Comput Ability Corp., 400000 Grand River, Suite 109, Movi, MI 48375

Hach Associates, P.O. Box 11754, Winston-Salem, NC 27116

Jordan & Associates, 1127 Oxford Ct., Neenah, WI 54956

Polytel Corp., 1287 Hammerwood Ave., Sunnyvale, CA 94089

Psychological Corp., 555 Academic Ct., San Antonio, TX 87204

Unicorn Engineering, 5221 Central Ave., Suite 205, Richmond, CA 94704

Words+, Inc., 4421 10th St. W., Suite L.P.O., Box 1229, Lancaster, CA 93535

Zygo Industries, Inc., P.O. Box 1008, Portland, OR 97207–1008

Taken with permission from Giordano, Leeper, and Siegel (1996), p. 95.

In a comprehensive list by Parrette (1996) several issues relating to the identification of effective AAC were identified. Although their questions were focused on children in school, many of the same issues will affect individuals in work environments as well. Individual issues were: strengths and needs, gender, preferences, past experiences, and academic/vocational goals. Technology issues included: availability, features, cost, dependability, repair costs, flexibility, trial usage, comfort, maintenance, and assembly difficulties. School or work concerns included: resources, funding, transport and protection of devices, and training requirements for people who work with these individuals. The family was also a concern to the selection of effective AAC devices. Family issues included family preferences, family activities, changes in routine, family interaction, time and training (adapted from Parette, 1996).

Facilitated Communication (FC)

One fairly recent and highly controversial alternative communication tool is Facilitated Communication. This method "consists of a trained facilitator who places his/her hand over the hand of the individual who then types out his/her own thoughts, ideas, and answers to questions" (Colman, Simpson, & Myles, 1996, p. 294). This method was originally pioneered in Australia (Crossley & Remington-Guerney, 1992), then furhter developed in the United States (Bilkin, 1992). The original research demonstrated that individuals with developmental disabilities could perform significantly better in communication literacy and comprehension than their cognitive abilities had been assessed. Unfortunately, in later studies when the facilitator was not given the same information as the individual with disabilities, these amazingly high results were not duplicated. Proponents still maintain that individuals with developmental disabilities are cognitively able people who just have physical communication limitations, and that FC can allow this communication to occur.

However, most of their research is based on anecdotal records. Critics are concerned that the attractiveness of this method may draw people away from more proven communication devices and methods. There is also a concern as to the feasibility of FC for each noncommunicative person with disabilities as a viable tool since the time and demands are enormous. The pervasive attitude toward FC and AAC is that future research is needed and some researchers have encouraged a "middle ground" to the debate where some of the research is questioned but the whole idea of FC is not dismissed altogether (Koppenhaver, Pierce & Yoder, 1995).

COMPUTER-ASSISTED INSTRUCTION (CAI)

Individuals with special needs can be assisted by computer-aided instruction because these programs are often self-paced and individualized to each student's area of needs. These computer programs allow for assessment, drill, practice, instruction, simulation, or creative productions (Siegel, Good, & Moore, 1996). Research has shown that computer-aided instruction motivates, teaches, and empowers special needs students, as well as helping to improve their communication skills (Bitter, 1993; Holzberg, 1994).

There are several types of software available for CAI. These can be divided into the following categories (Church & Bender, 1989): drill and practice, tutorials, games, simulations, and problem solving. Woodward and Gersten (1992) reviewed research studies indicating that in the United States and other developed countries, students with special needs spent comparable amounts of time on CAI, but their CAI use was significantly more drill and practice programs, as compared to their nondisabled peers. Cochran and Bull (1993) identified computers as assisting individuals with communication instruction in addition to AAC devices and evaluation. Computers can be a context for instruction, which can provide stimulus (text, audio, and visual) for interaction between instructors and students. (Giordano, Leeper, & Siegel, 1996).

There are also computer assessment tools for diagnostic purposes used with exceptional individuals, but these programs would not be technically considered CAI software, as they are often not directly associated with instruction. However, often the instructional programs in CAI allow for recording and modifiying of software to meet individual needs. This continuous assessment and data recording allows for improved programmed instruction by instructors and practitioners. Computer assessment will be discussed more in the next section of this chapter.

The use of CAI in education was reviewed by Roblyer (1989) and the research was found to be incomplete. Some interesting trends were noted in CAI that impacted their use with exceptional individuals. One result was that CAI showed significant results to improve students learning at all levels, though more prominently in postsecondary and with adults than in schools or with children. Ability level was not found impact learning with CAI. Additionally, a variety of curricular areas were taught with success using different types of computer programs for instruction. One trend of note was that drill and practice had some success with low-level skills, but the tutorials were better for the higher-level problem-solving skills (Roblyer, 1989). There have been a number of studies examining the use of CAI with children and adults with mental retardation. Although most of these studies show mild to moderate improvement in a variety of areas when using CAI, several studies demonstrated results with no gains in abilities. These studies are from different areas of the world and are examining a variety of software with diverse individuals, so a comparison of studies is difficult to accomplish.

Some studies reported success with children who have mental retardation with mathematics skills (in the Netherlands: Baltussen & Van Lieshout, 1991, and Jaspers & Van Lieshout, 1989; in Hong Kong: Leung, 1994a, 1994b; in the U.S.: Podell, Tournaki-Rein, & Lin, 1992), but in the study by Podell and his colleagues (1992) it was discussed that although CAI was more effective than paper-and-pencil prompting for arithmetic, children with mental disabilities still required more time than nondisabled peers to achieve automaticity. CAI instruction was successful with children with mental retardation in spelling (in Israel: Margalit & Roth, 1989), reading—using text to speech technology (in Canada: Leong, 1992), word recognition (in the U.S.: Plienis, 1987), typing (in the United States: Molcho, 1989), social skills (in Israel: Margalit, 1991), and music (in the U.S.: Spitzer, 1990). Communication skills were improved in two studies using CAI (in the United States: Iacono & Miller, 1989; Osguthorpe & Chang, 1988), but in a review of CAI for communication (Bull, Cochran, & Snell, 1988), it was suggested that AAC would be better for students than CAI for communication disorders or delays.

Some promising studies in the U.S. examined students' behavior with CAI and found that most students were more motivated to learn using CAI, versus adult prompts (Chen & Bernard-Opitz, 1993) and with students who practice task avoidance with adults, CAI was more effective (Plienis & Romanczyk, 1985). Additionally, the study by Chen and colleagues (1993) did not find improved learning rates, just improved behavior. Burg (1984) describes the microcomputer in her class as a "magical, useful but expensive toy." She claims that it could be used in her kindergarten classroom to promote self-esteem, problem-solving, and autonomy with her developmentally delayed students.

CAI has also been demonstrated to be effective in a few studies when used with adults with mental retardation. Spelling instruction was improved with CAI (Dube, McDonald, & McIlvane, 1991; Stromer, Mackay, & Flusser, 1996), and matching (Dube, Iennaco, Rocco, & Klendaras, 1992), as well as typing and word processing (Saka, 1985). Saka also found typing improvements from CAI led to additional job placements for several adults with developmental delays. There were no differences found in sight word acquisition of difference sight words using CAI versus traditional teaching (Baumgart & Van Wallingham, 1987).

The new developments in CAI are exciting in education. Schools are now using videodisks, compact disks, and other software that includes interaction with audio and video. In some cases, teachers can program questions or directions into the video to create an interactive activity that is customized for their students and their curriculum (Brosnan, 1995). Brosnan also gives some good examples of the types of "hypermedia" software that could make a significant difference in the classroom. She defines these as an "important breakthrough in making computers more compatible with human thinking." Hypermedia provides access to text, graphics, images, and sound on CD-ROM. Improved graphics, animation, sound, and real-time video can make subjects of study "come alive." Some of the current simulations such as frog dissections, continental drift, and chemical experiments can be used to conduct simple "virtual" experiences. The newest development has been the virtual reality software, where the visuals are a 3-D experience and often allow the user to interact with the virtual reality and creates the illusion of being there or doing the action. Examples include traveling along the Oregon Trail, flying a plane, and constructing a building. Although there is little research on the use of this simulation software with individuals with disabilities, the prospects are good for eventually creating virtual environments that can be modified to an individual's needs, response rate, and mode of communication.

There are some concerns with CAI. One concern is that teachers and practitioners who work with students with mental retardation are not being adequately trained to select appropriate CAI, use CAI effectively, or modify available programs for their student's individual needs (Siegel, Good, & Moore, 1996). Although it is unlikely that CAI will ever replace teachers, it is a concern that educators may automatize more and more of the educational and students will socialize with peers less and less. With the current isolation problems of individuals with mental retardation, it is a caution to practitioners that in their enthusiasm for embracing exciting instructional opportunities for students with disabilities, they do not segregate them into computer labs.

Access to CAI is also not equitable. Again, in many areas of the world this technology is not available, affordable, or in a language understandable to their population. The curricular designs and cultural compatibility of CAI has been determined by the publishers of the software, who more often design for market performance rather than educational purposes.

Finally, there is sometimes an incompatibility between computer-managed instruction (CMI) and computer-assisted instruction (CAI). One of the most positive qualities of original computer instruction was the ability to program the instruction toward individual progress as determined by continuous assessment. In recent years, the trend was to separate the assessment component and the instructional component of the educational computer use. It was proposed that the CAI should incorporate CMI and that technology-based assessment be integrated into CAI (Hanley, 1994).

TECHNOLOGY-BASED ASSESSMENT

Computer and other technology-based assessment is a current phenomena in education that has also impacted the assessment of students with mental retardation. There are several advantages to the use of computers with assessment. These advantages are: (a) the test administration is consistent, (b) there are improvements to standardization, (c) there is less possibility of examiner bias, (d) the keyboard can be made compatible to the individual, (e) there is quick scoring and feedback, and (f) results may be integrated into CAI (Sampson, 1995). One exciting use of technology in assessment has been the adaptation of technology for authentic assessments. Examples of authentic or performance assessments include computer simulations, multimedia or oral presentations, and videotaped performances (Bennett & Hawkins, 1992). There are some drawbacks to computer assessments. As with human examiners, there is always the possibilities of errors in scoring. But there is less likelihood of these errors being suspected or caught when due to programming errors. Also, the rich data acquired from observation by a test examiner is lost in a computerized testing situation and may compromise test interpretations. Finally, there is a possibility of some individuals being incompatible with computers, which may lead to invalid testing results (Sampson, 1995).

With individuals with disabilities, the technology-based assessments have been found to assist in many areas of special education assessment. In a special topics issue of *Exceptional Children*, Greenwood (1994) reviewed several studies that demonstrated exciting practices being done with technology-based special education assessments. There are assessments available that can be changed to the appropriate language with a click of a button, or video clips that can be reacted to by students in a real life problem-solving test. Also, test items can be selected based on whether or not a student was successful with previous items, and CAI can be administered even during the testing situation. Social skills can be modeled and reacted to by computer simulations, and data can be recorded in portable computers and analyzed quickly for decision making purposes (Greenwood, 1995). It is hoped that eventually general education assessments and special education assessment will be integrated, and include the use of technology based assessment with CAI (Hanley, 1995).

ON-LINE RESOURCES FOR MENTAL RETARDATION

On-line resources include the Internet, electronic mail, and discussion formats including listservs, newsgroups, and bulletin boards. The Internet is an computer access channel to a myriad of information posted by companies, organizations, and individuals. The advantage to the Internet is that information can be disseminated quickly, widely, and inexpensively. The disadvantage of this is that although on-line information is more current, it may not be as carefully edited and may have inaccuracies or misleading and confusing information (Giordano et al., 1996). Electronic mail and discussion formats have allowed any person with access to an on-line computer to get an account so that they can send and receive electronic mail, which is free of charge, easy to learn, and almost instantaneous. In addition, it allows access to individuals often considered difficult to reach. On-line discussions allow strangers from any where in the world to exchange ideas and information on their own time at a computer. Chat lines allow real-time discussion either in text or voice or even video, where individuals from different locations can discuss topics of mutual interest.

At the time of this publication, there were over 300,000 websites devoted to issues concerning individuals with mental retardation on the Internet. Additionally, there were hundred of on-line discussion groups available. On-line resources are continually expanding and adapting, so any comprehensive list of these is obsolete in a short period of time. Fortunately, major sites that are used frequently attempt to keep the same addresses so that they can be easily accessed. The following websites are considered useful sites that will enable anyone interested in mental retardation to obtain quick information and access to resources. They have been organized as basic information, organizations, electronic journals, and on-line discussions. There are also a multitude of related sites that are not included that can be accessed through these sites. Some of the related issues that had many locations were Down syndrome, autism, Assistive Technology, Facilitated Communication, Accessibility Support, ADA, and inclusion.

Basic Information

The following sites have excellent general information about mental retardation and they also include many links to disability related sites. Although there may be many other sources for information, many of the best links can be found through these websites.

Family Village

http://www.familyvillage.wisc.edu/
The Family Village website is an attempt to bring together valuable information for parents of individuals who have disabilities. This is an excellent, graphics-rich site that is well-organized and quite thorough. Please look under cognitive disability/mental retardation, but also Down syndrome, Fragile X syndrome, and Williams syndrome. This well-produced site is provided by the Waisman Center located at the University of Wisconsin-Madison.

Intellectual Disability Network

http://www.monash.edu.au/informatics/idcn.html
This fairly comprehensive resources site has information organized into the following categories: General Information on the Intellectual Disability Information Services, Medical Issues, Family, Development and Other Life Issues, Behavioral Issues, Legal and Ethical Issues, Accommodation, Employment of the Intellectually Disabled, Education and Educational services, Professional Development of Workers in the Field of Intellectual Disability, Sociocultural Issues in Intellectual Disability, Communication, Advocacy Issues, Computers and Disability, Leisure/Recreation, Funding for Research into Issues concerning the Intellectually Disabled, Other Issues Pertaining to Intellectual Disability, and Bulletin/Notice Boards.

Office of Special Education

http://teach.virginia.edu/go/cise/ose/categories/mr.html

This site has some good general information about mental retardation and has links organized as follows: Organizations, General Resources, Down Syndrome, Special Olympics, and Mental Retardation Centers and Departments.

Waisman Center's List of Web Sites
Related to Cognitive and Developmental Disabilities

http://waisman.wisc.edu/www/Mrsites.html
This list of links was quite comprehensive for websites related to mental retardation and related issues.

Organizations

The following organizations have well-constructed websites that provide resources and information for individuals with mental retardation, their families, and professionals who work with these individuals.

AAMR

http://www.aamr.org/#Services
Since 1876, AAMR has been providing leadership in the field of mental retardation. AAMR is the oldest and largest interdisciplinary organization of professionals and others concerned about mental retardation and related disabilities. Over 9,500 members in the U.S. and 55 other countries have chosen AAMR and their association. AAMR's mission is to advance the knowledge and skills of professionals in the field of mental retardation by exchanging information and ideas. This website has information about membership, periodicals, publications, conventions, training institutes, career opportunities, grants and fellowships, AAMR policies and positions, and a good list of links to other disability related websites.

The Arc

http://TheArc.org/welcome.html
With more than 1,100 affiliated chapters and 140,000 members across the United States, The Arc (formerly Association for Retarded Citizens of the United States) is the country's largest voluntary organization committed to the welfare of all children and adults with mental retardation and their families. The Arc, with its rich history in advocacy and services, is comprised of individuals with mental retardation, family members, professionals in the field of disability, and other concerned citizens. The Arc is a nonprofit organization that provides resources for mentally retarded persons and their families as well as conducting research and providing legislative advocacy. On their website, users will find information about the Arc and its services and resources. Each Arc department provides publications and resources from their work, such as government reports, pamphlets discussing topics such as Aging with Mental Retardation and Family Support, and information about the Arc's newspaper. A fact sheet about

disability information on the World Wide Web is also provided, as well as links to other disability web sites.

Disabled Peoples International

http://wpg-01.escape.ca/~dpi/frame.html

The purpose of DPI is to promote the Human Rights of People with Disabilities through full participation, equalization of opportunity, and development. DPI is a grassroots, cross-disability network with member organizations in over 110 countries, over half of which are in the developing world. DPI is administrated through their headquarters in Winnipeg, Canada and through eight Regional Development Offices. DPI has consultative status with the ECOSOC, UNESCO, WHO, and the ILO, and has official observer status at the United Nations General Assembly. The main functions of DPI are development, human rights, communications, advocacy, and public education. This website includes information on DPI publications, links to other disability-related sites, and international conference listings.

Electronic Journals

The following are samples of quality electronic journals that can be accessed online. As with all print media, one must check out publishing requirements before judging the quality of the information provided.

Disability International Online

http://www.escape.ca/~di/frameset.html

Disability International is published quarterly by Disabled Peoples' International, a cross-disability coalition of organizations of disabled people, consisting of over 120 national affiliates. The philosophy of DPI is that disabled persons are citizens with equal rights, and hence should achieve full participation and equality with their fellow citizens in all societies.

AAMR Periodicals

http://www.access.digex.net/~aamr/PerToc.htm

AAMR produces three periodicals, of which portions can be accessed on-line for no charge:

The American Journal on Mental Retardation (AJMR) is a leader in reporting original, quality research in biological, behavioral, and educational sciences for researchers, clinicians, and students in mental retardation and related disabilities.

Mental Retardation (MR) is a peer-reviewed multidisciplinary journal that provides information on the leading-edge policies, practices, and perspectives in mental retardation..

News and Notes is AAMR's bimonthly newsletter. Read updates on congressional activities, court decisions, innovative service models, research trends, special interest groups, conferences, expert opinions, and new resources.

On-Line Discussions

There are hundreds of listservs, newsgroups, bulletin boards, and chats available where individuals can ask questions, have discussions and interact with other individuals interested in the same topics. Rather than listing particular sites, the following are links to lists of available on-line discussion formats.

Listservs

These sites had lists of disability-related list serves (listservs), many related to mental retardation.
List of Lists: http://www.nas.com/downsyn/listserv.html
Family Village: http://www.familyvillage.wisc.edu/lists/longlist.htm

Newsgroups

These sites had lists of disability-related newsgroups, several devoted to mental retardation issues.
WNY Disability Forum: http://freenet.buffalo.edu/~wnydf/public/news.html
ADA Information Center Online: Newsgroups Page:
http://www.idir.net/%7Eadabbs/newsg.html

Bulletin Boards and Chats

These sites had lists of disability-related bulletin boards and chats, several devoted to mental retardation issues.
International Disability Network:
http://www.monash.edu.au/informatics/idcn.html#bulletin.notice
Family Village (Coffeeshop): http://www.familyvillage.wisc.edu/coffee.htm

FUTURE TECHNOLOGIES

Video Telephones

Video telephones have not become widespread in even developed countries at this time, but current computer video transfer (i.e., cuseeme) is becoming less expensive and more commonplace. Plus, the imaging technology is improving, so it is likely that video telephones will become a viable telecommunications tool in the next decade.

Brodin and her colleagues in Sweden (Brodin, Fahlin, & Nilsson, 1993; Brodin & Bjork-Akesson, 1995; Brodin & Thurfjell, 1995) have conducted several studies examining the use of video phones with individuals with mental retardation. They found that communication abilities may even increase with the use of a video phone and they predict this may lead to increased social integration of individuals with mental retardation. In one study (Brodin & Bjork-Akesson, 1995), they even state that video phones "may be a necessary support mechanism to support individuals with mental retardation access to telecommunications."

There are some drawbacks to the use of video phones. In another study, Brodin et al. (1993) reported that staff members were not sure how high a priority they should place on video phones, since it was a time-consuming task and the video image was quite poor. Although the technology has improved since these studies were conducted, video images still may be found with a variety of resolutions. The higher resolution images are still costly. Other countries have also researched the use of video phones, most often with the hearing impaired. In Portugal, a school was successful in teaching children with mental retardation how to use video phones. Research has also been conducted in Japan and Norway (Brodin & Maginussen, 1992 & 1993).

Future Trends

As society is in the midst of a technological revolution, the schools and workplaces are changing rapidly in developing countries. On-line resources are becoming more commonplace and computers exist in almost every classroom. Distance education is common at postsecondary schools and becoming used as an instructional delivery device in rural areas. It will be possible to receive instruction anywhere in the world, by any person, in any discipline, on a variety of levels, in different languages. Telecommunications now allows instant transmission of audio, video, documents, and computer images. Eventually this will be available everywhere through satellites, where even remote regions of the earth can be reached. "Increased access to resource centers all over the world can broaden students' appreciation of different cultures" (Brosnan, 1995). The simulations available now on CD-ROMs are already starting to exist on the Internet, where people can interact in a virtual world from computers located all over the world. Until the time that this technology is readily available everywhere, the gap between the technological influences on developed countries and nondeveloped ones will increase.

Although it may seem impossible to keep up with these continually changes, technology is getting easier to access, less expensive, and equipment is getting more standardized with easier upgrading abilities. So although one's technology might go obsolete, equipment can grow through several computer generations. Cost will always be a factor in discriminating who will have access to new technologies.

This is an exciting time for computers in education and the possibilities for individuals with mental retardation are only limited by the imagination. Technology will continue to grow and the opportunities for individuals with disabilities to be assisted by these advancements are endless.

Currently the technology is growing faster than the amount of research conducted to assess its affects. According to Roblyer:

Findings indicate that computer applications have an important role to play in the future of education, but the exact nature of that role has only begun to be explored. Opportunities for using technology to make an impact on education have never been greater, and neither have opportunities for research. The next decade must be a time for taking full advantage of both. (Roblyer, 1989)

This statement was accurate in 1989, and will continue to be true through the next decade as well. It is the hope of the practitioners and researchers that these advancements are made with an understanding that individuals with mental retardation should be further integrated into society.

REFERENCES

The Arc. (1993). *Assistive technology for people with mental retardation. The Arc Q & A.* Arlington, TX: Arc. (ERIC Document Reproduction Service No. ED 376 662)

The Arc. (1994). *How to evaluate and select assistive technology.* Arlington, TX: Arc. (ERIC Document Reproduction Service No. ED 376 664)

Baltussen, M. W., & Van Lieshout, E. C. (1991). Een foutencategorieen-systeem en zijn toepassing in een computer-gestuurde remediele rekentraining. [An error-classification system and its application in a computer-assisted remedial arithmetic training program]. *Tijdschrift voor Onderwijsresearch, 16*(5), 279–296.

Baumgart, D., & Van Walleghem, J. (1987). Teaching sight words : A comparison between computer-assisted and teacher-taught methods. *Education and Training in Mental Retardation, 22*(1), 56–65.

Bennett, D., & Hawkins, J. (1992). *News From the Center for Children and Technology and the Center for Technology in Education,* 1, (3).

Bigge, J. L. (1991). *Teaching individuals with physical and multiple disabilities* (3rd ed.). New York: Macmillan.

Bilkin, D. (1992). Typing to talk: Facilitated communication. *American Journal of Speech and Language Pathology, 1*(2), 15–17.

Bitter, G. G. (1993). *Using a microcomputer in the classroom* (3rd ed.). Needham Heights, MA: Allyn & Bacon.

Brodin, J., Fahlen, M., & Nilsson, S. H. (1993). *A limited study of the use of videotelephoney for people with moderate mental retardation* (Technology, Communication and Disability, Report No. 7). Stockholm, Sweden: University of Stockholm. (ERIC Document Reproduction Service No. ED 358 605)

Brodin, J., & Bjork-Akesson, E. (1995). Still picture telephone used by persons with profound mental retardation: A pilot study. *European Journal of Special Needs Education, 10*(1), 31–39.

Brodin, J., & Maginussen, M. (1992). *Videotelephones and mental retardation survey of results achieved and research in progress* (Report No. 92-1). Stockholm, Sweden: University of Stockholm. (ERIC Document Reproduction Service No. ED 348 777)

Brodin, J., & Thurfjell, F. (1995). Bedcomning Av Kommunikativ Formaga Hos Personer Med Utvecklingsstorning Teknik, Kommunikation, Handikapp Forskningsrapport nr 12 [Assessment of the Communicative Ability in Persons with Mental Retardation]. (Technology, Communication, Disability Research Report No. 12). TeleCommunity, RACE 2033 (Research in Advanced Communication Technologies in Europe).

Brosnan, P. A. (1995). *Learning about tasks computers can perform.* Columbus, OH: ERIC Clearinghouse for Science, Mathematics, and Environmental Education. (ERIC Document Reproduction Service No. ED 380 280)

Brown, C. C., & Cavalier, A. R. (1992). Voice recognition technology and persons with severe mental retardation and severe physical impairment: Learning, response differentiation and affect. *Journal of Special Education Technology, 11*(4), 196–206.

Brown, C., Sauer, M., Cavalier, A., Frische, E., & Wyatt, C. (1991). *The assistive dining device: A tool for mealtime independence.* Paper presented at the 14th annual conference of RESNA, Kansas City, MO.

Bull, G. L., Cochran, P. S., & Snell, M. E. (1988). Beyond CAI: Computers, language and persons with mental retardation. *Topics in Language Disorders, 84*(4), 55–76.

Burg, K. (1984). The microcomputer in the kindergarten: A magical, useful, expensive toy. *Young Children, 39*(3), 28–33.

Chen, S. H. A., & Bernard-Opitz, V. (1993). Comparison of personal and computer assisted instruction for children with autism. *Mental Retardation, 31*(6), 368–76.

Church, G., & Bender, M. (1989). *Teaching with computers: A curriculum for special educators.* Boston: College Hill.

Cochran, P. S., & Bull, G. L. (1993). Computers and individuals with speech and language disorders. In J. D. Lindsey (Ed.) *Computers and exceptional individuals.* (2nd ed., pp. 143–158). Austin, TX: PRO-ED.

Colman, M. C., Simpson, R., & Myles, B. (1996). Facilitated communication: Does it work? In M. C. Coleman (Ed.), *Emotional and behavioral disorders: Theory and practice* (3rd ed., pp. 294–295). Needham Heights, MA: Allyn & Bacon.

Copel, H. (1991). *Tech use guide: Students with moderate cognitive abilities* (Technical Report). Reston, VA: Center for Special Education Technology.

Crossley, R., & Remington-Guerney, J. (1992). Getting the words out: Facilitated communication training. *Topics in Language Disorders, 12*(4), 29–45.

Dube, W. V., McDonald, S. J., & McIlvene, W. J. (1991). Constructed-Response matching to sample and spelling instruction. *Journal of Applied Behavior Analysis, 24*(2), 305–317.

Dube, W. V., Iennaco, F. M., Rocco, F. J., & Klendaras, J. B. (1992). Microcomputer-based programmed instruction in identity matching to sample for persons with severe disability. *Journal of Behavioral Education, 2*(1), 29–51.

Giordano, G., Leeper, L., & Siegel, J. (1996). Computer assisted literacy programs. In G. Giordano (Ed.), *Literacy: Programs for adults with developmental disabilities.* San Diego: Singular Publishing.

Greenwood, C. (1994). Advances in technology-based assessment with special education. *Exceptional Children, 61*(2), 102–104.

Hanley, T. V. (1994). The need for technological advances in assessment related to national education reform. *Exceptional Children, 61*(3), 222–229.

Holzberg, C. S. (1994). Technology in special education. *Technology and Learning, 14*(7), 18–21.

Iacono, T. A., & Miller, J. F. (1989). Can microcomputers be used to teach communication skills to students with mental retardation? *Education and Training in Mental Retardation, 24*(1), 32–44.

Jaspers, M. W., & Van Lieshout, E. C. (1989). Een trainingsprogramma voor kinderen met leerproblemen gericht op het aanleren van concrete representaties voor redactieopgaven [A computer-assisted instruction program for children with learning problems aimed at the acquisition of external representations of arithmetic word problems]. *Pedagogische Studien, 66*(6), 240–255.

Kerka, S. (1994). *Life and work in a technological society* (ERIC Digest No. 147). (ERIC Document Reproduction Service No. ED 368 892)

Koenigsfeld, A. S., Beukelman, D. R., & Stoefen-Fisher, J. M. (1993). Attitudes of severely hearing impaired persons toward augmentative communication. *Volta Review, 95*(2), 109–124.

Koppenhaver, D. A., Pierce, P. L., & Yoder, D. E. (1995). AAC, FC, and the ABC's: Issues and Relationships. *American Journal of Speech Language Pathology, 4*(4), 5–14.

Leong, C. K. (1992). A framework for ameliorating reading disorders in children. *Developmental Disabilities Bulletin, 20*(1), 81–97.

Leung, J. P. (1994a). Teaching simple addition to children with mental retardation using a microcomputer. *Journal of Behavioral Education, 4*(3), 355–367.

Leung, J. P. (1994b). Improving simple addition efficiency in Chinese children with mental retardation. *Psychologia: An International Journal of Psychology in the Orient, 37*(1), 39–48.

Margalit, M. (1991). Promoting classroom adjustment and social skills for students with mental retardation within an experimental and control group design. *Exceptionality, 2*(4), 195–204.

Margalit, M., & Roth, Y. B. (1989). Strategic keyboard training and spelling improvement among children with learning disabilities and mental retardation. *Educational Psychology, 9*(4), 321–329.

Molcho, M. (1989). The effects of traditional instruction and game strategies on teaching selected typing skills to junior high school students with moderate to severe handicaps through computer-assisted instruction (CAI). *Dissertation Abstracts International, 50*(2-A), 347–348.

Morgan, R. L., Ames, H. N., & Taylor, M. J. (1995). Training for supported employment specialists and their supervisors: Identifying important training topics. *Education and Training in Mental Retardation and Developmental Disabilities, 30*(4), 229–307.

Osguthorpe, R. T., & Chang, L. I. (1988). The effects of computerized symbol processor instruction on the communication skills of non speaking students. *AAC: Augmentative & Alternative Communication, 4*(1), 23–24

Parette, H. P. (1991). The importance of technology in the education and training of persons with mental retardation. *Education and Training in Mental Retardation, 26*(2), 165–178.

Parette, H. P. (1994). *Augmentative and alternative communication (AAC) assessment and prescriptive practices for persons with mental retardation and developmental disabilities: Current practices and future issues.* Paper presented at the 4th Annual International Conference on Mental Retardation, Chicago, IL.

Parette, H. P. (1996, April). *Augmentative and alternative communication decision making strategies for IEP teams.* Paper presented at 74th Annual International Convention of the Council for Exceptional Children, Orlando, Florida.

Plienis, A. J. (1987). Sources and methods of instruction with atypical children: An investigation of stimulus fading and computer delivered instruction. *Dissertation Abstracts International, 47*(8-B), 3539.

Plienis, A. J., & Romanczyk, R. G. (1985). Analyses of performance, behavior, and predictors for severely disturbed children: A comparison of adult vs. computer instruction. *Analysis & Intervention in Developmental Disabilities, 5*(4), 345–356.

Podell, D. M., Tournaki-Rein, N., & Lin, A. (1992). Automatization of mathematics skills via computer-assisted instruction among students with mild mental handicaps. *Education and Training in Mental Retardation, 27*(3), 200–206.

Postman, N. (1992). *Technopoly: The surrender of culture to technology.* New York: Knopf.

Roblyer, M. D. (1989). *The impact of microcomputer-based instruction on teaching and learning: A review of recent research.* Syracuse, NY: ERIC Clearinghouse on Information Resources. (ERIC Document Reproduction Service No. ED 315 063)

Saka, T. T. (1985). Computer work skills training for persons with developmental disabilities. *Computers in Human Services, 1*(4) 39–51.

Sampson, J. P. (1995). *Computer-assisted testing in counseling and therapy.* Greensboro, NC: ERIC Clearinghouse on Counseling and Student Services. (ERIC Document Reproduction Service No. ED 391 983)

Schlosser, R.W., Belfiore, P. J., & Hetzroni, O. (1995). The effects of speech output technology in the learning of graphic symbols. *Journal of Applied Behavioral Analysis, 28*(4), 537–549

Selby, C. C. (1993).Technology: From myths to realities. *Phi Delta Kappan, 74*(9), 684–689.

Siegel, J., Good , K., & Moore, J. (1996). Integrating technology into Educating Pre-service Education Teachers. *Action in Teacher Education, 17*(4) 53–63.

Snyder, T. L. (1994). The effects of augmentative communication on vocabulary acquisition with primary age students with disabilities. *British Columbia Journal of Special Education, 18*(1), 14–23.

Soto, G., Belfiore, R. J., & Schlosser, R. W. (1993). Teaching specific requests: A comparative analysis of skill acquisition and preference using two augmented and alternative communication aids. *Education and Training in Mental Retardation, 8*(2), 169–178.

Spitzer, D. R. (1990). Computers and music therapy: An integrated approach: Four case studies. *Music Therapy Perspectives, 7,* 51–54.

Stromer, R., Mackay, H. R., & Flusser, D. (1996). Teaching computer-based spelling to individuals with developmental and hearing disabilities: Transfer of stimulus control to writing tasks. *Journal of Applied Behavioral Analysis, 29*(1), 25–42.

Venkatagiri, H. S. (1995). Techniques for enhancing communication productivity in AAC : A review of research. *American Journal of Speech Language Pathology, 4*(4), 36–45.

Woodward, J., & Gersten, R. (1992). Innovative technology for secondary students with learning disabilities. *Exceptional Children, 59,* 407–421.

CHAPTER 15

Sociocultural Factors Influencing Social and Vocational Inclusion of Persons With Mental Retardation: A Cross-Cultural Study

ROBERT L. SCHALOCK
CHRISTOPHER KELLY
Hastings College

People live in a number of systems that influence the development of their values, beliefs, behavior, and attitudes (Bernal, Bonilla, & Bellido, 1995; Bronfenbrenner, 1979; Hogg, 1996; Jahoda, 1992; Lonner & Malpass, 1994). According to Bronfenbrenner, for example, the systems that support human development and behavior can be seen as occurring at four levels, each nested within the next. The microsystem is the immediate social settings—such as family, the peer group, and the workplace—that directly affect a person's life. The mesosystem includes the links that connect one microsystem to another. Examples include job coaches, case managers, and natural support personnel. The exosystem includes neighborhood and community structures such as newspapers, television and public agencies that affect directly the functioning of smaller systems. Finally, the macrosystem includes the overarching patterns of culture, social-political trends, and economic systems. This overarching pattern of culture directly affects our values and assumptions, the meanings of words and concepts, and the potential universality of concepts.

Many countries are currently experiencing the realization that persons with disabilities can become productive members of society and live successfully within community-based residences (Hernes, 1991; Keith, 1996; Kiernan, Schalock, Butterworth, & Sailor, 1993; Konig & Schalock, 1991; Schalock, 1996; Tse, 1991). Past policies of segregation, isolation, and protective approaches to providing services for persons with disabilities are giving way to concepts of inclusion, integration, and heightened expectation. Past practices of viewing persons with disabilities from a categorical perspective are moving toward an emphasis on the unique abilities, needs, and interests of the individual. General economic and technology changes throughout the world have given rise to new employment and community living opportunities for persons previously denied these opportunities.

The purpose of this chapter is to discuss the influence that a number of socioeconomic factors have on the inclusion into community living and integrated employment of persons with disabilities. The chapter is divided into four major sections. The first two discuss the impact that values and contextual variables play in one's beliefs, behavior, and attitudes. The third section outlines briefly four cross-cultural research guidelines. The final section summarizes the results of a cross-cultural study just completed, which determined the influence that 10 values and 10 contextual variables have on the development of integrated employment and community living programs for persons with mental retardation and closely related conditions in seven countries. Throughout the chapter the reader will encounter a number of terms:

- Culture: a construct involving shared values, beliefs, behaviors, and attitudes (Matsumoto, 1994).
- Cross-cultural: frames of reference and comparison (Lynch & Hanson, 1992).
- Values: a conception held by an individual, or collectively by members of a group, of that which is desirable and which influences the selection of both means and ends of action from among available alternatives (Kluckhohn, 1951).
- Contextual variables: external factors that influence the development of human services programs (Schalock, 1995).
- Emics: principles that are culture-bound (Berry, 1969).
- Etics: universal principles (Berry, 1969).

THE IMPACT OF VALUES

Different value orientations and value emphases in various cultures account for both philosophical and psychological dimensions, including beliefs, values, assumptions, attitudes and behavior. For example, Honigmann (1967), in his book *Personality in Culture,* discusses the following six value orientations affected by one's culture: (1) human-supernature orientation, which involves value judgments about humans and the metaphysical environment including one's religious orientation and use of myths and symbols; (2) human-nature orientation, which involves concerns about one's environment and one's effect on it; (3) human-habitat orientation, which includes value judgments about how to design and create living/work environments such as parks and controlled developments; (4) human-relational orientation, which involves value judgments about how to conduct relationships between and among people; (5) human-activity orientation, which includes value judgments about the individual and group endeavors such as work and the need to keep busy; and (6) human-time orientation, which includes value judgments about how to use time, and whether one's time is oriented to the past or to the future. Similarly, Kluckhohn (1951; Kluckhohn & Srodtbeck, 1961) and others (Berry, Poortinga, Segall & Dasen, 1992; Ibrahim, 1993; Rokeach, 1973; Schwartz & Bilsky, 1990; Triandis, 1990, 1994) have proposed additional universal values (that is, etics) related to a general organized conception of human nature (referred to as "man-nature orientation"), social relationships ("relational orientation"), nature of man, time orientation, activity orientation, terminal values (equality, freedom, happiness, salvation, self-respect), and instrumental values (courageous, honest, polite, and responsible).

One of the primary purposes of the cross-cultural study described later in the chapter was to evaluate across seven countries the influence that values and value orientations have on the development of integrated employment and community living programs. Ten values were selected for inclusion in the study, based on the above-referenced work, plus that of Daniels & Hogg (1991); Feather (1994); Ibrahim (1993; 1995); Jordan (1993); Keith, Heal, & Schalock (1996); Keith, Yamamoto, Okita, & Schalock (1995); Leelakulthanit & Day (1993); Kuyken, Orley, Huelson, & Sartorius (1994); Schalock, Bartnik, Wu, Konig, Lee, & Reiter (1990); Skevington (1994); and Triandis, Bontempo, Villareal, Asai, & Lucca (1988). The 10 values that were hypothesized to have an effect on integrated employment and living programs are summarized in Table 15.1.

THE IMPACT OF CONTEXTUAL VARIABLES

The concept of community inclusion for persons with disabilities exists in an environment that is increasingly international (Fowers & Richardson, 1996; Mays, Rubin, Sabourin, & Walker, 1996; Rogoff & Chavajay, 1995). This global orientation necessitates increased cultural exchanges and greater cross-cultural research and understanding (Brislin, 1993). In the previous section, the potential role that values play on such inclusion was discussed. This section discusses the role that contextual variables may well play. As we approach a discussion of 10 contextual variables that are hypothesized to have an impact on the development of integrated employment and community living programs, one should keep four points clearly in mind (Hughes, Seidman, & Williams, 1993): First, all individuals develop in a cultural context; second, many aspects of culture are abstract in that they are not overtly or internally socialized; third, culture is evidenced in patterns and social regularities among members of a population within the larger ecological context; and fourth, the research process is influenced by the

TABLE 15.1
Values Potentially Influencing Integrated Employment
and Community Living Programs

Value	Descriptors
1. Relation with nature	Mastery over versus harmony with, change versus accepts
2. Time orientation	Future versus past or present, inflexible versus flexible, negotiable versus settled/permanent
3. Interpersonal relations	Competition versus cooperation, aggressiveness versus submission, respect for youth versus respect for elders, challenge authority versus conformity, nuclear family versus extended family, role flexibility versus role rigidity
4. Self	Individuality versus anonymity, assertive versus group, extroverted versus introverted, independence versus interdependence, being direct versus saving face, action oriented versus stoicism or patience, doing versus being
5. Use of wealth	Saving versus sharing, public versus private
6. Thinking style	Mind oriented versus heart oriented, analytical versus contemplative
7. Support systems	Formal (agencies or services) versus informal (family or friends)
8. Conception of disability	Normal versus abnormal, attractive versus ugly, sick versus well, educable versus non-educable
9. Locus of control	Source of control is within oneself versus external sources
10. Locus of responsibility	Source of responsibility is oneself (for example, "rugged individualism") versus others (for example, "social welfare mentality")

meanings and interpretations respondents attach to the research setting, constructs, and instruments.

Movements such as the inclusion of persons with mental retardation and closely related disabilities into the mainstream of society occur within a social and cultural context that varies widely from place to place (Schalock, 1996) Therefore, it was of interest to the present authors to identify cross-culturally some of the more important contextual variables influencing the development of integrated employment and community living programs for persons with disabilities. In this regard, the authors were influenced by the earlier work of Gaylord-Ross, who used a qualitative research approach to determine the influence of contextual variables in which one "attempts to understand the emerging program models in terms of an adaptive system whereby values, economic needs, and socialization patterns interact to form particular cultural artifacts" (1987, p. 533).

Some cross-cultural work regarding the impact of contextual variables has already been done. For example, Gaylord-Ross (1987) identified five contextual variables that influenced the development of integrated employment in Europe: political will (as reflected in public policy), charismatic leaders, model demonstration programs, instructional technology, and the economic state of the country. Similarly, Hernes (1991) found a number of contextual variables that impacted successful employment programs internationally: focus on integrated employment, outcomes related to environmental variables rather than client characteristics, habilitation processes that stress obtaining and maintaining a job, shifting from financial to other forms of support, establishing an individualized and flexible approach, emphasis on coordination and collaboration, personal follow-up and evaluation of outcomes, focus on psychosocial aspects of the workplace, responding to changes in job markets, and focusing on the person's strengths and possibilities.

Additionally, the senior author has compared measured quality of life scores across a number of different living and employment environments in five countries (Australia, Germany, Israel, the Republic of China (Taiwan), and the United States). The study (Schalock et al., 1990) involved administering the Quality of Life Questionnaire (Schalock & Keith, 1993) to a group of 92 individuals with mental retardation in the four countries and comparing their measured scores to the standardization sample of 552 persons with mental retardation in the United States. The average age of the sample was 32.6 years, with 46.9% female and 53.1% male. Their living status at the time of the study (across samples) was independent (19.9%), semi-independent (38%), or supervised (42.8%). Their employment status was competitive or supported (29.5%), sheltered (61.6%), or unemployed (8.9%). The major analysis involved summarizing quality of life scores across different living and work environments, collapsing across countries (hence, looking for etic properties). There was a clear trend across the five countries: quality of life scores increased as one lives and works in more normalized environments.

Table 15.2 summarizes the 10 contextual variables that were hypothesized in the present study to influence the development of integrated employment and community living programs. The variables were selected based on the above-referenced studies, plus the work of Bronfenbrenner (1979), Cole (1988), Lonner & Berry (1986), Rogoff & Chavajay (1995), and Schalock (1995).

RESEARCH GUIDELINES

The cross-cultural study to evaluate the influence of sociocultural factors on integrated employment and community living described in the following section was completed within the context of the following four cross-cultural research guidelines (Schalock, 1996): know the purpose of the study, demonstrate conceptual and linguistic equivalence, use well formulated research designs, and involve diverse people.

Know the Purpose of the Study

The primary purpose of the cross-cultural study was to gain a better understanding of the influence that 10 values and 10 contextual variables have on inte-

TABLE 15.2

Contextual Variables Potentially Influencing Integrated Employment
and Community Living Programs

Contextual Variable	Descriptors
1. Public policies	Laws or regulations related to integration, main-streaming, normalization, deinstitutionalization, quota systems, affirmative action
2. Funding tied to public policies	Consistency between the policy and the actual money spent on policy-targeted services
3. Economic status of the country	Gross national product, employment/unemployment rates, tax rates, housing expenses, population density
4. Coalitions	Business, unions, politicians, families, self-advocates, professionals
5. Technology	Systematic instruction, adaptive devices, applied behavior analysis, task analysis
6. Academic/professional Supports	Medical and rehabilitation personnel, teachers, psychologists, social workers
7. Teaching/rehabilitation staff	Direct service workers, job coaches, care providers
8. Research and development	Model programs, program evaluation, association with universities and colleges
9. Political movements	Trade unions, charismatic leaders, social welfare campaigns, leadership
10. Attitudes toward persons with disability	Normalcy, potential, person-centered, capable, risk-taking, labels, status, historical attitudes

grated employment and community living programs for persons with mental retardation and closely related disabilities. The primary focus of the study was on
etic (that is, universal) principles that might explain the development of these
programs. According to Berry (1969), characteristics of an etic approach include:
studying from a position outside the system, examining many cultures, using
structures created by the analyst, and developing criteria that are considered absolute or universal.

Our primary intent was to identify a minimum set of universal factors that
clarify the process. Only secondarily did we compare geographical regions. We
felt that this rationale was justifiable given the general consensus across cultures
that we have reported earlier for both quality of life concepts (Keith et al., 1996)
and quality of life scores (Schalock et al., 1990).

Demonstrate Conceptual and Linguistic Equivalence

The most basic question in cross-cultural research is whether the concepts under
study have both conceptual and linguistic equivalence (Hines, 1993). Conceptual

equivalence asks whether the concepts under study have equivalent meaning to the groups being considered; linguistic equivalence asks whether the terms and concepts have been translated accurately (Brislin, 1993). In reference to the latter, back translation provides the opportunity to examine the extent to which concepts "come through" in the translation, and can lend some credence to the assumption that the respective groups are talking about the same thing (Keith, 1996). In the present study, back translation was used.

In addition to conceptual and linguistic equivalence, Lonner (1985, 1990) also discusses functional and metric equivalence. In functional equivalence, the role or function that the behavior plays in different cultures needs to be considered. For example, one may not assume that public policy is the same across all cultures. Metric equivalence asks whether the scale measures the same constructs in different cultures. In addition, even if assured of conceptual, linguistic, functional, and metric equivalence, one needs to be concerned in cross-cultural research about the universality of the indicators used, the relevance of the topics being investigated, the comparability of the measurements used, and the acceptance of the task (Hines, 1993).

Use Well-Formulated Research Designs

Even if the researcher is assured of conceptual and linguistic equivalence, different methods may be required to measure the concept/construct under investigation. Indeed, the current movement towards combining qualitative and quantitative research methods promises to provide significant information corresponding to the underlying thought processes of respondents (Hughes et al., 1993; Schalock, 1995). The use of multiple research methods should also help the research community meet the three commonly accepted criteria for cross-cultural research: replication of factor structure, discrimination among cultures, and correlation with existing criteria (Funkhouser, 1993).

The cross-cultural study described in the next section used a within-subjects design and a quantitative (that is, written survey) approach to data collection. Whereas qualitative research provides an emic (that is, culture-bound) perspective to a group's experience, quantitative methods emphasize empiricism, hypothesis testing, and etic/universal properties (Hughes et al., 1993).

Involve Diverse People

A frequently overlooked research guideline is to involve representatives from the cultural or ethnic group(s) under consideration. In addition to increasing the probability of a successful cross-cultural study, the involvement of persons who have a stake in the study will force one to keep focused on two key cross-cultural research principles (Keith, 1996): Comparative studies that illuminate key characteristics of cultures are likely to contribute to cross-cultural understanding and communication in important ways; and we must recognize and overcome our propensity to project our own norms on people of other cultures. National coordinators were used in the following study to ensure the involvement of persons who were very familiar with the MR/DD service delivery system in their respective country.

INFLUENCE OF VALUES AND CONTEXTUAL VARIABLES: A CROSS-CULTURAL STUDY

Research Questions

The two research questions investigated were:

1. Across the seven respondent countries, are there similarities in the values and contextual variables that influence the development of integrated employment and community living programs?
2. Do countries within geographical regions attribute different importance to some values and contextual variables than others?

General Procedure

Contact was made with colleagues in each of the following seven countries: Canada, England, Japan, the Netherlands, Poland, Republic of China (Taiwan), and the United States. Under their direction, the questionnaire entitled "A Cross-Cultural Study to Evaluate the Influence of Sociocultural Factors on Integrated Employment and Community Living" was translated into the respective language, then back-translated into English to verify meaning (Brislin, 1993; Keith, 1996). Each country coordinator gave the translated questionnaire to a minimum of 10 persons working in the field of mental retardation/developmental disabilities, with the request that they select persons who "had interest, expertise, knowledge, and involvement in the MR/DD service network in their country."

The Questionnaire

The authors developed the questionnaire based on the research on values and contextual variables reviewed previously. The questionnaire, which used a five-point Likert rating scale, was field tested in the United States on 25 professionals in the field of MR/DD. Instructions and definitions (see Tables 15.1 and 15.2) were clarified as necessary based on the field test data. Final instructions and scoring categories included:

• *Instructions.* Think about the factors that have influenced the development of integrated employment and community living programs in your country for persons with mental retardation and closely related conditions. Integrated Employment includes supported and competitive employment; Community Living includes supported (group homes or apartments) or independent living.

- *Scoring Scale:*

5 = Factor has had a significant positive influence on the development of services.

4 = Factor has had a somewhat positive influence on the development of services.

3 = Factor has had neither a positive nor a negative influence on the development of services.

2 = Factor has had a somewhat negative influence on the development of services.

1 = Factor has had a significant negative influence on the development of services.

NA = Not applicable in your country or unfamiliar to you.

Participants

The study included 172 persons working actively in the field of MR/DD (or "intellectual disability" in England). The number of respondents by country were: Canada (21), England (29), Japan (27), the Netherlands (13), Poland (18), the Republic of China (46), and the United States (18). A summary of the major demographic variables (averaging across the 172 respondents) included 50.6% female, 49.4% male; average age, 38.9 years; educational levels included Ph.D./M.D./Ed.D. (26.2%), M.A./M.S.W. (10.8%), B.A./B.S./B.Ed. (51.5%), A.A./Junior College (3.8%), and high school (7.7%); and primary positions (based on job title) included research/training (21.1%), direct service (27.8%), administration (18.0%), advocacy (2.2%), or professional services including psychology, nursing, teaching, or rehabilitation counseling (30.8%). Patterns on these demographic variables across countries were quite similar.

RESULTS

Combined Mean Rating

The first research question (similarities across countries) was addressed by computing mean scores for each of the 10 values and 10 contextual variables, averaging across the seven countries. These "combined" means are presented in Figure 15.1. Three trends are apparent in this data. First, there were definite differences in the importance assigned to the values and contextual variables. Specifically, there were three values and five contextual variables that were rated higher, suggesting their importance across respondent groups in the development of integrated employment and community living programs in these seven countries. The three values were interpersonal relations (item 3), self/person (item 4), and

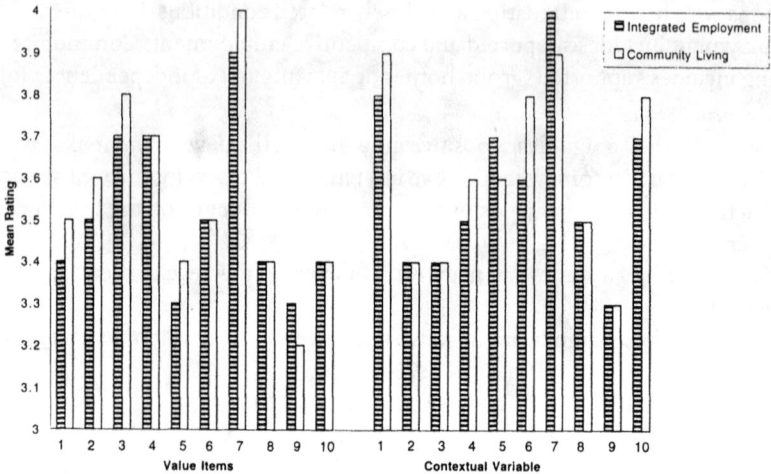

FIG 15.1.   Mean ratings on value items and contextual variables influencing integrated employment and community living programs.

support systems (item 7). The five contextual variables were public policies (item 1), technology (item 4), academic/professional support (item 6), teaching/rehabilitation staff (item 7), and attitudes towards persons with disabilities (item 10). As shown, the highest rated value was support systems, and the highest contextual variable was teaching/rehabilitation (that is, direct support) staff.

The second trend was a high degree of communality among ratings. Specifically, if the factor was rated important for the development of integrated employment, it was also rated high for the development of community living. Similarly, the importance assigned to the values and the contextual variables was not different for integrated employment and community living. Specifically, the total mean for values was 3.5 for integrated employment and 3.6 for community living; for contextual variables, both means were 3.6.

The third trend was that all of the ratings were above 3 (neutral), which makes sense given that the values and contextual variables evaluated have been shown to influence persons' attitudes and behaviors. This result is consistent with a recent study (Keith et al., 1996) evaluating cross-culturally the meaning of key quality of life concepts. In this study, all of the concepts were also rated above neutral on the three semantic dimensions.

Regional Mean Ratings

The second research question (differences among regions) was addressed by comparing mean scores for each of three geographical regions: Asia/Pacific (Japan and the Republic of China), Europe (England, the Netherlands, Poland), and

North America (Canada and the United States). These regional means per item are summarized in Table 15.3. As shown, item means across the three regions are generally similar for both value and contextual variables, with two exceptions. First, North American respondents had lower mean scores on values than the other two regions (3.25 vs. 3.65 for Asia/Pacific and Europe). These lower scores were especially true for values related to use of wealth (item 5), conception of disability (item 8), locus of control (item 9), and locus of responsibility (item 10). And second, North American respondents also had lower mean scores on the contextual variables (3.4 vs. 3.65 for Asia/Pacific and Europe). The lower score was especially true for funding tied to public policies (item 2).

TABLE 15.3

Regional Mean Ratings on Value Items and Contextual Variables Influencing
Integrated Employment (IE) and Community Living (CL) Programs

Factor/Item	Regional Mean Ratings					
	Asia/Pacific		Europe		North America	
Values	IE	CL	IE	CL	IE	CL
1. Relation with nature	3.5	3.6	3.4	3.4	3.3	3.6
2. Time orientation	3.7	3.6	3.6	3.7	3.2	3.6
3. Interpersonal relations	4.1	3.9	3.7	3.9	3.2	3.6
4. Self	3.6	3.5	3.9	4.0	3.7	3.6
5. Use of wealth	3.6	3.7	3.5	3.5	2.8	2.9
6. Thinking style	3.6	3.4	3.5	3.6	3.4	3.4
7. Support systems	4.3	4.2	3.7	4.1	3.6	3.5
8. Conception of disability	3.6	3.5	3.6	3.5	2.8	3.0
9. Locus of control	3.5	3.3	3.3	3.3	2.7	2.8
10. Locus of responsibility	3.6	3.6	3.7	3.6	2.9	2.9
Total mean	3.7	3.6	3.6	3.7	3.2	3.3
Contextual Variables	IE	CL	IE	CL	IE	CL
1. Public policies	3.8	3.8	3.8	3.9	3.7	3.9
2. Funding tied to public policies	3.7	3.7	3.4	3.5	3.0	2.9
3. Economic status of country	3.8	3.8	3.3	3.4	3.2	3.3
4. Coalitions	3.7	3.8	3.5	3.6	3.4	3.3
5. Technology	3.8	3.6	3.6	3.5	3.5	3.5
6. Academic/professional supports	3.8	3.7	3.6	4.1	3.3	3.4
7. Teaching/rehabilitation staff	4.1	3.8	4.0	4.1	3.8	3.8
8. Research and development	3.5	3.4	3.5	3.6	3.5	3.5
9. Political movements	3.4	3.4	3.5	3.4	3.0	3.2
10. Attitudes toward persons with disabilities	3.6	3.6	3.9	4.1	3.3	3.5
Total mean	3.7	3.6	3.6	3.7	3.4	3.4

DISCUSSION

In regard to the etic properties of these factors (research question number 1), there was general agreement across the seven countries in the importance that particular values (interpersonal relations, self/person, and support systems) and contextual variables (public policies, technology, academic/professional supports, teaching/rehabilitation [direct support] staff, and attitudes towards people with disabilities) have on the development of integrated employment and community living programs. These results, which support the etic (universal) properties of these factors, are consistent with a growing body of literature supporting the etic nature of key quality of life concepts (Heal, 1996; Jordan, 1993; Keith et al., 1996), enhanced measured quality of life associated with more independent and integrated environments (Schalock et al., 1990), and with factors underlying meaningful judgments (Osgood, May, & Miron, 1975; Osgood & Sebeok, 1965).

Although there were few differences among the three regions, the North American respondents ascribed less importance than the other two regions to four values and one contextual variable. The lower scores assigned to values related to the use of wealth and conception of disability could be due to the current social/political environment within North America (and especially the United States) regarding the concern over the impact of managed care and capitated services. Similarly, the lower scores associated with locus of control and responsibility might well be related to the potential decrease of person-centered planning in a strict market economy (Ashbaugh & Smith, 1996). The lower importance assigned to the contextual variable of funding tied to public policies is easily understood, at least in the United States, where there has been a definite trend for funding not to be tied to public policies in both employment (Kiernan & Schalock, 1997) and residential placement/options (Braddock & Hemp, 1996).

There are always a number of concerns when one does cross-cultural research. Four of these were discussed earlier in the chapter under "Research Guidelines." The first of these concerns relates to conceptual (i.e., do concepts have equivocal meaning?) and linguistic (have terms and concepts been translated accurately?) equivalence. This study is not without some concern in this regard. For example, a number of respondents indicated that some of the values were difficult to understand and rate. Those mentioned the most often were relation with nature, time orientation, thinking style, locus of control, and locus of responsibility. Although these values potentially influence one's work view (Ibrahim, 1993) and other behaviors (Markus & Kitayama, 1991), they may not be all that relevant to the development of integrated employment and community living programs.

To determine empirically whether there was conceptual and linguistic equivalence, the questionnaire did allow for respondents to indicate (with a NA) whether the item was either not applicable in their country or was unfamiliar to the respondent. A total of 117 items (out of 6880; 1.7%) were evaluated NA. Of these, 88 (75.2%) related to relation with nature (13.6%), thinking style (13.6%), locus of control (11.4%), and locus of responsibility (20.5%); 29 (24.8%) related to two contextual variables (research and development, 24.1%, and political movements, 41.9%). In analyzing the NA responses further, it was found that 10 respondents were responsible for 120 of the 172 (69%) NAs. This fact, plus the small percent (1.7) of items overall rated as NA, suggests that the items were both understandable and comprehensive. In reference to the latter, only five additional values (self determination, civil rights, caring society, use of medical personnel, and communication) and three contextual variables (inclusion/integration, social and economic policy research, and learning from other countries) were added by the respondents.

The second concern relates to the research design that one uses. The present study used a within subjects design and a quantitative approach to data collection, which maximizes the possibility of determining etic properties and providing substantive illumination rather than hypothesis testing (Sanders, 1994). Our use of a quantitative design might also explain differences between our data and that reported by Gaylord-Ross (1987), who drew his conclusions based on a five-month period of observations, interviews, and document reviews. Based on this work, he found considerable importance to political movements, charismatic leaders, and demonstration sites in the development of integrated employment in Europe, but found less importance to public policies, which were rated high in the current study.

The third concern relates to the use of diverse people in the study. Concern about this factor was lessened by using national coordinators who were familiar with the respondents who were on-site persons familiar with their respective MR/DD system. Additionally, the fairly even split among positions and professionals would suggest a good cross-section of respondents.

In conclusion, we may be experiencing universality of the movement towards integrated employment and community living throughout the world. Although this may not be true of other concepts and phenomena, the concepts of normalization, inclusion, supported living/employment, and quality of life are increasingly becoming popular around the world (Goode, 1994; Schalock, 1997). The major result of the cross-cultural study reported in this chapter is that there may well be some universal values and contextual variables that are significant factors in the development of integrated employment and community living programs throughout the world. Among the most important of these factors are support systems, direct service workers, and public policies. Each of these factors is basic to the currently popular supports paradigm that is universally a primary sociocultural factor, if not *the* factor, influencing the social and vocational inclusion of persons with mental retardation into the mainstream of their society.

ACKNOWLEDGMENTS

The authors thank each of the following national coordinators (and the respondents whom they recruited) for making this study possible: in Canada: Ivan Brown and Patricia Minnes; in England: John Bottomley, Nick Bouras, and John Lobley; in Japan: Masako Iwasaki and Kanji Watanebe; in the Netherlands: Anthony A. J. Millenaar; in Poland: Andrzej Juros and Wojciech Otrebski; and in the Republic of China: Hung-Chih Lin, Kuo-yu Wang, and Tien-Miau Wang. We also thank Ann Podraza for her excellent technical assistance in the preparation of the manuscript.

REFERENCES

Ashbaugh, J., & Smith, G. (1996, June). Beware the managed health-care companies. *Mental Retardation*, 189–193.

Bernal, G., Bonilla, J., & Bellido, C. (1995). Ecological validity and cultural sensitivity for outcome research: Issues for the cultural adaptation and development of psychosocial treatments with Hispanics. *Journal of Abnormal Child Psychology, 23*(1), 67–82.

Berry, J. W. (1969). On cross-cultural comparability. *International Journal of Psychology, 4,* 119–128.

Berry, J. W., Poortinga, Y. H., Segall, M. H., & Dasen, P. R. (1992). *Cross-cultural psychology: Research and applications.* New York: Cambridge University Press.

Braddock, D., & Hemp, R. (1996). Medicaid spending reductions and developmental disabilities. *Journal of Disability Policy Studies, 7*(1), 1–31.

Brislin, R. W. (1993). *Understanding culture's influence on behavior.* Fort Worth, TX: Harcourt Brace Jovanovich.

Bronfenbrenner, U. (1979). *The ecology of human development: Experiments by nature and design.* Cambridge: Harvard University Press.

Cole, M. (1988). Cross-cultural research in the sociohistorical tradition. *Human Development, 31,* 137–152.

Daniels, H., & Hogg, B. (1991). An intercultural comparison of the quality of life of children and youth with handicaps in Denmark, Italy, the United Kingdom and Germany. *Education and Child Psychology, 8*(4), 74–83.

Feather, N. T. (1994). Values and culture. In W. J. Lonner & R. Malpass (Eds.), *Psychology and culture* (pp. 183–189). Boston: Allyn & Bacon.

Fowers, B. J., & Richardson, F. C. (1996). Why is multiculturalism good? *American Psychologist, 51*(6), 609–621.

Funkhouser, G. R. (1993). A self-anchoring instrument and analytical procedure for reducing cultural bias in cross-cultural research. *Journal of Social Psychology, 133*(5), 661–673.

Gaylord-Ross, R. (1987). Vocational integration for persons with mental handicaps: A cross-cultural perspective. *Research in Developmental Disabilities, 8,* 532–548.

Goode, D. A. (Ed.). (1994). *Quality of life for persons with disabilities: International perspectives and issues.* Boston: Brookline Books.

Heal, L. W. (1996). [Review of the book *Quality of life of persons with disabilities: International perspectives and issues*]. *American Journal on Mental Retardation, 100,* 557–560.

Hernes, T. (1991, October). *Trends and challenges in vocational rehabilitation: An international perspective.* Paper presented at "Charting a New Course" International Conference on Transition from School to Working Life of Young People with Disabilities. Experts meeting. Genoa, Italy.

Hines, A. M. (1993). Linking qualitative and quantitative methods in cross-cultural survey research: Techniques from cognitive science. *American Journal of Community Psychology, 21*(6), 729–746.

Hogg, J. (1996, July). *Intellectual disability and aging: Ecological perspectives from recent research.* Paper presented at the 10th Annual IASSID Conference, Helsinki, Finland.

Honigman, J. (1967). *Personality in culture.* New York: Harper & Row.

Hughes, D., Seidman, E., & Williams, N. (1993). Cultural phenomena and the research enterprise: Toward a culturally anchored methodology. *American Journal of Community Psychology, 21*(6), 687–703.

Ibrahim, F. A. (1993). Existential worldview theory: Applications in transcultural counseling. In J. McFadden (Ed.), *Transcultural counseling: Bilateral and international perspectives* (pp. 25–58). Alexandria, VA: ACA Press.

Ibrahim, F. A. (1995). Multicultural influences on rehabilitation training and services: The shift to valuing nondominant cultures. In O. C. Karan & S. Greenspan (Eds.), *Community rehabilitation services for people with disabilities* (pp. 187–207). Boston: Butterworth-Heinemann.

Jahoda, G. (1992). *Crossroads between culture and mind: Continuities and change in theories of human nature.* London: Harvester Wheatsheaf.

Jordan, T. E. (1993). Estimating the quality of life for children around the world: NICQL '92. *Social Indicators Research, 30*(1), 17–38.

Keith, K. D. (1996). Measuring quality of life across cultures. In R. L. Schalock (Ed.), *Quality of life: Volume I: Conceptualization and measurement* (pp. 73–82). Washington, DC: American Association on Mental Retardation.

Keith, K. D., Heal, L. W., & Schalock, R. L. (1996). Cross-cultural measurement of critical quality of life concepts. *Journal of Intellectual and Developmental Disability, 21*(4), 273–293.

Keith, K. D., Yamamoto, M., Okita, N., & Schalock, R. L. (1995). Cross-cultural quality of life: Japanese and American college students. *Social Behavior and Personality, 23*(2), 163–170.

Kiernan, W. E., & Schalock, R. L. (Eds.). (1997). *Integrated employment: Today and tomorrow.* Washington, DC: American Association on Mental Retardation.

Kiernan, W. E., Schalock, R. L., Butterworth, J., & Sailor, W. (1993). *Enhancing the use of natural supports for people with severe disabilities: An international perspective.* Boston: Training and Research Institute for People with Disabilities, The Children's Hospital.

Kluckhohn, C. (1951). Values and value orientations in the theory of action. In R. Parsons & E. Skils (Eds.), *Toward a general theory of action* (pp. 388–433). Cambridge: Harvard University Press.

Kluckhohn, C., & Srodtbeck, F. (1961). *Variations in value orientations.* Evanston, IL: Row, Peterson.

Konig, A., & Schalock, R. L. (1991). Supported employment: Equal opportunities for severely disabled men and women. *International Labour Review, 130*(1), 21–37.

Kuyken, W., Orley, J., Huelson, P., & Sartorius, N. (1994). Quality of life assessment across cultures. *International Journal of Mental Health, 23*(2), 5–27.

Leelakulthanit, O., & Day, R. (1993). Cross cultural comparisons of quality of life of Thais and Americans. *Social Indicators Research, 30*(1), 49–70.

Lonner, W. J. (1985). Issues in testing and assessment in cross-cultural counseling. *Counseling Psychologist, 13*, 599–614.

Lonner, W. J. (1990). An overview of cross-cultural testing and assessment. In R. W. Brislin (Ed.), *Applied Cross-Cultural Psychology: Cross-Cultural Research and Methodology, 14*, 56–76.

Lonner, W. J., & Berry, J. W. (1986). *Field methods in cross-cultural research.* Beverly Hills, CA: Sage Publications.

Lonner, W. J., & Malpass, R. (1994). *Psychology and culture.* Boston: Allyn & Bacon.

Lynch, E. W., & Hanson, M. J. (1992). *Developing cross-cultural competence: A guide for working with young children and their families.* Baltimore: Paul H. Brookes.

Markus, H. R., & Kitayama, S. (1991). Culture and self: Implications for cognition, emotion, and motivation. *Psychological Review, 98*(2), 224–253.

Matsumoto, D. (1994). *People: Psychology from a cultural perspective.* Pacific Grove, CA: Brooks/Cole.

Mays, V. M., Rubin, J., Sabourin, M., & Walker, L. (1996). Moving toward a global psychology: Changing theories and practice to meet the needs of a changing world. *American Psychologist, 51*(5), 485–487.

Osgood, C. E., May, W. H., & Miron, M. S. (1975). *Cross cultural universals of affective meaning.* Urbana: University of Illinois Press.

Osgood, C. E., & Sebeok, T. A. (1965). *Psycholinguistics: A survey of theory and research problems.* Bloomington: Indiana University Press.

Rogoff, B., & Chavajay, P. (1995). What's becoming of research on the cultural basis of cognitive development? *American Psychologist, 50*(10), 859–879.

Rokeach, M. (1973). *The nature of human values.* New York: Free Press.

Sanders, D. (1994). Methodological considerations in comparative cross-national research. *International Social Science Journal, 46*(4), 513–521.

Schalock, R. L. (1995). *Outcome-based evaluation.* New York: Plenum.

Schalock, R. L. (1996). Considering one's culture in the application of quality of life. In R. L. Schalock (Ed.), *Quality of life: Application to persons with disabilities* (pp. 225–244). Washington, DC: American Association on Mental Retardation.

Schalock, R. L. (1997). The conceptualization and measurement of quality of life: Current status and future considerations. *Journal on Developmental Disabilities, 5*(2), 1–21.

Schalock, R. L., Bartnik, E., Wu, F., Konig, A., Lee, C. S., & Reiter, S. (1990, May). *An international perspective on quality of life measurement and use.* Paper presented at the meeting of the American Association on Mental Retardation, Atlanta, GA.

Schalock, R. L., & Keith, K. D. (1993). *Quality of life questionnaire.* Worthington, OH: IDS Publishing.

Schwartz, S. H., & Bilsky, W. (1990). Toward a theory of the universal content and structure of values: Extensions and cross-cultural replications. *Journal of Personality and Social Psychology, 58,* 878–891.

Skevington, S. M. (1994). Social comparison in cross-cultural quality of life assessment. *International Journal of Mental Health, 23*(2), 29–47.

Triandis, H. C. (1990). Cross-cultural studies of individualism and collectivism. In G. Jahoda, H. C. Triandis, C. Kagitcibasi, J. Berry, et al. (Eds.), *Cross-cultural perspectives: Nebraska Symposium on Motivation: 1989* (pp. 41–131). Lincoln: University of Nebraska Press.

Triandis, H. C. (1994). Culture and social behavior. In W. J. Loner & R. Malpass (Eds.), *Psychology and culture* (pp. 169–173). Boston: Allyn & Bacon.

Triandis, H. C., Bontempo, R., Villareal, M.J., Asai, M., & Lucca, N. (1988). Individualism and collectivism: Cross-cultural perspectives on self-group relationships. *Journal of Personality and Social Psychology, 54,* 323–338.

Tse, J. W. (1991). Directions in the field of mental retardation in the 1990s: An Asian perspective. *International Social Work, 34*(4), 339–352.

CHAPTER 16

Conclusion: Cross-Cultural Perspectives — Diversity and Universalism

SHUNIT REITER
University of Haifa

With modern telecommunications and computer technology, the world is becoming "one big village." This window to the world allows anyone to know, in real time, what is happening in the homes of others. The present book provides us with another world window, which looks specifically at the policies and programs for people with disabilities. Chapters in the present book come under the umbrella title of "cross-cultural" studies, including diverse reports concerning ethnic diversity, racial differences, and comparisons between nations and between continents. The term "culture," which we used in the present book, is the definition suggested by Pitman, Eisikovits, and Dobbert (1989), which is that junior members of a society learn whole patterns of behavior within the contexts of everyday life and in personal action. They individualize and adapt these patterns by varying some of the elements and recreating new ones. This definition assumes a holistic interactive view of culture. The assumption is that there are universal and biological substrata shared by all human beings and that differences between groups are not human ultimate potentials or competencies, but rather are structures and processes that make up the specific patterns of interaction typical of each culture. Cross-cultural studies in special education and rehabilitation tackle such questions as:

1. What are the different meanings attached to disability?

2. Do different countries face similar issues regarding services for persons with disabilities?

3. Are there similarities and differences in the meanings of policies regarding the disabled? Are any of these meanings based on attitudes that affect the implementation of policies and services?

4. What are the different cultural approaches of goals regarding services provided for the disabled?
5. What are some of the alternative ways for solving problems in the area of disabilities? What are the differences in practice between cultures?

By answering these and similar questions, it is hoped that better communication can be achieved between different cultural groups. Indeed, despite the multiculturalism of immigrant countries such as the United States, Australia, Israel, and the fact that many European countries are host to large ethnic groups of foreign workers and families, one general trend has recently arisen based on the normalization principle. However, it seems that professionals, although they recognize gross differences, often fail to appreciate the subtle cultural differences between subgroups. This is especially evident in the area of belief systems and by different meanings attached to these belief systems in which a difference in meaning becomes attached to the same concept. Fernald (1995) demonstrated this when he made comparisons regarding disability language preferences among English-speaking countries. He stated "some terminology that Americans assume to be sensitive and stigma-free was, in fact, offensive to British colleagues" (p. 99).

From an international perspective, cross-cultural studies have provided us with an important cautionary message regarding the simple transfer of policies and services from one country to another or from one social group to another. There is often a tendency for visiting professionals, who are impressed by what they see in a hosting country/group, to return home trying to implement the policies and services they observed during their visit. However, what is useful in one culture may not be very useful in another. This over-reliance on foreign perspectives and research data for domestic decision-making may be misleading. Furthermore, knowing only one system can result in one country's recommendation for domestic reform in other countries, but not in their own. This single-sided perspective could actually represent serious policy limitations for that country (Moberg, 1997; Safran, 1989).

On the other hand, cross-cultural joint projects and research can enrich participants' self-evaluation and self-analysis. A more clear understanding of ones' own system can be achieved by learning about other social and philosophical systems in other countries. This point is nicely illustrated in a cross-cultural study of vocational rehabilitation centers in the U.S. and Israel (Bryen, Newman, Reiter, & Hakim, 1987). As pointed out by the authors, "embedded in one's own culture, it is easy to arrive at narrow ideas, perspectives, and conclusions regarding the nature of a problem. First, one learns about one's own cultural assumptions, which influence the very ways in which problems are defined and solutions are sought and evaluated. Sensitization to these embedded assumptions often results in a broader and more critical view of the nature of the problem in one's own culture and its potential solutions."

This process of an enhanced self-awareness was further demonstrated in a multidisciplinary exchange and research program involving communities in Denmark, Germany, Italy, and the United Kingdom (Daniels & Hogg, 1991). This project focused on the issue of the quality of life for children and youths with disabilities in a variety of educational contexts. It examined the relationships between theory, local practices and policies, and national legislation. The study highlighted these local practices and perceptions and also on the decision-making process in each community. Enriched by the visits and comparisons made with other communities, this research resulted in better services in the local community and in each country according to its own traditions, and in line with its culture.

Therefore, cross-cultural studies not only have an international, global perspective but often a practical value that can be applied to professional work. The contribution of such studies is becoming especially relevant as client-centered approaches and trends towards empowerment are becoming valued mediums of service. The diversity in conceptual interpretations and practices has raised demands for more cultural sensitivity among professionals working in the field of disability.

Bridging the gap between professionals and clients that come from different ethnic groups is, therefore, another important aim of cross-cultural accounts, studies, and projects (Hanline & Daley, 1992). Hampson, Beavers, and Hulgus (1990) pointed out that the interpretation of behavior may be skewed in pathological ways in that the observer does not understand the ethnic group being observed. Further, demographic factors and social class differences can be confounded with differences in ethnicity (p. 307). Hampson and colleagues concluded that "these data encourage the view that for families of all ethnic backgrounds, subtle ethnic and social class differences exist, and imposing one's own ethnically influenced standards regarding clarity of expression, autonomy, egalitarianism, and even sex-role standards may limit therapeutic efficacy. Appreciation of a variety of manifestations of family competence and style are necessary for effective interventions, rather than relying on a single concept of family therapy" (p. 318).

The process by which services for persons with disabilities are formed can be described in a model representing the overlay between the international and the particular in three areas:

1. Basic human rights
2. Cultural diversity
3. Outcomes.

In Figure 16.1, this process is presented. The general philosophy concerning people with disabilities is implemented in practice that leads to certain accepted outcomes as defined by human rights. This general outline of the flow from philosophy to practice to outcome is only a skeletal view of the process. The principle that people with disabilities have a right to lead a normal life and the principle that they are entitled to lead a life of quality serve as the two outer points of the diagram. Between these two points are the cultural groups that are made up of

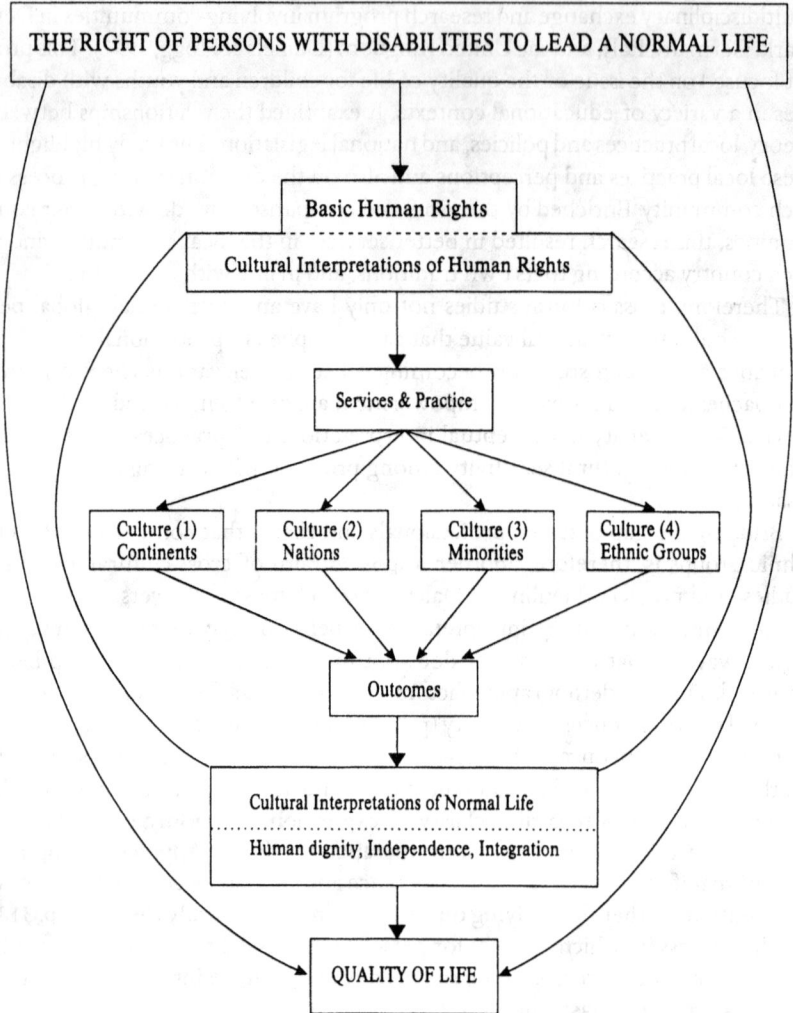

FIG. 16.1. The process of the development of services: The interplay between international and local/cultural variables.

nations, ethnic groups, minorities, and social classes. Each cultural group interprets differently basic human rights and the means and ways to implement them into practice.

Figure 16.1 encompasses two circles. The outer is the international sphere. This represents the direct link between the rights of persons with disabilities to lead a normal life and the responsibility of services to assist them to enhance the quality of their lives. The inner circle is the particular sphere, and this represents the diversity between cultures.

From the chapters presented here and from other cross-cultural studies, it appears that in spite of diversity in cultural orientations and belief systems, there seems to be a universal consensus regarding people with disabilities. This consensus is based on the principles that people with disabilities are entitled to lead a decent life in the community, living with dignity, sharing normal standards, and having quality of life. Further, that governments have the responsibility to make sure that conditions will enable them to do so (Bryen et al., 1987; Daniels & Hogg, 1991; Walton, Rosenquist, & Sandling, 1989). We witness a move away from the rhetoric of segregation to the rhetoric of integration; a move away from provisions in which individuals become dependent on services to support systems that emphasize empowerment and enable them to lead as much as possible an independent and autonomous life.

Not only is there an agreement on the philosophy that people with disabilities should not be segregated in large faraway institutions, but we also witness a genuine interest in different countries to try out new programs and projects in order to achieve this aim. Daniels and Hogg (1991) point out that the consensus regarding the emphasis on integration and on quality of life leads to other necessary by-products. Some of the by-products include recognition of the importance of partnership with parents and of an interdisciplinary collaboration, the rise of self-help organizations, self-advocacy and policy and administrative collaboration at national, regional, and local levels in the development of integration policies and practices. These trends seem to be accompanied by attitudinal changes such as a move away from a consideration of individual deficiency to more situational and ecological analysis and improving the decision-making process.

The consensus also lends support to the anthropological tenet that there are common biological and psychological factors that are characteristic of human beings, wherever they are and whatever their culture that affect the way they experience disability. It appears that the condition of disability touches a most basic issue of human existence, which present similar pressures and needs in every human society.

However, the universal consensus on the issue of disability presents only the challenge, or the trigger for different solutions to the same basic problems. Indeed, the specific interpretation of concepts such as integration, independence, work, quality of life, and the governments' responsibility are culturally and politically bound. The policy of inclusion, though wide-spread, has different roots and different forms of implementation in each country (Moberg, 1997). The inner circle in Figure 16.1 describes the process by which different cultures develop different services. Here diversity is the key word. Cross-cultural studies show that diversity exists already in the first phase of philosophy. this diversity is not so much expressed in the use of different concepts regarding human rights—to the contrary, values such as respect, integration, independence are used by most people regarding persons with disabilities. However, the interpretation and meanings attached to these values and concepts can be different. How one defines dignity and respect for persons can vary greatly from one culture to another. One of the most significant aspects of any culture is the meaning that is attached to the concept of "person" in that culture. The interpretation of human rights will, therefore, be done according to the different ways cultures define what is normal and what is not. Consequently, these interpretations will affect not only differences in practice but ultimately differences in outcomes.

In this volume, each of the chapters seems to address one or more variables that appear in the above chart. Mitchell's chapter on the transfer of beliefs, knowledge, and experiences between countries most directly addresses the issue of universalism. Mitchell opens the chapter with this statement: "In recent years, beliefs, principles, knowledge, and practices relating to special education and rehabilitation increasingly have been transferred between countries, with the result that there is a remarkable degree of convergence, both in ideology and in practices, across all types of nations." This affects a trend for globalization or for the emergence of a "transitional world" and the expansion of global economy and cultural links.

The chapters by Schalock and Kelly, Corbet, and MacNeil and Anderson address universal issues, as well. Schalock and Kelly state, "We may be experiencing universality of the movement towards integrated employment and community living throughout the world . . . that the concepts of normalization, inclusion, supported living/employment, and quality of life are increasingly becoming popular around the world." MacNeil and Anderson address another issue that has global implications, as it focuses on a basic human activity—that of leisure. The authors suggest a universally valid operational definition of leisure: "We may conceive of leisure as an emotional condition within satisfaction. This condition is characterized by feelings of mastery, achievement, success, personal worth, and pleasure. The underlying characteristic of leisure experience is the perception of personal control." This definition of leisure can be applied within any cultural milieu. However, while the processes might be regarded as typical for any human being, the patterns, contents, and style of leisure activities will be different according to cultural interpretations.

These chapters lend support to the variables in Figure 16.1 that compose the outer circle of the chart; that is, the seemingly worldwide consensus regarding the rights of persons with disabilities to lead a normal life. In recent years, "normal life" is understood to mean "quality of life" and not simply regular or conventional life. To the contrary, persons with disabilities are seen as having the right to make their own choices concerning the style of life they choose. This could be a style that is not necessarily congruent with what professionals perceive to be a "normal lifestyle."

Corbet presents the issue of the discrepancies among cultural interpretations very vividly in her chapter. Specifically, we see a discrepancy in the principle of normalizations "being like everybody else" and the concept of the "quality of life" that implies the right to be different and to choose a way of life that might include a "not-normal" circle of friends. Corbet describes British self-help groups of disabled persons who gather together around the shared interest in arts and literature. Corbet indicates: "while it might be argued that disabled people should ideally be participating in mainstream arts programs, the reality is that fierce competition for inclusion is likely to limit them to either minimal participation or a stereotyped role in which their scope for development is severely constrained." Corbet's statement tells us that "quality of life" means that any person should be free to pursue any activity that is both meaningful and enriching. This includes participation in special groups where people share not only the same interests but also similar disabilities.

The final chapter of the book by Siegel on the utilization of technology of inclusion points to the possibility of enhancing quality of life in global terms. The international aspect of computer technology is evident on two levels, the technical and the personal. At the technical level, the world of computers has increased the availability of devices that can be used by all. On the personal level, computer technology has afforded the individual person with connections, communications and "windows" to other countries around the world. These devices and open lines of communication can contribute tremendously to combating the sense of loneliness many persons with disabilities struggle with, making them not only members of their own communities but also citizens of the world.

Earlier we indicated that the outer circle of the figure addresses global issues concerning the convergence of beliefs and attitudes towards people with disabilities, and that the inner circle represents diversity. Schalock and Kelly provide the link between the universal and local cultural interpretations of human rights. They provide a list of value dimensions with which every society seems to struggle with and suggest different meanings by which to interpret these dimensions.

The way different belief systems, values, and attitudes lead to differences in terms of policies and practice is presented by several chapters of the book. An international view is presented in the chapter by Rojewski, which describes and compares vocational preparation and employment options for adults with disabilities in different regions: America, Western Europe, Eastern Europe, Asia, and India. Saul and Ling's chapter describes policy and practice concerning disability in Australia, and Wehman's chapter describes policy and practice in the U.S. and Europe on transition to employment. The two chapters provide us with a detailed look at the way concepts such as integration, employment, and independent living are understood by different countries. The manner in which these and related terms are interpreted and expressed are exhibited in national policies, and consequently in services and practice. The authors are critical of the discrepancies found between national politics that give lip service to human welfare and that which actually affects policies and services—economical and political power gains.

Can differences between nationals be bridged in both theory and practice?

Ramot and Gitelman's chapter on the application of a Western orientation towards services for the disabled in Eastern European nation address this issue. The authors state, "we believe that the combination of factors, including timing, resources, appropriate professional and personal contacts and partnerships, and basic common human needs and concerns that characterize all societies have made it possible to transfer and adapt experiences and approaches from one society and culture to another."

The problem of the application of services initiated in one culture to another happens not only at an international level but also on a more particular level of different minority groups and ethnic groups within the same culture. Chapters by Herr and Young, Pedroza, and Kavanaugh focus on minority and ethnic issues concerning services and special education. Herr describes new immigrants with disabilities and the legal issue around their absorption in the mainstream of Israeli society. The chapter by Young, Pedroza, and Kavanaugh tells us of the conflicting attitudes between American professionals and Mexican parents of children with disabilities.

In terms of outcomes, the chapter by Garber and Osher provide us with one example of the way professionals can bridge the gap between cultures by creating parent-student-teacher partnerships. As the authors point out, "Families differ in their structure, culture, resources, and values. School-based outreach to empower parents may be provided in different forms to accommodate the individual needs and build upon the strengths of different families." The methods suggested are: information brokerage, parent support groups, and individual counseling. The authors conclude that the key to overcoming barriers of cultural diversity is the establishment of communication links between parents and teachers. We would add that communication is the key to any meeting between service providers and service recipients, between professionals in the fields of special education and rehabilitation, and persons with disabilities and their families. Outcomes of services should lead to the integration of persons with disabilities into society, enabling them to lead an independent and dignified life. What is normal for them will depend on the specific meanings attached to normal life, including such variables as role expectations, style and patterns of communications among individuals, conventional mores, technology, beliefs, and values. In this sphere we can envision two levels of stress, one that relates to discrepancies between the specific cultural milieu of the individual and mainstream society, and another that relates to the discrepancy between individual needs and his or her cultural norms. Shaughnessy, Glover, Green, and Coy address the issue of parents with mental retardation in their chapter and demonstrate these dual discrepancies. From the beginning, we have pointed out that there is a global consensus on the rights of individuals with mental retardation to enjoy the same basic human rights as other members of the community. However, the issue of marriage and family involves religious beliefs, medical advice, social welfare services, and other considerations that might be contradictory to the needs and desires of a person with mental retardation. Normalization means that they have the right to be like everybody else. However, if we consider (as these authors point out in their conclusion) that the ultimate concern of services is the welfare of all children, in all nations, of all parents, then we can address issues regarding quality of life.

SUMMARY

Cultural diversity is an inherent feature of human life. The forces that lead to diversity and the strengthening of local cultural identities will continue to exist in spite of, and along with, the forces leading towards universalism. This raises several philosophical issues concerning what is meant by the concepts of integration, dignity, and independence.

In most Western countries, the first breakthroughs in reform concerning people with disabilities were due to the spread of the principle of normalization. Their greatest contribution was in enhancing advanced legislation concerning the legal rights of people by mainstream society. However, the interpretation of the normalization principle has been found to be an oversimplification. Normalization is more than just "being normal," or being adjusted to a life according to socially accepted standards and norms based on conformity and on "making" the disabled adjust to conventions. Not only has this interpretation of normalization been oversimplified, but also it has been detrimental to the quality of life for many people with disabilities. Indeed, a conflicting message was given to the disabled. On one hand, normalization meant respect for each person as a human being of worth; on the other hand, conformity meant disregard for the unique individual and his/her specific characteristics. This incongruence has been expressed by people with disabilities who, at times, simply tell us "Let me be what I want to be, not what either you or my society wants me to be."

For this reason, concepts such as *integration, dignity,* and *independence* are being reinterpreted and replaced by the terms such as *inclusion* and *interdependency.* These terms demand respect for the unique personality of each individual with a disability, regarding him or her as a subject. It also calls for autonomy; that is, inner independence. Integration, civil dignity, and independence were found to be necessary but not sufficient conditions for quality of life.

This book calls for cultural sensitivity and raises the issue as to what extent do professionals, when dealing with clients coming from different cultural milieus, adhere to the simplified interpretation of normalization. Do professionals consent to any cultural orientation towards disability and make adjustments for the person with a disability in regard to the norms and standards of his or her society? Or should the professional express their own conception of what quality of life means?

Knowing more about another culture does not always mean that one accepts its interpretation of human dignity, independence, and social integration. Professionals have a right to be at odds with cultural interpretations that seem to be contrary to human rights and detrimental to their clients' quality of life. Conflicts between different cultural values should not be ignored or made trivial, or lead professionals to inhibit their own point of view for the sake of cultural sensitivity. Respect for the client means that he or she also has an opinion, a recommendation, a vision. Cultural sensitivity should lead to a dialogue based on mutual respect and open communication and assist in avoiding any power struggles.

What is called for here is not a one-sided, client-centered approach, in which the practitioners or professionals "listen" only to the client and accommodate their responses according to the clients' belief system and practices, but instead it is a dialogue. In a dialogue, the professional has the right and the responsibility to express clearly his or her own point of view and philosophy. Furthermore, according to this philosophy, professionals should outline what has best practical value and the desired outcomes. Cultural sensitivity, a client-centered approach, and empowerment do not mean that the professional's responsibility is only to serve as a mirror to clients. The professional is there on an educational mission too: to provide people with disabilities and their parents alternative interpretations.

However, the balance between cultural relativism in the area of services for persons with disabilities and between universalism of philosophy and outcomes will probably be a continual professional dilemma. Modern societies seem to show two parallel trends. One trend leads towards universalism, towards one Western culture with its emphasis on the individual and civil legal rights, and material and technological gains. Another trend is towards cultural diversity, with an emphasis on ethnic mores and norms and on a particular ethnic identity. As shown in this book, the two general trends moving towards opposite poles are also expressed in the areas of special education and rehabilitation and will demand our attention in the coming decade. The present book is one small contribution to the future of dilemma of the global versus the particular. It raises more questions than it answers.

REFERENCES

Bryen, D., Newman, E., Reiter, S., & Hakim, S. (1987). *Barriers to employability of persons with handicaps: A bi-national study in the United States and Israel.* Philadelphia: Temple University Developmental Disabilities Center.

Daniels, H., & Hogg, B. (1991). An intercultural comparison of quality of life of children and youth with handicaps in Denmark, Italy, the United Kindom and Germany. *Educational and Child Psychology, 8,* 74–83.

Fernald, C. D. (1995). When in London . . . : Differences in disability language preferences among English-speaking countries. *Mental Retardation, 33,* 99–103.

Hampson, R. B., Beavers, W. R., & Hulgus, Y. (1990). Cross-ethnic family differences: Interactional assessment of White, Black, and Mexican-American families. *Journal of Marital and Family Therapy, 16,* 307–319.

Hanline, M. F., & Daley, S. E. (1992). Family coping strategies and strengths in Hispanic, African-American, and Caucasian families of young children. *Topics in Early Childhood Special Education, 12,* 351–366.

Moberg, S. (1997). Inclusive educational practices as perceived by prospective special education teachers in Estonia, Finland, and the United States. *International Journal of Rehabilitation Research, 20,* 29–40.

Pitman, M. A., Eisikovits, R. A., & Dobbert, M. L., (Eds.). (1989). *Culture acquistion: A holistic approach to human learning.* New York: Praeger.

Safran, S. P. (1989). Special education in Australia and the United States: A cross-cultural analysis. *Journal of Special Education, 23,* 330–341.

Super, C. M. (Ed.). (1987). *The role of culture in developmental disorders.* New York: Academic Press, Harcourt Brace Jovanovich.

Walton, W. T., Rosenquist, J., & Sandling, I. (1989). A comparative study of special education contrasting Denmark, Sweden, and the United States of America. *Educational and Psychological Interactions, 99,* 1–29.

Author Index

Subject Index

A

Academics, *see* Education
Adjustment to life as an adult, 5, 34, 42, 125, 131, 136, 195
   self-image, 8, 19, 326
Adult education, *see* Rehabilitation, Education
Advocacy training, *see* Empowerment
Affirmative action, *see* Legislation for disabled persons
African American students with disabilities, 34
AKIM, 195, *199*
American Humane Association, 36, *54*
American Jewish Joint Distribution Committee, 167, *169*
American Share Foundation, 235, *254*
Americans with Disabilities Act (ADA) (1990), *see also* Legislation on disabled persons, 11, 18, *29*, 154, *199*, 230, 231, 290
Arc (formerly Association of Retarded Citizens), 289–292, 301, *305*
Architectural barriers, *see* Recreation
Arkansas Research and Training Center in Vocational Rehabilitation, 230, 234, 235, *254*
Arts for disabled persons, *see* Disability arts
Asia, *see also* China, Hong Kong, India, Japan, 265
Asia Pacific Decade of the Disabled (1993–2002), 265
Assistive devices, *see* Assistive technology
Assistive technology, *see also* Computer-aided instruction, Computer-managed instruction, Assistive Technology Evaluation Checklist, 273, 287–295, 331
   future, 303, 304
Assistive Technology Evaluation Checklist, 292, 293

Association for Civil Rights in Israel (ACRI), 188, 193
Attributional analysis, 136
Augmented and Alternative Communication (AAC), *see* Assistive technology
Australia
   affirmative industry, 246
   disability policy and practice, 103–120, 138, 150, 206
   legislation on disability employment, 230
   vocational education, 205

B

Barriers to recreation, *see* Recreation

C

Canada, 138, 150
   legislation on disability employment, 230
Career education, *see* Education
Case management, *see* Education
Central America
   vocational services, 241, 242, 247
Challenge, 25, *30*
China
   vocational rehabilitation, 238, 239, 250
Clearinghouse on Disability Information, 234, 235, *254*
Collaboration, *see* Cooperative relationships
Commissie Dualisering, 226
Commonwealth of Australia, 106, 107, 115, *120*
Commonwealth/State Disability Agreement (CSDA) (1991), 107
Communication, *see* Language
Communication barriers, *see* Recreation
Communication devices, *see* Assistive technology
Community-based rehabilitation, *see* Rehabilitation

347

For Product Safety Concerns and Information please contact our EU
representative GPSR@taylorandfrancis.com
Taylor & Francis Verlag GmbH, Kaufingerstraße 24, 80331 München, Germany

www.ingramcontent.com/pod-product-compliance
Lightning Source LLC
Chambersburg PA
CBHW070546270326
41926CB00013B/2219